KETO
ANSWERS

KETO ANSWERS

Simplifying Everything
You Need to Know about the
World's Most Confusing Diet

**DR. ANTHONY GUSTIN, DC, MS
AND CHRIS IRVIN, MS**

four pillar **health**

KETO ANSWERS
Simplifying Everything You Need to Know about
the World's Most Confusing Diet

ISBN   978-1-5445-0464-3   *Hardcover*
       978-1-5445-0462-9   *Paperback*
       978-1-5445-0463-6   *Ebook*

CONTENTS

HOW DID WE GET HERE?

You can't avoid health recommendations. They're on TV, littered on your social media feed, and all over your Google searches. Even worse, all of the recommendations conflict! One day eating bacon is the cure to heart disease, the next day fat will give you a heart attack. Yesterday exercise was the key to health, and tomorrow a glass of wine will be just as good as that exercise. What is going on?

One of the reasons we are so confused about how to improve our health is the outdated and misinformed recommendations made by governing bodies, especially nutrition recommendations. This confusion is nothing new, and it's rooted in old—and incorrect—dietary advice.

If we take a brief look at history, we see a rising and falling of dietary trends, some of which have made a much greater impact than others. Historically, research has driven nutritional recommendations. In fact, one of the most important characters in the tale of why we are where we are with our health and nutrition recommendations is Ancel Keys, a very successful scientist who led the charge on demonizing fat as a cause for heart disease. Despite the fact that the data Ancel used to support his hypothesis was bogus and has since been debunked, which we will get into more in the coming chapters, his findings were used to spark the movement of low-fat diets meant to improve overall health and reduce our risk for disease. Where did those recommendations get us? If you consider the continued rise in obesity, heart disease, and type 2 diabetes, surely it hasn't helped!

Why is this such a big deal? If you go to the American Heart Association's website right now, you'll still see low dietary fat recommendations, especially low saturated fat, and not much mention of animal meat. Go ahead, take a look. That's why this is a big deal: decades later this misinformation is still being used to shape dietary recommendations.

Today we still see a lot of bad research or misinterpretations of research. However, now social media allows us to easily share that bad or misinterpreted research and provide our own opinions on it, even if we are not qualified to do so. Even worse, these opinions on misinterpreted research are commented on and shared, leading to a nasty cycle of spreading bad nutrition recommendations. On top of this, we also see a lot of click-bait articles on nutrition that are used to market at us, not to educate us. And don't even get us started on the fitness industry!

The explosive growth of the fitness industry has had a pretty substantial impact on nutrition as a whole. One of the problems with the fitness industry is that it has made a bad habit of focusing more on the way we look and less on actually improving our health. Don't believe us? Check out how much

IIFYM has blown up over the last few years. If It Fits Your Macros, or IIFYM, is a type of eating focused only on hitting your recommended macronutrients to achieve body composition goals. This nutrition strategy is plastered all over social media and is why we see so many fitness influencers eating pizza and Pop-Tarts. There is a lot more to health than just aesthetics; unfortunately, the fitness industry has failed to emphasize that.

So, where are we now? Confused. We don't know which foods are good, which ones are bad, or if we can even trust the quality of foods we are supposed to put in our body. We go from fad diet to fad diet for thirty days, we see some progress, and we go right back to our old habits. The perpetual cycle called yo-yo dieting that can lead to poor health and not to mention poor relationships with food.

This is why we see so many people who are sick, unhappy, and unhealthy. Common nutrition recommendations are a mess, reliable information is hard to come by, and oh, yeah, a lot of doctors don't know squat about nutrition.

ROLE OF NUTRITION IN HEALTH AND DISEASE PREVENTION

Another reason why our diets are so out of whack is because a lot of us fail to realize that what we put in our body actually impacts our health and the way we feel! If you drank twelve beers and felt like heck the next day, you would blame it on the beer, right? Why don't we look at food the same way? Instead, we tend to point our fingers toward things like diseases or various conditions that we think require medicine when really—this is where nutrition is supposed to come in. You may have heard the famous quote from Hippocrates:

"Let food be thy medicine and let medicine be thy food."

Hippocrates was right; what you put in your body matters! This is why functional medicine exists. In case you are not familiar with functional medicine, here is a Wikipedia definition.

Functional medicine is a form of alternative medicine, which proponents say focuses on interactions between the environment and the gastrointestinal, endocrine, and immune systems, but opponents have described it as "pseudoscientific silliness" and quackery.

Opponents say it's fake. We thought it was fake, too, until we started reading more research on nutrition. Again, what you put in your body matters. It's fuel. It's what determines how you look, feel, function, and live. If you have chronic conditions, the food you eat is either *fueling* or *fighting* those conditions. Taking control of the foods you eat allows you to take control of your health.

In fact, taking control of the foods you eat can impact your life in far more ways than you may realize. If you have no energy, changing the way you eat can help you not spend $50 a week on sugary Starbucks coffee. If you are overweight, changing the way you eat can make your body burn more fat (notice we said you still get to eat). If you have diabetes, changing the way you eat can reduce or even completely remove the need for medication. If you have cancer, changing the way you eat could starve cancer, improve outcomes from standard treatments, and maybe even prevent the nearly inevitable return of cancer after remission.

To date, we haven't taken control of our health, and that is why we are in the obesity/diabetic/overweight/sick epidemic we are in. We rely on doctors to prescribe medication when we aren't feeling well or have a disease. Most times these medications only address side effects; rarely do they address the root cause of a particular condition. Interestingly enough, as you will see throughout this book, your nutrition can actually impact the root cause of certain conditions. Doesn't that sound better than taking medication?

WHY KETO NOW

Taking control of your health isn't just about nutrition. There are actually four aspects to health that we think are most important: nutrition, movement, sleep quality, and stress management. We refer to these as the Four Pillars of Health. Each plays a vital role in overall health and wellness, as well as disease prevention and management.

The 4 Pillars of Health

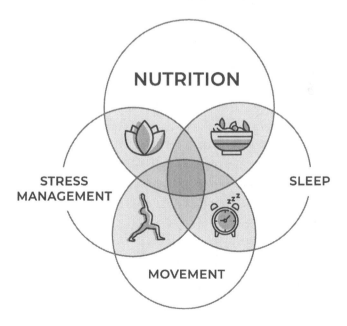

NUTRITION

STRESS MANAGEMENT

SLEEP

MOVEMENT

While each is important, nutrition is at the top because we believe it has the largest impact on our overall health and wellness. In fact, our diet plays a big role in each pillar and is at the core of taking control of your health. You can't control everything, but you can control what you put in your body. That is why the focus of this book is keto. Keto has an ability to impact our health through multiple facets, and can even target some of the common drivers of our most popular chronic diseases. But keto isn't the only thing that is important in nutrition. There is even a wrong and a right way to do keto, which is another purpose of this book.

The goal behind this book is to tell you what you need to do to take control of your health—with a keto diet providing the foundation—along with numerous other nutrition and lifestyle strategies. We challenge anyone who picks up this book to read through it with the goal of having your life changed. Be ready, once you have completed this book, to tackle this lifestyle change and start your journey toward a happier, healthier, and better functioning human being. Let's get you in the driver's seat!

HOW TO READ THIS BOOK

Keto Answers has been created to help provide information on all of the questions that a beginner may have regarding the ketogenic lifestyle. The intention is that this book can be used as a resource for those interested in starting keto, those who want to be able to speak more fluently about keto, and those who are trying to help others start keto.

What is unique about Keto Answers is that we created it in a question and answer format. When first outlining this book, we sat down and interviewed individuals who were at different stages of their ketogenic journeys. Beginners, longtime dieters, those using it for disease management, those using it for performance, and everything in between. Taking this approach not only allowed us to incorporate a ton of questions into this book, but it also allows the book to be consumed in a couple of different ways.

For those who are new to keto or are looking to expand their knowledge base, we recommend reading this book from start to finish. You do not have to be an expert to follow a ketogenic diet; however, having a fundamental understanding of the diet is a powerful tool, because it provides a why that we have seen dramatically improve adherence to this ketogenic lifestyle. Keto Answers will provide you with a knowledge base, allowing you to do just that.

The Q&A format of this book also presents the ability to use this book as a keto encyclopedia. Simply flip to the index located in the back of this book and search for your question, to find the chapter associated with that question to get your answer. This is a great technique for any practitioners out there who are looking to prescribe or recommend keto to others. Regardless of how you use this book, we just want you to use it.

PART

1

KETO 101

The purpose of Part 1 is to lay the foundation required for you to improve your understanding of not only the ketogenic diet, but nutrition as a whole. To do this, we are going to first start by answering the most common questions asked by those first introduced to keto. This will provide you with the base knowledge you will need as you continue to progress through this book. Remember, being an expert isn't necessary to succeed on a ketogenic diet; however, we have seen that having a basic understanding of the diet and how it works will improve dietary adherence. After all, a diet is only as strong as your ability to adhere to it.

Once you learn more about the basics of a ketogenic diet, naturally you will have a lot of questions based on previously held nutrition beliefs that have been ingrained in you. For this same reason, it is expected that you will experience resistance to some of the principles the keto diet is based on. Debunking these nutrition beliefs will be the focus of Chapter 2.

These first couple of chapters may seem a bit elementary if you already have a strong understanding of the ketogenic diet. We strongly encourage you to read these chapters regardless, since we have a different outlook on this diet compared to most and understanding this outlook will be imperative to getting the most out of this book.

CHAPTER 1

UNDERSTANDING KETO

C hris first heard about the ketogenic diet at a conference in January of 2015 from two scientists we will be mentioning frequently throughout this book: Dr. Jeff Volek and Dr. Dominic D'Agostino. At the time, the diet was not as mainstream as it is today. There were not a bunch of social media accounts created to spread awareness on the diet, there were only a couple of websites spreading relevant information, and accessing and understanding the research on the diet was a lot more challenging.

Now several years later there is a lot more information available. You can learn about keto on Instagram, through books, or from your uncle who just heard about the diet on the 7 o'clock news and has decided to spread his "wealth" of knowledge to you. While access to information is typically perceived as a good thing, it is important that the information is correct. What you first learn about keto will help shape your understanding of the diet moving forward. This is why it is so important to lay that strong foundation with credible knowledge.

Our understanding of keto is different from many others and has changed over the years as we have continued to research, learn, and experiment with this lifestyle. This chapter will provide you with our understanding to serve as a knowledge base for the rest of this book and your ketogenic lifestyle.

⑦ WHAT IS A KETO DIET?

> *Short Answer:* The ketogenic diet is a very low-carbohydrate, adequate protein and fat diet that transitions your body to using fat and producing ketones for energy in replacement of glucose coming from carbohydrates.

The ketogenic or keto diet is a variation of a low-carb diet that is popularly used for weight loss and improving energy levels; however, the keto diet has much more to offer. Low-carb diets are becoming more popular because research, and our current health epidemic, have begun to demonstrate that chronic high-carbohydrate consumption can lead to many health impairments, promote obesity, insulin resistance, and contribute to the progression of numerous diseases.

What we eat determines how and what energy source is available to the body to use to carry out its various functions. The energy source being used also plays a critical role in the outcome of our overall health. For most diets, carbohydrates are the primary energy source or fuel. On a ketogenic diet, carbohydrates are restricted to a degree that triggers a response in the body to find a different fuel source to replace carbohydrates. This different source of fuel comes from our stored fat and the fat we eat. However, the brain cannot use fat directly for energy, so under these conditions the body must produce another fuel source known as ketones or ketone bodies. Ketone bodies are produced in the liver from the breakdown of fat stored in the body. When the body is producing ketones, it is in a state of ketosis, putting the "keto" in ketogenic diet.

Interestingly, this metabolic state of ketosis is also what occurs when the body is under conditions of fasting or starvation. Under these conditions, this transition to using stored energy to meet the energy demands of the body exists for survival. However, on a keto diet, you are not starving. Instead, you are replacing carbohydrates with fat and protein, which allows you to still nourish your body but also achieve ketosis and mimic this state of starvation, which has so many proposed benefits. A snapshot of a keto diet done properly (yes, there are improper ways to do keto) consists of meat, eggs, vegetables, nuts, few fruits, and healthy oils.

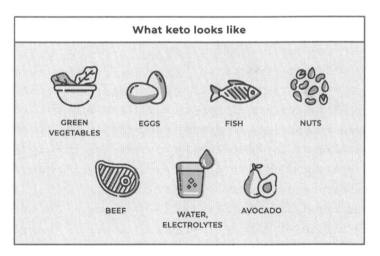

What keto looks like

GREEN VEGETABLES   EGGS   FISH   NUTS

BEEF   WATER, ELECTROLYTES   AVOCADO

There are numerous benefits of keto, which we will get into more in the coming chapters. Here are a few of the most notable:

- More Energy
- Improved Brain Health/Function
- Fat Loss
- Improved Insulin Sensitivity
- Lowered Inflammation
- Improved Blood Sugar Control
- Improved Mood
- Disease Prevention and Management

(?) ISN'T KETO JUST SOME FAD DIET?

Short answer: No. Ketosis is a state of metabolism that has existed throughout all of human history.

Get out of here! We told you in the intro we aren't into fad diets! But we get it, keto does seem to be a fad diet. Its popularity has been booming the last couple of years, leading many to think that it is just a trend that will soon go away. What many people don't realize is that modern keto has actually been around for nearly a century, and the biological state of ketosis has been around for as long as humans have walked on two legs.

The keto diet was actually first studied in the 1920s as a therapeutic intervention, not a weight loss diet. In 1921, Dr. Rollin Woodyatt made a unique observation: ketones appeared in the blood of those who were eating "too much fat" and "not enough carbohydrates." During this same time, Dr. Russell Wilder from the Mayo Clinic made the observation that these ketone bodies were reducing seizure activity similar to fasting in children with epilepsy (fasting was a commonly used treatment option for children suffering from drug-resistant epilepsy). Together this led to the hypothesis that a diet that mimics fasting, such as this "too much fat" and "not enough carbohydrate" diet, may be a viable alternative to fasting for epilepsy, allowing the patient to follow the treatment for longer than they previously could with fasting. Wilder ran a study, found that this diet was successful, and coined the term ketogenic diet.[1]

The keto diet was widely used during the 20s and the 30s therapeutically, and up until the 80s could be found in most textbooks on pediatric epilepsy. But most people only recognized keto for its antiepileptic effects, so after the discovery (and profit) of antiepileptic drugs the diet was largely forgotten. If you couple this development with the war on dietary fat from our government, which we will get into in a bit, you can see why the keto diet never picked up traction in the modern nutrition world. This lack of traction meant that there was limited quality research being done on the benefits of the keto diet.

Now that keto is resurfacing and gaining popularity, many people view it as a fad diet. However, just because ketosis can be a great tool for losing fat doesn't make it a fad or a trend. In fact, humans have been burning ketones for as long as they've walked upright.

For much of human history we either ate a very low-carbohydrate (and thus ketogenic) diet, or we fasted because there wasn't an endless buffet of food. If we relied on burning carbohydrates alone and couldn't switch into a state of burning fat and ketones for energy, we'd be dead within days. Luckily, that didn't happen, and the species has survived long enough for us to write this book.

Hell, babies are born in a state of ketosis. Are all babies trendsetters right out of the womb, or is keto just a normal metabolic process? You can argue that a selection of certain superfoods

---

1   James W. Wheless, "History of the Ketogenic Diet," *Epilepsia* 49 (2008): 3-5.

are fads that come and go, but your metabolism and cellular machinery has stood the test of time.

? IS KETO JUST A LOW-CARB DIET?

Short Answer: All ketogenic diets are low-carb diets, but not all low-carb diets are ketogenic. On a keto diet, carbohydrates must be restricted enough for the body to start actually producing and utilizing ketones.

While the keto diet is a low-carb diet, there are many differences between keto and all other low-carb diets, which we are going to be highlighting throughout this book. One of the biggest differences between other low-carb diets and keto is this metabolic state of ketosis where the body is producing these unique energy molecules known as ketones.

Ketones, which can be used by nearly all cells in the body, are produced through a process known as ketogenesis, which again occurs when carb intake is low enough. The degree of carbohydrate restriction necessary for ketogenesis to occur is dependent on the individual but is much greater than what we typically see on other low-carb diets. In fact, below you'll see a study that shows how different amounts of carbohydrate intake can affect ketone levels.[2]

As you can see from this study, to get your body into a state of ketosis, carbs need to be severely restricted and like this study demonstrates, it is typically recommended that carb

---

[2] Charlotte Young, Sonia S. Scanlan, Hae Sook Im, and Leo Lutwak. "Effect on Body Composition and Other Parameters in Obese Young Men of Carbohydrate Level of Reduction Diet," *The American Journal of Clinical Nutrition* 24, no. 3 (1971): 290-296.

intake be less than 30 g per day to do so. This number is different for everyone, but we'll try to provide you a framework that will work for you later in the book.

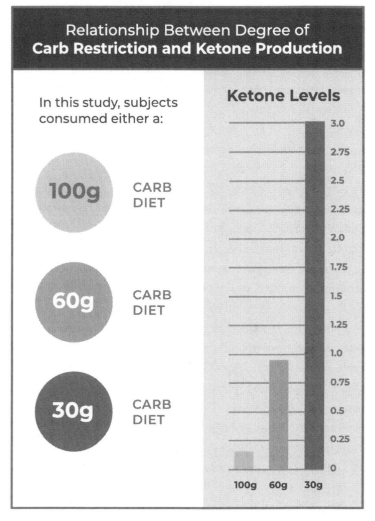

In addition to carbohydrate restriction, fat intake is typically higher on a ketogenic diet compared to many other low-carb diets where the emphasis is simply on keeping carb intake low. This is important since dietary fat is a great source of energy, which is helpful when the body's typical energy source of carbohydrates is being restricted.

? HOW IS KETO DIFFERENT FROM THE ATKINS DIET?

> *Short Answer:* Both Atkins and keto restrict carbs to similar levels, but Atkins fails to recognize the metabolic change to utilizing ketones for fuel.

When you say you've been eating low-carb, most Americans will imagine you're doing some sort of "Atkins" diet, made popular by Dr. Robert Atkins in the 1990s. Dr. Atkins published great work about using a moderate-fat, high-protein, and low-carbohydrate diet to improve various aspects of health. His approach is certainly low-carb, but again, that does not make it ketogenic. Just aimlessly reducing carbohydrates without knowing if you're in a state of ketosis isn't enough.

Another primary difference between Atkins and keto is protein and fat intake. The Atkins approach typically calls for replacing carbs with more protein and not fat. The problem is that protein is not a great source of energy, so if the bulk of your food is protein, there is not much available fuel for the rest of your body.

There are more calories per gram of fat (9 calories per gram), compared to protein (4 calories per gram) which is why the Atkins Diet can become too low-calorie and promote low energy and hunger. These factors together can lead to poor health, diet adherence, and easier regained fat.

Another common problem with Atkins (and keto) is the failure to emphasize food quality. The diet has been ridiculed, and fairly, for imagery of people stuffing down ten overcooked grain-fed burgers topped with processed bacon and fluorescent cheese. They call themselves healthy because they skipped the bun. That's not healthy no matter what you call it, but that's also a mistake we commonly see on keto, too.

Typical keto diets fail to promote food quality as well, which is why we'll get into what we call Keto+ shortly to make sure you make this the healthiest version of keto possible.

Finally, the Atkins Diet also plans for carbohydrate reintroduction. Since ketosis is one of the goals of a keto diet, there is no planned reintroduction of carbohydrates. That does not mean you have to stay keto forever (don't worry, we will get into that, too), but it does mean that you are not starting keto with the goal of returning to carbohydrates as a primary fuel source.

Later in the book we will discuss the different variations of a keto diet, one of which is Modified Atkins, which is closer to traditional Atkins in that it is higher protein but still contains more fat, emphasizes food quality, and is done with certain goals in mind.

? DOES THAT MEAN KETO IS THE SAME AS PALEO?

Short Answer: While there are some similarities, the main differences between keto and paleo is that paleo doesn't inherently limit carbohydrates and is far more focused on food quality.

Keto is also often confused with the paleo diet. The main difference between the two is once again the degree of carbohydrate restriction. Fruit and starchy vegetables, which are accepted on a paleo diet, are the primary drivers of this difference in carbohydrate intake. Paleo dieters eat fruit and sweet potatoes. Keto dieters avoid nearly all fruits and carbs.

Paleo is also much more focused on food quality and is essentially based on the idea that we should eat what our ancestors ate, and we don't mean your grandfather, who probably had a thing for Triscuits and Swanson TV dinners. If you eat paleo, you generally eat at a pre-agricultural level. Rather than eating carbohydrate-rich foods that people would have farmed, such as grains and tubers, paleo means eating foods that our hunter-gatherer ancestors would recognize: animal products, vegetables, fruits, nuts, and seeds. This eliminates much of what causes insulin resistance, chronic inflammation, and preventable diseases: grains, trans fats, and vegetable oils, sugars, and other Frankenfoods.

Many preventable modern diseases, such as cancer, heart disease, and diabetes, grew in significance during and after the Agricultural Revolution, when we lived in cities and had to figure out how to grow just a few staples, then process and store food to feed many people. The revolution worked; we have eliminated starvation. But the system we built is killing us slowly, through chronic disease brought on by what we have done to the food we are eating.

Contrary to what you might believe, wheat and other grains are processed foods. If you tried to eat a raw wheat kernel, you'd probably break your teeth. But we're humans, so we decided we should have machines help us make our food.

The Agricultural Revolution combined with the Industrial Revolution and capitalism to create the food system we have now, and thus the poor-health epidemic we have now. We feed food that isn't real to sick animals, then slaughter them to feed sick humans, who also eat food that isn't real. This toxic system and processed carbohydrates are the root causes of a massive increase in obesity, diabetes, heart disease, cancer, neurological disease, and more.

Our modern food system is starkly different from our ancestors' habits of eating hundreds of different plants and hunting wild game. Research done on populations of humans that still eat and live life according to our ancestors' ways shows they have lifespans similar to ours, yet live rich lives free of most preventable diseases. Adults stay lean late in life, they don't demonstrate a lot of neurodegeneration, they don't have heart disease, and they don't get "hangry" if they don't have a snack every sixty minutes. Sound impossible? It's not.

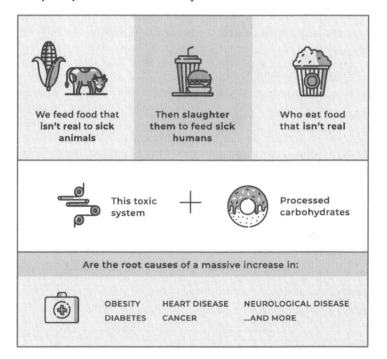

We feed food that isn't real to sick animals

Then slaughter them to feed sick humans

Who eat food that isn't real

This toxic system + Processed carbohydrates

Are the root causes of a massive increase in:

OBESITY   HEART DISEASE   NEUROLOGICAL DISEASE

DIABETES   CANCER   ...AND MORE

Paleo and keto are interconnected but different. Since not all paleo foods are low-carb, you can be on a paleo diet but not be in ketosis. And since there are many low-quality processed foods out there that are still low-carb, you can be in ketosis without being paleo.

We think the best approach combines both paleo and keto, which is a main tenet of Keto+ and is often referred to in research as the paleolithic ketogenic diet. After all, the goal is optimal health, so you want to be in ketosis, *and* you want to get there by eating *real food*s that are the basis of the paleo diet—not junk. An exclusive focus on maintaining ketosis leads some people to eat a lot of fat, few carbohydrates, and some proteins but ignore the main benefit of the paleo approach: a framework for eating real, quality foods.

You are literally what you eat. Every single cell in your body is made from the food you eat, so quality must be paramount. You can burn low-quality fats for fuel, but that doesn't mean you're going to build a resilient body.

? HOW DOES KETOSIS WORK?

Short Answer: Ketosis occurs when carbohydrate intake is restricted enough to cause low blood sugar and insulin levels, which stimulates the burning of stored fat and the production of ketones in the liver.

Thus far we have really driven the point home that ketosis is what makes a keto diet unique. Understanding how ketosis works can be a great way to understand the changes that are going on in your body. However, to understand how ketosis works, we have to first discuss how carbohydrate metabolism works. When you consume carbohydrates, those carbohydrates are broken down to glucose and released into the bloodstream. Glucose is a type of sugar, and in this case is what we know as blood sugar.

This increase of blood sugar, from the breakdown of carbohydrates, causes the pancreas to secrete a hormone known as insulin, which binds to cells in the body to open the door for glucose to enter the cell and go through a process known as glycolysis. Glycolysis further breaks glucose down into a substrate that can be used by the cell to produce energy or scientifically speaking, ATP (adenosine triphosphate).

Since carbohydrates can be broken down very quickly, whenever they are present (which for a lot of people is all the time), they are the primary fuel source for the body.

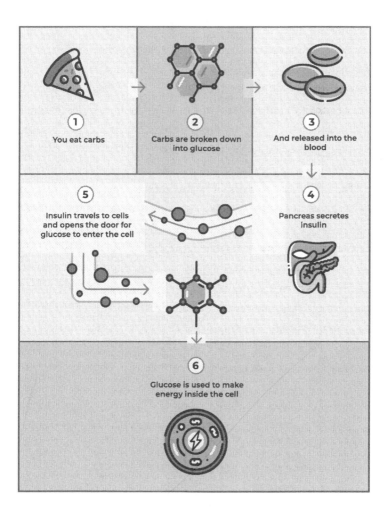

1. You eat carbs

2. Carbs are broken down into glucose

3. And released into the blood

4. Pancreas secretes insulin

5. Insulin travels to cells and opens the door for glucose to enter the cell

6. Glucose is used to make energy inside the cell

However, if we restrict our carb intake enough, as we would on a keto diet, we see a decrease in blood sugar, which means that the need for insulin decreases, so insulin levels also lower. When we have low levels of glucose and insulin, our pancreas secretes another hormone known as glucagon. Glucagon has many functions, one of which is to interact with our adipose tissue or fat cells to release stored fat into our bloodstream where it can be used by cells for energy. But that's not quite enough.

Interestingly, while most of our body can run on fat for fuel, the brain cannot. This is why we possess this unique metabolic mechanism of ketosis. The liver can break down fat and use it to make little energy molecules known as ketones or ketone bodies. However, the liver does not possess the necessary enzymes to use ketones for fuel, so these little energy soldiers are shuttled out of the liver and into the blood, where they are able to travel to cells and tissues and be taken in and used for energy.

Research has found that many cells in the body will skip using ketones for fuel and use fat instead, allowing the ketones zooming through the bloodstream to be taken in and used by the brain.[3] Remember, the brain can't effectively use fat, which is why this adaptation of the body is crucial.

Your body being in a state of ketosis is what differentiates keto from other low-carb diets *and* makes it superior. One of the problems with other low-carb diets is brain fog and lack of energy. This is because these diets do not allow enough carbs to meet the demands of the brain and body, yet do not restrict

3   Alexandre Courchesne-Loyer, Etienne Croteau, Christian-Alexandre Castellano, Valerie St-Pierre, Marie Hennebelle, and Stephen C. Cunnane, "Inverse Relationship Between Brain Glucose and Ketone Metabolism in Adults During Short-term Moderate Dietary Ketosis: a Dual Tracer Quantitative Positron Emission Tomography Study," *Journal of Cerebral Blood Flow & Metabolism* 37, no. 7 (2017): 2485-2493.

carbs enough to stimulate more fat burning and trigger ketone production to meet the needs of the brain.

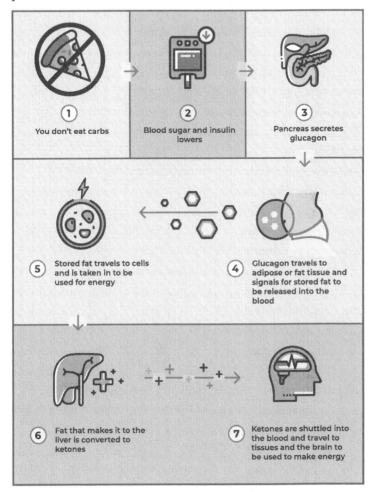

Most people think that eating fat is required to stimulate ketone production, but that isn't necessarily the case. Here's a brief science lesson. Note that there is a difference between the fat that we eat and the fat in our body. Ketones are made when stored fatty acids are mobilized and delivered to the liver.

Ketones are not made from the fat you eat with the exception of MCTs, which we will be covering later in this book.

The fat that we eat gets absorbed in our digestive tract and packaged into little carriers known as *chylomicrons*. Chylomicrons travel through our bloodstream and are roped in by muscle and adipose tissue where they can then dump off the fatty acids they are carrying into cells to be used for energy or stored for later use. However, chylomicrons only go to the liver to be disposed of after they have dumped their fatty acids, meaning they are not able to deliver significant amounts of dietary fat to the liver for ketone production. That means that the fat we eat will preferentially be used for energy by our tissues and not for ketone production. Do not fall victim to the misconception that eating more fat will get your ketones higher or that it is necessary to be in a state of ketosis.

At this point, some of you may be wondering about "macros"—that is, how much fat, protein, and carbohydrate you should consume. After all, to get your body into a state of burning ketones for energy, following a particular macronutrient range plays a critical role. We will discuss macros on keto in much greater depth in Part III. For now, it is important to note that the emphasis is not just on macros. Cutting carbs is important, but so are numerous other factors. Let's keep going!

? WHAT ARE KETONES?

Short Answer: Ketones are energy molecules that are produced in the liver from the breakdown of fat. Once produced, ketones can leave the liver and travel to places like the brain to be used for energy.

The body actually produces three different types of ketone bodies. They are referred to as acetone, acetoacetate (AcAc), and beta-hydroxybutyrate (BHB).

Technically, BHB is not a ketone body, due to a difference in its chemical structure, but is considered one for the purpose of energy metabolism. That is because BHB is the primary ketone body that is the end product of ketogenesis in the liver, meaning it is also the ketone that we see circulating in the blood, ready to be taken in by cells and used to convert to energy.

When stored fat, mobilized by glucagon, makes it to the liver, it is broken down to acetyl-CoA. Acetyl-CoA can then either enter the mitochondria of the cell to be used for energy, or it can be shuttled through another process known as ketogenesis. If shuttled toward ketogenesis, acetyl-CoA then goes through several steps leading to the production of AcAc, which is further converted to BHB, with acetone being made as a by-product.

Then BHB is released into the blood, where it can circulate through the body, be taken up by cells, and undergo a reverse process of being broken back down to AcAc and eventually acetyl-CoA, where it can now enter the mitochondria and be used for energy.

While some research suggests that acetone could also be used for energy, it is common for this ketone to be excreted as a waste product in our urine or breath.[4]

In addition to the ketones our body creates, we can also take what is known as exogenous ketones, which are supplemental

---

4   K. Musa-Veloso, S. Likhodii, E. Rarama, S. Benoit, Y.M.C. Liu, D. Chartrand, and S. Cunnane, "Breath Acetone Predicts Plasma Ketone Bodies in Children With Epilepsy on a Ketogenic Diet," *Nutrition*, 22, no.1 (2006): 1-8.

ketones that, when ingested, can lead to an acute increase in blood ketones. While exogenous ketones aren't magic erasers for carbohydrates, they can be a great complement to a ketogenic diet or healthy nutrition plan. We will give you a better breakdown of exogenous ketones and how they can be used in coming chapters.

? IS KETOSIS SAFE?

> *Short Answer:* Yes, ketosis is a safe and natural metabolic state that serves a purpose within our body. The keto diet has been evaluated and deemed safe for many different populations.

Yes, of course, Anthony is a doctor! Definitely kidding! To be clear, just because someone is a doctor does not mean that they are educated on nutrition. In fact, most MD programs contain very little nutrition training. This is one of the reasons why you should be doing your own research (that's right, keep reading).

Anyway, back to the question: yes, ketosis is safe. Do you think our ancestors had the chance to eat every sixty to ninety minutes while roaming the savannah for millions of years? Nope. We fasted a lot and ate measly amounts of carbohydrates. If we only ran on carbohydrates, we would have died off very easily by fasting just for two to three days. We literally would not have lasted more than a few generations as a species, but here we are writing this book in a coffee shop on our MacBooks. All thanks to metabolic flexibility and being able to transition from using carbs as fuel to fats as fuel, or *ketosis*. So, not only is ketosis safe, it's necessary.

In addition, the use of the keto diet has been researched and generally accepted in many populations, including pediatric, athletic, obese, diseased, and elderly. For the vast majority of people, the keto diet is safe. There are, however, a few conditions where using a keto diet may not be advised, such as pyruvate carboxylase deficiency, porphyria, and other fat metabolism disorders.

Fat consumption is the primary reason why keto is thought by some observers to be unsafe; however, it is now being recognized that the consumption of healthy fat does not pose the same risk we once thought it did. In fact, fat actually has a lot of benefits. We will get into both the negative perception of fat, and the health benefits of fat, in a bit.

Another reason why someone, especially your doctor, may think that the keto diet is unsafe is because they may confuse it with diabetic ketoacidosis (DKA). We will discuss the difference between DKA and nutritional ketosis in the next chapter but for now, it should be known that they are not the same thing, and nutritional ketosis has been deemed as a safe metabolic state. If you ask your doctor about keto and they shake you off, make sure he or she knows the difference between nutritional ketosis and DKA, and probably take the hint to go find a new doctor.

? IS KETOSIS HEALTHY?

> *Short Answer:* Ketosis can lead to many health improvements and help prevent and manage symptoms of many diseases. One of the primary reasons why keto can do this is its ability to target insulin resistance and inflammation. But unfortunately, ketosis can be unhealthy, if done improperly.

Not only is keto safe, it can also make a huge impact on overall health and wellness, if done properly. Additionally, as more and more research comes out, we are seeing that the diet offers therapeutic potential for numerous diseases. Keto's impact on so many different aspects of health can lead many to see the diet as a panacea. While this is not necessarily the case, the keto diet is able to target some of the primary contributors to many health impairments, allowing the diet to insert its benefits in many different situations.

There are two primary health-destroying aspects that keto targets, allowing the diet to provide such robust benefits: *insulin resistance* and *inflammation*. These two factors play a huge role in how we feel and perform. They are also two of the most important factors to the onset and progression of most common chronic diseases. The standard Western diet, high in carbs and processed food, promotes both insulin resistance and inflammation. It should come as no surprise that when we flip the script to a ketogenic lifestyle, it can save the day.

KETO TARGETS:	
Insulin resistance Inflammation	
WHICH CONTRIBUTE TO:	
Obesity	PCOS
Cancer	Arthritis
Alzheimer's Disease	Traumatic Brain Injury
Autism	Mental Disorders
Diabetes	Hormonal Problems
Cardiovascular Disease	And More

We have already mentioned insulin numerous times because it is an extremely important hormone, which is why we are going to take a bit of a deep dive on it here. You have probably heard of insulin as something that type 2 diabetics take to control their symptoms. However, it is actually a vital hormone secreted by the pancreas in all healthy humans.

Simply put, insulin's job is to manage the nutrients you digest and absorb from food and plays a role in carbohydrate and fat metabolism. Remember, when you eat carbs, they are broken down into glucose and released into your bloodstream (known as blood sugar). Increases in blood sugar signal the pancreas to secrete insulin. Insulin interacts with the cells of your body to "open the door" for glucose to enter the cell into your cellular "gas tanks," where it can be burned as energy right away or shuttled toward glucose storage called glycogen. The problem is that most people have too much fuel. If you are overeating carbs and/or don't exercise and move your body, you're going to constantly have a full tank of gas.

What happens when the gas tank is full and there's still glucose in the bloodstream? The body has to convert the sugar to something else. This something else is fat, which occurs through a process known as de novo lipogenesis. The fat created during this process is fat that can *actually* cause damage in the body and contribute to fat storage.

This is essentially what most people do every day by eating the large quantities of carbohydrates included in the standard American diet. To stick with the car analogy, every single day they go to the gas station to fill up on fuel, but their tanks are full, so they fill gas can after gas can and load them into the trunk.

The worse news is that if this trend continues, the overconsumption of carbs causes your cells to stop responding to the signals from insulin. This is known as reduced insulin sensitivity or insulin resistance. Insulin sensitivity is how easily your body responds to insulin. You are considered insulin sensitive if your body only needs to secrete a small amount of insulin to deposit glucose into the cells. The more insulin sensitive you are, generally the healthier you are.

Insulin resistance occurs when your blood sugar is constantly elevated, so your pancreas continues to secrete insulin. Over time this chronic high level of insulin, or hyperinsulinemia, results in the cells of your body no longer responding to insulin, a.k.a. insulin resistance.

When you become insulin resistant, your pancreas continues releasing more insulin in the attempt to decrease blood sugar levels. This is a dangerous cycle that can result in numerous health complications, most notably, type 2 diabetes.

Diabetes is not the only disease caused by insulin resistance though. As mentioned, insulin resistance plays a big role in many of the most common chronic diseases we see today. It appears that as we age, our bodies lose their effectiveness at utilizing glucose. This trend seems to be accelerated by lifestyle factors, including the chronic overconsumption of carbohydrates. This is why we should stop neglecting nutrition's role in the treatment *and* prevention of disease.

Another reason why insulin resistance is so damaging to our health is because when insulin is elevated, the body does not burn fat. In fact, under conditions of high insulin, fat consumed is shuttled toward storage in combination with the fat created from excess carbohydrates. Furthermore, insulin prevents the burning of stored fat, so if you are insulin resistant, stored fat burning is also going to be hindered. This not only leads to obesity, which is a huge contributor to poor health, but it also drives up inflammation and other contributors to poor health and disease.

We are not saying that carbs alone will kill you. The problem is that we consume too many of them, and in forms that are not what our body needs. It's pretty simple; if you are insulin resistant, you don't use carbohydrates well and continuing to consume them is damaging to your body. If you are younger and more insulin sensitive, don't ruin that by flooding your body with carbohydrates until you lose that sensitivity. Under both of these conditions, it seems like a better idea is to cut the carbs and allow your body to transition to a different fuel source (fat and ketones) that will not lead to the same complications. Ketones can be taken in by cells through pathways that are independent of insulin, so despite any insulin dysfunction, ketones can still be utilized as fuel. This is extremely important because of the energy crisis that is created by insulin resistance, which further contributes to the progression of many diseases. Another problem with insulin resistance is that it is a prime driver of the other factor that plays a key role in our overall health: inflammation.

As for inflammation, there are two kinds: acute and chronic. Acute inflammation is your friend. If you cut your hand trying to slice the perfect avocado, you want your acute inflammatory pathway activated immediately. This is your body's way of sending reinforcements to take care of a problem. You may notice a little swelling, a little redness in the area—and this is normal.

Chronic inflammation is an entirely different animal. This is the low-grade response by your body to having to continually repair tissues or combat foreign invaders from your diet and environment. If you are slowly and constantly damaging cells, your body will be in a consistent, slow repair process at all times. This results in chronic inflammation, another great landscape for chronic disease to build on. Interestingly, consuming too many carbs and being insulin resistant can promote chronic inflammation, so going keto also breaks this cycle.

We cannot say this enough; the majority of health impairments and modern chronic diseases are rooted in insulin resistance and chronic inflammation. Address these and you are taking a huge step toward improving your health and addressing the root causes of chronic disease, rather than just treating symptoms. One of the best ways you can do this is by cutting out those carbs, especially processed carbs, and running on an entirely different energy system. This is what makes keto so special.

The unfortunate bit here is that you can eat really terrible quality food and still be in a state of ketosis. Remember the Atkins cliché of fried food, void of nutrients and full of chemicals, just without the bun? This can lead to your body producing ketones for energy molecules, but that's not all that matters for health. You need to eat the right foods that both allow for proper cellular function as well as ketone production, if you want the true benefits of ketosis. Think Keto+!

? SO, WHAT DO I EAT ON KETO?

Technically, as long as you limit carbohydrates enough, you can be in ketosis. That's not the option that will keep you healthy long term though. Later in the book we will get more into the specifics of what foods you should be eating on your keto diet to follow Keto+. As an introduction, here are some of the foods you'll be eating to both be in ketosis and be healthy:

- Meat (beef, pork, poultry, etc.)
- Fish
- Eggs
- Avocados

- Leafy green vegetables
- Nuts/Seeds
- Minimal amount of cheese
- Quality oils like MCT, coconut, and avocado oil
- Few low-glycemic fruits such as blueberries

Now you can probably start to see the "low-carb, high-fat" description of a keto diet. This is as far as most people get in terms of understanding keto. However, we look at keto a lot differently. This is not just a fat-loss diet; it is a healthy lifestyle change.

That means that the quality of food that you are putting in your body is also important, so on keto you will not only be avoiding things like bread, pasta, oats, and fruits, you will also want to avoid low-quality processed meats and vegetable oils. But we are getting ahead of ourselves—we will get more into the *how* to do keto later in the book!

IF I'M A VEGETARIAN OR A VEGAN, CAN I DO KETO?

Many people consider keto to be a restrictive diet. We actually don't see it that way, but for a vegetarian or a vegan it can be. Typically, the foods used to replace meat on a standard vegan or vegetarian diet contains carbohydrate replacements making them not keto-friendly. This means that the approved keto food list for vegans and vegetarians is a lot smaller and thus restrictive.

That makes following keto as a vegetarian or vegan a lot harder. You can still consume plenty of fats if you stick to healthy oils, nuts/nut butters, avocados, seeds/seed butters, and coconut as your sources, but making sure you get enough protein in can be a little more challenging. But that doesn't mean it can't be done, and in fact, there are numerous people reporting that they do follow a vegetarian keto diet.

In truth, we do not believe that a vegetarian or vegan lifestyle is the best thing for your overall health. While these diets are gaining more and more traction, long term it appears they are not a good idea for your overall health and can cause many side effects due to various nutrient deficiencies. However, if you're a vegan or vegetarian, stay with us here!

The concept of a ketogenic diet does not have to be challenging. Cut out the carbohydrates because you do not need them, and replace them with high-quality fat and protein to fuel your body and allow it to produce ketones naturally. Now that you know a little more about what a ketogenic diet is, we are guessing you have a lot of questions and concerns based on what you have been told about nutrition your whole life. That's good—we want you to question everything so we can help debunk those previously held beliefs!

CHAPTER 2

DEBUNKING NUTRITION MYTHS

I f you are new to the concept of keto, then chances are that last chapter challenged a lot of previously held beliefs you may have had. You may even be a little skeptical and likely have tons of questions. That's part of the process and is something we encourage. Question everything.

When both of us were first introduced to the keto diet, we were skeptical. In school we were both taught that carbohydrates were essential, and that fat was bad. Cholesterol should be avoided, and red meat is dangerous. However, very rarely are these views ever supported with clear evidence.

In fact, if you take a close look at the research used to support our current dietary guidelines, you will find that the evidence isn't there. Yet this lack of evidence fails to bring questions to our dietary guidelines and the myths used to support our current nutrition advice. Every five years, the US Department of Health and Human Services (HHS) and the US Department of Agriculture (USDA) publish the Dietary Guidelines for Americans. These guidelines are created by a committee and are supposed to be supported by available research. However, most of the studies used to make these recommendations are epidemiological studies that are flawed and cannot provide enough information to make a definitive claim about anything.

At the time when this book was written, the current dietary guidelines have failed to address the real research that supports low-carb diets, studies that are a lot stronger than what is being used to make the guidelines. What impact does this have? Besides encouraging people to follow diets with no scientific evidence of improving health, it also leads to a flawed medical system.

At a conference, nutrition journalist Nina Teicholz told a story about a student who reached out to share an experience she had in medical school. After a lecture on nutrition and dietary guidelines, the student approached her professor to ask if the professor had any idea of the research that was out on low-carb diets. The professor's response was astonishing. The professor was actually following the ketogenic diet, recommends the ketogenic diet, but was not allowed to teach this to his students because he was obligated to teach according to the current dietary guidelines. In case you didn't catch that, the future doctors of America are being taught the wrong information by educators who do not believe in what they are being forced to teach. That is a broken system.

The way we have been looking at nutrition the last few decades has not proven to be beneficial. It's time to question everything and challenge the status quo, which we will be doing in this chapter as we help debunk some of the most commonly held nutrition beliefs.

? DOES THE BODY NEED CARBS?

> *Short Answer:* No, the body can produce the glucose it needs
> naturally without the consumption of carbohydrates.

As you now know, the body can replace the need for carbohydrates with fat and ketones. Despite this, the body does still
need glucose, a product of carbohydrate digestion, which leads
many to believe that carbs must be consumed to meet demand.
But this thinking is a little flawed.

There are some cells in the body, such as red blood cells and
even certain portions of the brain, that can *only* use glucose for
fuel. Even on a keto diet, the need for glucose by these cells
remains. The secret is, you don't have to eat the carbs to fuel
these cells!

Our body possesses a unique metabolic process known as
gluconeogenesis (GNG), a word that some ketogenic dieters
fear for reasons we'll investigate later. GNG is the creation of
glucose from non-glucose substrate, like amino acids from protein and even from the fat you burn for fuel. No, that does not
mean that when you eat a steak high in protein that it turns
into a donut inside our body. It means that your body has a regulatory process in place to ensure that these cells that consume
only glucose have the fuel they need. This is a demand-driven
process, meaning your body does this as it needs glucose, and
doesn't when it has enough.

This process is also the reason why your blood glucose does
not go to zero when you follow a low- or no-carb diet or fast for
more than a few hours. Don't believe us? Test your blood sugar on
a multi-day fast and watch your blood sugar stabilize quite nicely.

We will get into the fear of GNG later in the book, but for
the purpose of answering this question, you do not need to

worry about the need for carbs since our body has an innate ability to replace the need for them.

? ARE CARBS BAD THEN?

> *Short Answer:* No, carbs are not necessarily bad, but they are not essential, and people eat far too many of them and from bad sources.

It is often perceived that those in favor of low-carb diets think that carbs are bad. While many keto advocates do fall victim to this line of thinking, it should be noted that carbohydrates are not inherently evil (with the exception of processed carbs). The problem is that we consume way too many carbs, especially those fake food, processed carbohydrates.

Seventy percent of US adults are obese or overweight and over 100 million (?!) are diabetic or prediabetic.[5] If someone is obese/overweight or diabetic/prediabetic, they are suffering from some degree of insulin resistance. In fact, if you recall from Chapter 1, many diseases are rooted in insulin resistance which occurs from the chronic overconsumption of carbohydrates.

If someone is insulin resistant, they no longer effectively utilize carbohydrates so consuming them does not make sense. Additionally, research has shown that as we age, we begin to lose our ability to effectively utilize carbs.[6] Furthermore, as we addressed in the last question, our body can make all of the

---

5   "Adult Obesity Facts," CDC: Centers for Disease Control and Prevention, Last Updated August 13, 2018, https://www.cdc.gov/obesity/data/adult.html.

6   Mayer B. Davidson, "The Effect of Aging on Carbohydrate Metabolism: A Review of the English Literature and a Practical Approach to The Diagnosis of Diabetes Mellitus in the Elderly," *Metabolism* 28, no. 6 (1979): 688-705.

glucose it needs without carbohydrate consumption so while they may not be bad, they are not necessary. In fact, there is no such thing as an essential carbohydrate.

To put another way, carbohydrates are not evil, but they are not essential, and we've abused them and fake foods for so long that as a society we may not tolerate them very well. As we age our ability to effectively utilize carbs for energy can become impaired, which is accelerated by the chronic overconsumption of carbohydrates. If you align with this thinking, then you should be able to see how low-carb diets can also promote disease prevention, but we will get into that later!

? IF I AM EATING "CLEAN" CARBS THEN THAT'S OKAY, RIGHT?

It's true that some carb sources are better than others. Certain carbs may have a lower glycemic response, meaning they can be digested slower, leading to a milder increase in blood glucose. Certainly, some carb sources may also contain a lot more nutrients compared to others (that doesn't mean you can access those nutrients, but we are getting ahead of ourselves again).

For someone who was raised eating only real foods, with strong exercise, sleep, and stress standards, eating "clean" or "good" carbohydrates may be well tolerated. The problem is quite a few of us have metabolic damage, excessive fat, and never-ending inflammation. If you are metabolically damaged and suffering from some degree of insulin resistance, you no longer effectively utilize carbohydrates whether they are "good" or "bad."

Even fruit, whole grains, brown rice, and sweet potatoes are broken down to glucose and remember, having chronically elevated levels of blood glucose can lead to your health spiraling out of control. Furthermore, if your goal is to achieve ketosis, spiking blood sugar will prevent this so on a ketogenic diet, even the "clean" carbs have to go. This does not mean you will never eat these foods again, which we will discuss in greater detail later.

? BUT I THOUGHT FRUIT WAS GOOD FOR YOU?

> *Short Answer:* While fruit may contain some vitamins and minerals, it also contains a lot of sugar in the form of fructose, which in excess is not healthy and should be limited or avoided on a keto diet.

This can't be a myth—what about that timeless folk wisdom, "An apple a day keeps the doctor away." Wasn't your mother right when she told you this? Many people believe fruit is a health food and, therefore, it doesn't matter how much you eat, right? Er, not quite.

Fruit also contains a lot of sugar, so consuming it can keep you out of ketosis, negatively impact weight loss efforts, and hinder your ability to develop healthy habits. How?

The sugar in fruit causes a big increase in blood sugar, followed by a big crash in blood sugar, leading to a hungry and tired you. When you eat fruit as a stand-alone snack, you'll probably feel full for half an hour. After that, hunger sets in again. Fruit doesn't have enough fat or protein to keep you satiated. Although fruit does contain fiber, which can help keep cravings at bay, it's usually not enough to prevent the inevitable blood sugar crash. Once that blood sugar starts crashing, the hunger and cravings begin to surface again.

Fruit doesn't just contain any sugar; it contains a special sugar known as fructose, a sugar that most people refer to as a "healthy sugar," because, well, it is found in fruit. Here's the problem: fructose fails to trigger the release of hormones and neurotransmitters in your brain to signal that you're full. Did you ever bring home a container of grapes or pineapple, eat a few pieces, and suddenly the entire container was gone? You're not alone. The combination of sneaky fructose and blood sugar spikes (followed by dips) is a recipe for disaster. This inadvertently prevents weight loss for many people.

Fructose is also known to cause bloating since it is not efficiently absorbed by the small intestine. This leads to gas and abdominal discomfort—something quite frustrating for someone trying to get healthy. And thanks to the magic of agricultural research and development, today's fruits are bigger and sweeter than ever. Have you noticed that some apples are the size of a baby's head, and you can buy table grapes that seem almost as big as kiwis? They are just bags of wet sugar with little to no actual nutrition. Beware.

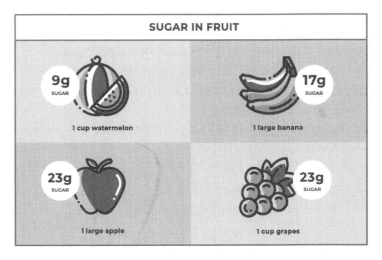

SUGAR IN FRUIT

9g SUGAR — 1 cup watermelon

17g SUGAR — 1 large banana

23g SUGAR — 1 large apple

23g SUGAR — 1 cup grapes

If that wasn't enough, there is also some research out there stating that fructose can activate an inflammatory cascade in the body, which can wreak havoc on your health. Furthermore, there is speculation that fructose may be a culprit in non-alcoholic fatty liver disease, a recent health epidemic, despite fat catching much of the blame.

One last thought about the supposed health benefits of eating a lot of fruit comes from a meta-analysis looking at fruit and vegetable consumption in relation to breast cancer risk. Findings showed vegetable consumption was associated with a reduced risk of breast cancer—but not fruit.[7] Why? Maybe because sugar fuels cancer, but we will get into that later too!

? BUT WAIT, ISN'T FRUIT HIGH IN VITAMINS AND MINERALS? HOW AM I GOING TO GET THOSE IN?

Yes, fruits contain some micronutrients, also called vitamins and minerals. Yes, it is very important to get enough of these in your diet. But fruit isn't your only option, or even close to the best option. There's nothing you get from fruit that you can't also get from foods on a ketogenic diet (except for all that sugar). Below are just a few of the ways you can increase micronutrient intake on a keto diet (we'll get into these in detail in the following chapters):

- Keto-friendly non-starchy vegetables
- 100 percent grass-fed meats and organ meats
- Nutrient-dense poultry and seafood
- Properly made greens powders

---

7 S. Gandini, H. Merzenich, C. Robertson, and P. Boyle, "Meta-Analysis Of Studies on Breast Cancer Risk and Diet: The Role of Fruit and Vegetable Consumption and the Intake of Associated Micronutrients," *European Journal of Cancer* 36, no. 5 (2000): 636-646.

These foods provide everything you need to increase your health and help combat disease—without causing unnecessary spikes in blood sugar and insulin levels.

It is also worth mentioning that there are a couple keto-approved fruits that we will be mentioning later like certain berries and avocados. These are lower glycemic fruits meaning they do not cause as much of a blood sugar spike, thus making them more acceptable on a ketogenic diet.

As a final point to put the need for fruit to rest. Many do not realize that while fruit does contain a lot of micronutrients, humans are not able to absorb these micronutrients very well. In fact, micronutrients found in meat are much more bioavailable, a term used to describe how well something can be absorbed, to humans compared to micronutrients of plant origin. For example, vitamin A has been found to be 15-20 times more bioavailable in meat compared to plant sources.[8] Iron from meat origin is three times more bioavailable compared to iron from plant sources.[9] As nutrition expert Dr. Georgia Ede says, "Just because a food contains a nutrient does not mean we can access it." If you are worried about your micronutrients, eat more meat!

---

8 Marjory J. Haskell, "The Challenge to Reach Nutritional Adequacy for Vitamin A: B-Carotene Bioavailability and Conversion—Evidence in Humans," *The American Journal of Clinical Nutrition* 96, no. 5 (2012): 1193S-1203S.

9 Lichen Yang, Yuhui Zhang, Jun Wang, Zhengwu Huang, Lingyan Gou, Zhilin Wang, Tongxiang Ren, Jianhua Piao, and Xiaoguang Yang. "Non-Heme Iron Absorption And Utilization from Typical Whole Chinese Diets in Young Chinese Urban Men Measured by a Double-Labeled Stable Isotope Technique," *PloS One* 11, no. 4 (2016): e0153885.

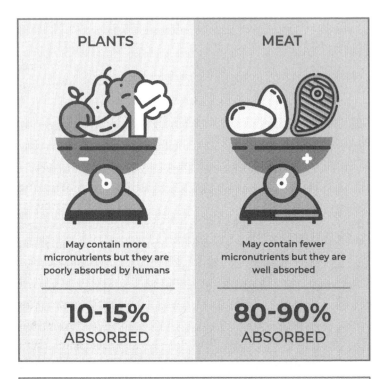

PLANTS	MEAT
May contain more micronutrients but they are poorly absorbed by humans	May contain fewer micronutrients but they are well absorbed
10-15% ABSORBED	**80-90%** ABSORBED

KETO FRUIT

Did you know that an avocado is a fruit? This is one of the reasons why we say that on a keto diet you will be avoiding *most* fruits. Avocados are rich in quality fat, high in fiber, low in net carbs, and contain many essential micronutrients.

Interestingly, an avocado actually contains much more potassium than a banana, making it a superior choice for potassium replenishment, which as we will discuss in more detail later, is a crucial component to a successful keto diet!

? IS CONSUMING MORE FAT EVEN SAFE?

Short Answer: Yep! A great deal of our body is made of fat and needs fat to thrive.

Despite what you have been told your whole life, eating fat is not bad. In *The Big Fat Surprise* by investigative journalist Nina Teicholz, you can read a pretty detailed description of the history that has driven a lot of the recommendations we have against dietary fat today, most of which was a result of research from Ancel Keys. While it is easy to poke holes in his research, it did still make quite the boom, and now today we are still struggling to combat the bad name given to dietary fat in the name of his research.

The truth is that it is actually more efficient for the body to metabolize fat than it is for it to metabolize carbs. We are not going to get overly complex with the biochemistry here, but what this means is that when your body is using fat and ketones as its primary fuel source, less oxidative stress is produced, resulting in reduced inflammation and improved cellular health. When your body is metabolizing primarily carbs for fuel, the opposite occurs.

If this is true, then why do we think fat is bad? Well, besides the easily debunked work of Ancel Keys, the problem is that a lot of studies that find that fat is bad are actually using low-quality fat in conjunction with high-carb consumption, just like the Standard American Diet (think burger and fries). Remember, when carbs are present the body will metabolize them first. This not only drives up inflammation, but also prevents fat from being metabolized and pushes it more toward storage. Additionally, the combination of high-fat and high-carb can promote a harmful shift in blood lipids and evokes a greater inflammatory response.

However, when carbs are out of the picture, the body preferentially utilizes the fat we eat for energy, cell structure, and various bodily functions, which is not dangerous. In simple terms, remove the bun and swap those fries for some greens and that burger meal becomes health promoting rather than a cheat meal.

? DOESN'T EATING FAT MAKE YOU FAT?

Short Answer: There is a difference between the fat you eat and the fat in your body. When you consume dietary fat without carbs, your body uses that fat for energy.

Now that is a good question! Fat is fat, right? Eating more fat should cause you to get fat, right? Seems to make sense, and that is what we have been told for a long time now. However, this is not the case.

It is important to distinguish the difference between fat in the body and fat we eat. Just because we can consume fat does not mean that eating it will lead to a higher body fat percentage. Let's take a look at how fat accumulation occurs:

Adipose tissue is what you are seeing when you are looking at things like your visceral or belly fat, but it is also found in many other places throughout the body. Many people think of adipose tissue as a sack of fat with no purpose other than making our pants not fit. However, adipose tissue actually plays a crucial role in communicating with other fat cells, immune cells, neurons, stem cells, and much more.

Adipose tissues are made up of adipose cells (adipocytes), and there are two different types of adipose cells: brown and white. Brown fat burns calories, while white fat cells are for storage, storing triglycerides until they are called on for energy production.

Remember that when we eat fat, it is packaged into chylomicrons and carried around the blood where it can dump off fatty acids to cells to be used for energy or stored for later use. When fat is consumed without carbohydrates, it is used for energy because it is the primary fuel available.

However, when we eat fat and carbs together the story goes a little differently. If you recall from Chapter 1, when carbohydrates are consumed the pancreas responds by secreting insulin. Insulin is commonly referred to as a storage hormone, because it drives energy-producing nutrients into cells to be used for energy or saved for later use.

Carbs are considered our body's primary fuel source because it is very easy for cells to use glucose for fuel, thus, when available, glucose will be burned ahead of fat. That means that when carbs are consumed with fat, the insulin secreted will result in fatty acids being pushed more toward storage, since glucose will be the primary energy source lowering the demand for those fatty acids. Pair this with the fact that the overconsumption of carbs can stimulate fatty acid production (through de novo lipogenesis) and when insulin is elevated, fat burning is halted, and you can see that dietary fat is not the cause of obesity.

The moral of the story here is that over-consuming carbs and pairing a high-fat intake with high-carb intake can lead to a cascade of events resulting in adipocyte hypertrophy or the growth of our fat tissue. This can start the path toward inflammation due to adipose tissues' ability to stimulate the release of cytokines and other inflammatory markers.

As we'll discuss later in the book, this doesn't mean you should eat an unlimited amount of fat on a ketogenic diet. Everything has its place and we'll help you decide how much fat works for your goals later on.

? OKAY, FINE ON THE FAT, BUT I'M SURE I SHOULDN'T EAT RED MEAT, RIGHT?

> *Short Answer:* Many people think red meat is bad due to saturated fat; however, saturated fat also provides many benefits to the body and is not dangerous when consumed without carbohydrates.

Red meat is often thought to be harmful because first, it is an animal product, and second, it contains saturated fat. Saturated fat has received more negative press than any other fat, mostly because of misunderstandings or misrepresentation of research. There is no actual evidence in the research demonstrating saturated fat being dangerous. Additionally, it has been determined that saturated fat intake does not correlate with saturated fat levels in the body. All of the research that points toward saturated fat intake and any complications of health are just weak epidemiological studies based on correlation.

Correlation does not equal causation. What does that mean? Well, just because a study finds a correlation for something causing another thing, does not mean that thing is the cause. Let's look at an example. Have you ever seen an article title like this?

"Red Meat Consumption Increases Risk of Cancer"

Everyone likes to take this title and run with it. In most cases, if you take a look at the actual study you will find that they are observational studies. Observational studies occur when a population is measured or surveyed as it is. Many of these studies are conducted via dietary recall surveys where in the instance of the above example, a group of people diagnosed with cancer would be asked to recall their diet through very vague questions like, "Over the last year, how many meals containing beef did you eat per week?" If the data reported high to red meat consumption, then it could be observed that red meat consumption correlates with a higher risk of cancer.

Let me ask you a question. If you interviewed people who just got diagnosed with cancer and found out that many of them have cats, would we assume that cats cause cancer? No, you would not. A single factor that does not take anything else into consideration can hardly be blamed for the cause of something. In the example of the above study, what about the carbs? Did they ask if these men were putting the bun on those red meat burgers? Or if they were having potatoes with that steak? No, they didn't, or at least they didn't report it. That is why we cannot take these studies to heart.

Yes, saturated fat can become harmful but not because it is fat, and not because it is saturated. When you have a gut problem, as you would if you were eating a diet high in processed carbohydrates, your body takes carbohydrates and makes these things called lipopolysaccharides, or LPS. These tiny molecules can hitch a ride into your bloodstream, where they lead to a cascade of inflammatory problems. However, LPS can't cause this mischief alone. It has to hitch a ride on saturated fat to get into your bloodstream, via those chylomicrons we talked about earlier.

So, the theme remains, saturated fat in the presence of carbohydrates *and* gut dysfunction leads to inflammation and all its associated chronic health problems. The root cause isn't saturated fat alone so, again, when we cut out the carbs and restore our gut health, which begins to happen as a result of keto dieting, then saturated fats are able to be used as they should be and provide their benefits to the body.

Besides carbohydrates, another real way red meat could actually be a concern is the manufacturing process, which can lead to low-quality meat that has lost much of its beneficial nutrients and is loaded with more pro-inflammatory fats. That is why the source of your food is so important, which we will get into more later in the book.

If you actually take a look at the available evidence, like this review of forty-nine observational and randomized controlled trials did, you will find that there is no link between saturated fat consumption and heart disease or death.[10] The truth is, saturated fat actually is essential in our body for numerous reasons, most notably for brain health and hormone production.

? I HEAR PEOPLE EAT BUTTER; THAT CAN'T BE GOOD FOR YOU?

Actually, butter, if it is the right quality, isn't bad for you...but that doesn't mean you have to pour it on and in everything, you fat-mongers.

Ultimately the same problem occurs with the demonizing of butter as all animal products—saturated fat content. As we just mentioned, you shouldn't be worrying about saturated fat. Grass-fed butter can actually be rich in fat-soluble vitamins and other nutrients like conjugated linoleic acid (CLA). This doesn't mean you need to start wearing T-shirts with sticks of butter on them and eating them like candy bars.

The keto community has done quite the number on butter. We now see pictures on social media of people putting loads of

---

10   Rajiv Chowdhury, Samantha Warnakula, Setor Kunutsor, Francesca Crowe, Heather A. Ward, Laura Johnson, Oscar H. Franco, et al. "Association of Dietary, Circulating, and Supplement Fatty Acids with Coronary Risk: A Systematic Review and Meta-Analysis," *Annals of Internal Medicine* 160, no. 6 (2014): 398-406.

butter in their coffee or spreading butter thickly onto whatever keto food they are eating. Just because you can have butter on a keto diet does not mean that you have to consume it with absolutely no regard.

Butter is still a dairy product, and as we will get into more depth later, dairy can be a common inflammatory trigger for many people, although less offensive than most dairy sources due to the high fat content. Don't fall victim to the notion that putting butter on everything makes you keto, which automatically makes you healthy.

? OKAY, FINE, BUT WE CAN AT LEAST AGREE THAT ANIMAL PRODUCTS ARE BAD FOR THE ENVIRONMENT, RIGHT?

Since research has now debunked many of the myths against animal fats, the lack of environmental sustainability is now the last thing that advocates for plant-based diets hold onto for justification. We have all heard it, right? "Animal meat production is not sustainable, and after all, cows release a lot of methane which is detrimental to our environment." Wrong again.

Peter Ballerstedt, an expert in agronomy (the science of soil management and crop production), looks at sustainability differently. He says that true sustainability should be a "multifaceted topic that should consist of societal, economic, and ecological aspects." Chronic illness has put quite the financial strain on our economy and should be taken into consideration when talking about sustainability, especially since a diet high in quality animal proteins appears to be one of the target methods for treating or improving symptoms of so many chronic diseases. Peter further explains his outlook by saying:

The production of high-quality animal protein and animal fat by ruminants from feed resources humans cannot directly utilize will be fundamental to feeding a growing population. What's more, this essential food production can preserve and enhance the diverse environments where it takes place. We need a revolution in our thinking of what constitutes a healthy diet, of what causes chronic illness, of the vital role that animal product play in the human diet, and the essential nature of ruminant animal agriculture in meeting humanity's needs. This will mean overthrowing established policies and institutions and confronting vested belief systems. In addition, we need an effort, analogous to the Green Revolution, to develop and deploy the knowledge and technology necessary to meet the mid-21st Century demand for ruminant animal products while preserving and enhancing the environments in which they're produced.

Truthfully, a lot of the evidence suggesting that meat is bad for the environment really isn't backed by science. However, the way animals are treated in the food industry is worth talking about. By no means are we animal rights activists but the way animals are treated is not only a form of animal cruelty, but it also leads to the production of a lower quality food source.

This can be avoided by shopping local through farmers markets, which as we will get into in Chapter 6, will also lead to higher quality meat. Shopping local is a way to support with your dollars a more sustainable method of acquiring higher quality meat while treating animals better in the process. If you want to learn more about sustainability, we suggest checking out more of Peter's work and if you get a chance to hear him talk, we suggest doing that, too—he's hilarious!

⑦ BUT SURELY, I SHOULD LIMIT MY CHOLESTEROL INTAKE, RIGHT?

Ah, we thought you'd ask that. That's okay, Mr. Keys made all of this very confusing for us. Bear with us on these next few questions, because they are going to be a little more science-based as we take a deeper look at cholesterol.

Cholesterol is a type of fat (also known as a lipid) that is found in many animal foods like beef, lamb, pork, eggs, and sardines, and is also produced by your liver. Cholesterol, despite getting a bad reputation, is extremely important and required for numerous processes in the body. Cholesterol is used to support cellular membranes, it's used to make hormones, it helps your body produce vitamin D, it is used to protect our intestinal tract, it is important to repairing damaged cells, it helps your body produce bile, and it plays a vital role in combating inflammation. Would you be surprised if I told you that cholesterol makes up 25 percent percent of your brain? Cholesterol is extremely important for proper brain function and low cholesterol levels may even contribute to neurodegeneration.

You may be wondering, if cholesterol has so many purposes in the body, why is it so often feared? Besides the fact that cholesterol is a fat and fat is feared, high levels of cholesterol in the body have been associated with high risk for various diseases, particularly heart disease. The problem here is that when you are testing cholesterol in the blood, you aren't actually directly testing cholesterol. Let us explain.

Earlier we talked about chylomicrons and how they had to carry fat from the diet through the blood. The same is true for all lipids that need to be transported in the blood. Unlike sugar and other components of the food you eat, which can mingle in your bloodstream, cholesterol is also a lipid and doesn't mix well with the watery nature of your blood (you know what they say about oil and water). Therefore, for cholesterol to make its rounds throughout your body, it needs to climb into a "boat" to sail your bloodstream in style.

These vessels are known as lipoproteins. Lipoproteins, like they sound, are lipid-carrying proteins. One of the primary jobs of lipoproteins is delivering cholesterol to the cells and organs that need it the most. There are five different types of lipoproteins, but the ones you hear about most are low-density lipoprotein (LDL), frequently referred to as "bad" cholesterol, and high-density lipoprotein (HDL), which has been labeled a "good" guy.

To be clear, HDL and LDL are not actual types of cholesterol, only the lipoproteins that transport cholesterol throughout your body. This is important because when you are getting total cholesterol measured at your doctor's office, you are just getting your lipoprotein levels measured or the combination of HDL and LDL. The problem with this measure is that HDL and LDL both have different functions in the body and lipoproteins carry other things besides cholesterol, including triglycerides, phospholipids, fat-soluble vitamins, and even various proteins. The amount of each of these contained within a lipoprotein varies and is dependent on numerous factors, such as the composition of your diet and your activity level.

The moral of the story here is that when we are measuring for cholesterol, we are essentially just correlating the number of lipoproteins in the blood with a predicted amount of cholesterol. That's like trying to predict how many people are traveling a highway just by counting the number of cars. What about the number of people in each car? Now you can see why saying elevated levels of cholesterol in the body is the cause of disease seems a little fishy. How can we be certain?

Regardless of whether or not we can measure it well, most of us have been told that we need to avoid cholesterol, and this is what shapes our dietary recommendations. In fact, recently Chris' grandpa's doctor recommended that he eat no more than one egg per week to keep his cholesterol levels low. There are two big problems with this recommendation. The first is that the foods you eat only contribute to about 20 percent of the cholesterol in your body, the other 80 percent comes from your liver. The second is that cholesterol is important and necessary for a healthy, properly functioning body!

The take home message is consuming cholesterol should not be feared and measuring total cholesterol as a risk factor for disease is far too simplistic.

? WHAT'S THE DIFFERENCE BETWEEN THIS GOOD AND BAD CHOLESTEROL?

HDL and LDL, the two primary lipoproteins discussed in the previous question, are commonly referred to as good and bad cholesterol. The two primary problems with this label are that they are not actually cholesterol—they only carry it—and they both serve different and equally as important roles in the function of the human body. Furthermore, cholesterol isn't bad, it just depends where it ends up in the body and this is regulated by the different types of lipoproteins and numerous other factors.

HDL is produced by the liver and is commonly referred to as the good cholesterol. HDL wears many hats as it relates to our human physiology, the most notable being its ability to scavenge the body looking for cholesterol to pack on board and deliver back to the liver, where it can be eliminated. Additionally, HDL particles have anti-oxidant, anti-inflammatory, anti-thrombotic, and anti-apoptotic properties.[11] For this reason, higher HDL levels have been associated with superior cardiovascular health.

LDL, commonly referred to as the bad cholesterol, also wears many hats. In fact, LDL is the primary lipoprotein that carries cholesterol and triglycerides to the cells to be used for energy or other functions like cellular repair. The chylomicrons we have been mentioning are actually a type of LDL, are produced by cells that line our digestive tract, and is responsible for carrying fats and other components from the foods we eat. VLDL, another type of LDL, are particles that are produced by your liver to carry cholesterol and triglycerides, made by the body, to the cells. Once VLDL has deposited its triglycerides to be used for energy, it turns into LDL and is made up primarily of cholesterol. Nearly 70 percent of circulating LDL is cleared through the liver while the rest is utilized throughout the body based on demand.

Now are you a little confused on why people consider LDL to be such a bad thing? Does it sound like LDL is necessary to make sure our cells have everything they need for energy and repair? Does it sound like LDL levels may have to go up on a high-fat diet since fat is the primary energy source and needs to be transported? You are correct. Like most of the lipid-related topics we have discussed, LDL has been falsely accused for contributing to poor heart health. How did this happen?

LDL is perceived negatively because we see elevated levels of it in many chronic diseases, diseases characterized by inflammation and cellular degeneration—which is one

---

11   Kenneth R Feingold and Carl Grunfeld. "Introduction to Lipids and Lipoproteins," in *Endotext*, K.R. Feingold, B. Anawait, A. Boyce, et al., ed. (South Dartmouth, MA: MDText.com Inc, 2000).

of the reasons we actually see elevated LDL in these conditions. Remember, LDL functions to transport cholesterol, triglycerides, and other useful material to cells to provide energy and help repair damage. If you are suffering from a sickness, disease, or have cell damage occurring, it should not come as a surprise that you would see elevated levels of LDL; your body is trying to repair itself. Just because something is present doesn't mean it's the cause.

Let's use a real-world example. If you came home and your house was on fire and you saw firemen there, would you assume the fireman started the fire? No, you would know, based on their job description, that they are there to help. Why don't we look at LDL like this? Probably because the function of LDL is typically not discussed, it is just referred to as "bad," and that's the end of the story.

Remember though, LDL does carry cholesterol and, as we alluded to earlier in this question, cholesterol is only harmful if it ends up where it isn't supposed to. Atherosclerosis, the hardening of our arteries, is a major contributor to poor cardiovascular health and disease. Cholesterol is one of the reasons why atherosclerosis occurs.

WHAT?! I THOUGHT YOU SAID CHOLESTEROL WAS COOL.

Don't worry, it is, let us explain. The lining of our blood vessels contains several layers of defense. When any of these layers become damaged, LDL will travel to the wreckage zone to help clean it up, primarily through the use of cholesterol. But LDL and cholesterol can get trapped inside our arterial cell walls. When this happens repeatedly, hardening occurs—atherosclerosis. Your next logical question *should* be, what causes the damage to the arterial wall and how does LDL get trapped inside? That's probably the issue, right? Bingo!

Inflammation, especially chronic inflammation, is one of the primary reasons we see damaged arterial walls. This starts with the glycocalyx. (A mouthful, we know.) The glycocalyx is a thick, gel-like layer that lines the inner wall of our healthy blood vessels. The glycocalyx has many functions, one of its primaries being the first line of defense for the lining of our blood vessels. Inflammation and oxidative stress can destroy our glycocalyx. Interestingly, at Low-Carb Houston 2018, chemical engineer and nutrition expert Ivor Cummins showed a pretty shocking picture of what happens to the glycocalyx following a high-carb meal. It looked something like this:

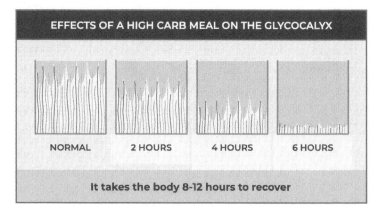

As you can see after a single high-carb meal, the glycocalyx, our first line of defense, is completely destroyed. Now the first line of defense is down, and the endothelium is exposed. That means LDL can have access to this area for repair. If this is done through a process known as endocytosis, this is fine. This process means that the endothelium is taking in the lipoprotein, allowing repair, and spitting what's left back out. The problem is that with chronic inflammation we see an increased occurrence of *transcytosis*, which occurs when the LDL goes a little deeper than it should and enters the intima proteogly-cans, where something like 25 percent of it can get trapped and become oxidized by macrophages. It is this oxidized LDL that is the primary contributor to atherosclerosis.

Now, notice something. Consuming carbohydrates can de-stroy your glycocalyx. Also, worth noting is that a high-carb diet can result in smaller LDL particle sizes, more likely to get trapped in blood vessels. Chronically consuming carbs can dramatically increase inflammation, and inflammation can damage our arterial walls, requiring LDL to come fix things up. Here it can be trapped, leading to atherosclerosis. Seems like carbs may be more of the problem here, doesn't it?

If you are looking for a take-home message, this is it. LDL is likely not a problem if everything else is in check. Here's an analogy: rain is a good thing (unless you're 10 and you have a big baseball game that day), but if you treat your house like crap and have holes in your ceiling, then that rain can become a problem. When you think about it like this, trying to lower your LDL is like doing a rain-go-away dance, rather than patch-ing up the holes.

Moral of the story: cut the carbs and let cholesterol do its thing.

❓ YOU MENTIONED TRIGLYCERIDES, AREN'T THOSE BAD?

We figured some of you would say that. Triglycerides have been demonized, along with red meat and cholesterol, making up a trifecta of bad things that will be sure to kill you. But if you take a closer look, you will see that triglycerides are just fats found in food and in the body.

Triglycerides, just as they sound, are three fatty acids with a glycerol backbone. Triglycerides are the fats we find circulating throughout our body and can either be synthesized by the body or they can be acquired through the consumption of dietary fat. The point here is that triglycerides in and of themselves are not bad, especially on a ketogenic diet when fat is our primary fuel source!

However, when it comes to measuring triglycerides in your blood, having very high triglycerides could be harmful. It is worth noting that recommended blood triglyceride levels may differ on a keto diet; however, we would still expect your triglyceride levels to lower overtime because the cells in your body should be soaking up these triglycerides for fuel rather than letting them circulate in your blood for a long time.

Of course, the time you test your blood matters. If you were to test your blood after eating a high-fat meal, we would speculate that your triglycerides would be higher since you just consumed fat. However, if you are measuring your blood fasted in the morning like you should, triglyceride levels should be decreasing on a keto because of better triglyceride usage. If this does not occur, it could be a result of too high carbohydrate consumption or consuming alcohol in the days leading up to your test.

? CAN YOU FOLLOW KETO LONG TERM?

> *Short Answer:* There is no reason to think that consuming a keto diet long term is dangerous and any theories that state so are not backed by credible science.

Some "experts" in the ketogenic space have strict plans in which you must "carb up" to intentionally kick your body out of ketosis. Long-term ketosis, they say, isn't healthy. For evidence they'll point to a theory that ketosis can lower certain hormone levels, but this is far too simplistic.

As we will discuss later in this book, our need for certain hormones may decrease while on a ketogenic diet so to say that having low levels of certain ones is far too simplistic of a view.

Currently, there are not many studies looking at long term uses of a ketogenic diet. While we do have research on the use of the diet for extended periods of time, we do not have studies looking at several years or more. These studies are hard to come by. However, there is no biological reason to think that following a keto diet long term is unsafe. Your body is being replenished with nutrition that is combating common contributors to many chronic diseases—where is the harm?

My answer to people who ask me how long they should be on a ketogenic diet is "as long as you are reaching your goals." If you feel best on a ketogenic diet, feel free to continue that indefinitely. However, a ketogenic state isn't the answer for everyone. If you notice a subjective or objective measure that is clearly going the wrong direction *and* you are doing everything the right way, ketosis might not be for you, and that's completely fine. An individual approach is essential. Find what works for you.

Alternatively, you also don't have to be in a state of ketosis forever. If you decide to start eating (real food) carbs again here or there after you've reached your goals and you aren't always in ketosis, you will not immediately die. Trust us on this one. No way of eating is worth becoming obsessed with.

To wrap up this question, it is worth mentioning that long term keto could become a problem if food quality is constantly poor or if chronic severe calorie restriction occurs. While short term calorie restriction can be beneficial, chronic undereating can be harmful to health and should be paid attention to since lack of hunger is a common side effect of a ketogenic diet.

? MY DOCTOR TOLD ME KETOSIS IS DANGEROUS, IS THAT TRUE?

> *Short Answer:* Ketosis is a safe metabolic state that should not be confused with diabetic ketoacidosis because it is not the same thing.

Many people (including some doctors who may have skipped biochemistry in med school—or forgot it) confuse the healthy state of nutritional ketosis with a harmful, more extreme condition known as diabetic ketoacidosis (DKA). Do not confuse these and don't let your doctor, either! Remember, ketosis is a natural process resulting from carbohydrate restriction and fasting. Diabetic ketoacidosis is an extremely dangerous metabolic state that is most commonly seen in people with Type 1 diabetes (and sometimes Type 2 diabetes).

DKA is often the first sign someone has diabetes. During DKA, the amount of ketones in the blood is extremely high, causing the blood to turn acidic, coupled with low insulin and high blood glucose levels. This is much different from nutritional ketosis.

DKA is commonly a product of poor diabetes management, including not getting enough insulin. However, other possible triggers for DKA include:

- Starvation combined with alcoholism
- An overactive thyroid
- Alcoholism
- Acute major diseases like pancreatitis or sepsis
- Illness or infections like urinary tract infections and pneumonia
- Medications that may inhibit proper use of insulin

- Drug abuse
- Stress
- Heart attack

DKA often involves some of the following symptoms:

- Excessive urination
- Dehydration
- Extreme thirst
- Hyperglycemia
- Vomiting
- Nausea or stomach pain
- Shortness of breath or gasping
- Fruit-smelling breath
- Feeling overly tired
- Feeling confused

Those with diabetes should use caution if they experience any of the triggers above and should see their doctor immediately if they have any of the symptoms of DKA.

Nutritional ketosis, brought about through carbohydrate restriction and eating a well-balanced keto diet, will only produce low levels of ketones *and* low insulin and blood glucose levels that are safe for the average person and not a cause for concern.

If you don't have Type I diabetes and your body produces even small amounts of insulin, it is actually a physiological impossibility to be in the dangerous state of ketoacidosis while following the keto diet. The normal quantity of measurable ketones in your blood on nutritional ketosis is about 0.5–3.0 (and sometimes as high as 5-6) mmol, not even remotely close to the amount you would have in diabetic ketoacidosis.

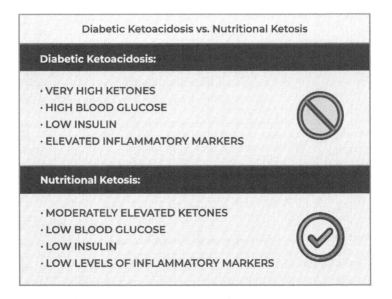

A KETO DIET SEEMS LIKE IT HAS A LOT OF PROTEIN, ISN'T THAT BAD FOR MY KIDNEYS?

How many people have you seen have health problems from consuming a protein shake? The reason many people think that protein could cause kidney damage is from increasing glomerular pressure and hyperfiltration. For those of you who don't know what that is, it doesn't matter. What matters is research has found no significant evidence for any harmful effect of high protein consumption on renal (kidney) function in individuals with healthy kidneys.[12]

---

12   Michaela C. Devries, Arjun Sithamparapillai, K. Scott Brimble, Laura Banfield, Robert W. Morton, and Stuart M. Phillips, "Changes in Kidney Function do not Differ between Healthy Adults Consuming Higher-Compared with Lower-Or Normal-Protein Diets: A Systematic Review and Meta-Analysis," *The Journal of Nutrition* 148, no. 11 (2018): 1760-1775.

Notice here that we are talking about the healthy population. For those suffering from chronic kidney disease, restricting protein consumption may be useful for preventing progression of the disease. Regardless, a keto diet is not necessarily a high protein diet and some research even suggests it could provide benefit to those suffering from impaired kidney health.[13]

? IS KETO JUST A WEIGHT LOSS DIET?

You beat us to the punch. The next section highlights all of the benefits of keto, and later in the book we will break down all of the therapeutic benefits. But remember, keto targets two of the biggest contributors to chronic disease: inflammation and insulin resistance. It just so happens that these two benefits, amongst several other physiological benefits of keto, can lead to profound weight loss as a nice "side effect." However, to say keto is just a weight loss diet doesn't do it justice.

? SO, IF I GET INTO KETOSIS, THEN I'LL BE HEALTHY?

Just because your body is breaking fat down and running on ketones, does *not* mean you are healthy. You can get into ketosis on a diet of cheese sticks, pork rinds, vegetable-oil-roasted nuts, and low-carb protein bars. You tell me—does that seem like a path to optimal health?

Yes, part of this diet is getting your body running on ketones and keeping blood glucose and insulin low, but that

---

13   Michal M Poplawski, Jason W. Mastaitis, Fumiko Isoda, Fabrizio Grosjean, Feng Zheng, and Charles V. Mobbs, "Reversal of Diabetic Nephropathy by a Ketogenic Diet," *PloS One* 6, no. 4 (2011): e18604.

alone does not cover all of the bases. Food quality and selection are also important considerations for optimal health. This is one of the reasons we see such different responses to keto in the real world and research settings. You may be following a keto diet where you are focusing on quality, well-sourced, nutrient-dense foods cooked in health-optimizing oils—this is a good approach to keto. On the other hand, we may be following a "keto diet" consisting of low-quality bunless burgers cooked in vegetable oils, topped with processed cheese and contaminated greens. Despite the fact that both of us may be in ketosis, these are two drastically different diets.

Remember the paleo-keto combo we call Keto+? This approach will not only get you in ketosis, it will also get you eating real, high-quality, nutrient-dense, low-carb foods. Combine this with a little movement, stress management, and quality sleep, and now you have a recipe for health!

? I HEARD IF YOU STOP KETO YOU JUST GO RIGHT BACK TO HOW YOU WERE. IS THAT TRUE?

At Low-Carb Houston in 2018, Dr. Andreas Eenfeldt, known as the Diet Doctor, gave everyone a good laugh when he said something along the lines of, "If you started working out really hard, put on some muscle, then stopped working out and you lost muscle, would you say, 'I tried that working out thing, it doesn't work, when I stopped I lost my muscle.' Or even, better if you stopped showering and started smelling, would you tell people, 'I tried that showering thing, it doesn't work, when I stopped, I started smelling.'"

On a serious note, yes, it is probable that if you come off of keto by binge eating carbohydrates or by returning to your previous lifestyle, you will likely see many of these benefits seen on the diet disappear. Of course, they will; your blood sugar and insulin are elevated and you are no longer in ketosis. You are no longer providing your body with that more efficient fuel source you once were. Additionally, the increase in insulin production as a result of the carbs will slow fat burning and increase water retention, both of which would contribute to real and perceived weight gain.

It is worth noting that this does not mean that you have to do keto forever. Again, we will get into that more later in the book, but for now we are just focused on being in ketosis, not getting out of it!

? IS SALT BAD FOR ME?

What are you, Chris' grandpa's doctor? Seriously, his doctor told him that he had to cut out salt, even though he had him on a statin that was depleting his glutathione levels and making him drop massive amounts of water, leading to electrolyte deficiencies and leg cramps. Sorry for the rant, that still pisses me off.

But no, salt is not bad for you. This question may seem a little out of the blue but we will be discussing sodium frequently throughout this book, because it is something that needs to be replaced on keto. Low insulin levels, a positive benefit that comes with keto dieting, causes your body to excrete water and electrolytes like sodium. The side effects of sodium deficiency can range from brain fog to muscle cramps to heart arrhythmia—not something you want to or have to deal with.

It is also worth pointing out that your kidneys possess the power to very rapidly regulate sodium levels, preventing any concern about over-consuming sodium. This is one of the reasons why we have actually seen some governing bodies loosen their restrictions on sodium intake.[14]

We know this chapter may have been difficult for some. It is very hard to change your mind about beliefs that you have had drilled into your head for such a long time. Don't worry, we had a hard time with this when we first started researching and following keto, too. The remainder of this book will continue to question conventional wisdom and in particular the current dietary guidelines. After seeing how wrong both of these are, we hope that you are ready to start this journey of taking control of your own health.

Now that we have spent some time debunking a lot of nutrition myths, let's get back to ketogenic dieting and all of the benefits associated with this lifestyle! After all, that is why you are thinking about starting this diet!

---

14 Niels Graudal, Gesche Jürgens, Bo Baslund, and Michael H. Alderman, "Compared with Usual Sodium Intake, Low-and Excessive-sodium Diets are Associated with Increased Mortality: a Meta-analysis," *American Journal of Hypertension* 27, no. 9 (2014): 1129-1137.

PART 2

KETOSIS IN ACTION

Many people first hear about the ketogenic diet for its potent weight loss ability; however, the diet offers a lot more than just making your pants fit better. In fact, the ketogenic diet has so many health benefits that it can often appear to be a panacea, leading many to be skeptical. As we stated earlier in the book, one of the reasons we see this is because keto can target two major contributors to poor health—insulin resistance and inflammation—allowing it to insert its benefits in many different ways.

You have likely heard many of the benefits that we will cover, which is likely why you are considering this diet in the first place. The purpose of this section will be to provide the why behind those benefits and introduce some benefits that you may not have known about!

During this section of the book we will be covering the numerous benefits you can experience through a ketogenic diet. We are going to start first with the general wellness benefits that occur while on a ketogenic diet, followed by benefits relating to body composition, and finish up with the physical performance benefits of the diet.

CHAPTER 3

WELLNESS BENEFITS OF KETO

When we were first introduced to keto, it was difficult to not just consider the diet a weight loss diet. At the time not many people were discussing the numerous non-scale related benefits. After a little more research, we found that there was more than meets the eye with keto and decided to give it a try. In doing so, we were able to experience the power of the diet first hand.

The truth is that keto can lead to many outcomes that promote a better overall quality of life. While some of these outcomes are a result of losing weight, as you will see in this chapter, there are several other mechanisms involved. The benefits discussed in this chapter are the biggest reasons why we are still followers of the keto diet. The diet has given us more energy, better focus, and improved mood, which has led to better relationships, stronger work, a way better quality of life, and, of course, improved health.

When outlining this book, we decided not to start with body composition related benefits first, because we think it is important to highlight the non-scale related ways keto will improve your life first. The best part is that when you dive into the science, you realize that it's not too good to be true!

? WHAT ARE THE WELLNESS BENEFITS OF A KETOGENIC DIET?

In some cases, these general wellness benefits of keto are the primary reasons someone may decide to start a keto diet. They are benefits that tend to be most noticeable and contribute to a better overall life. The most notable are:

- Increased Energy Levels
- Reduced Hunger/Cravings
- Improved Mood
- Improved Brain Health and Function
- Disease Prevention/Management

? HOW DO THESE BENEFITS OCCUR?

In short, by combating the big two problems in modern health care: insulin resistance and inflammation. Are you sick of hearing that yet? Sorry, it is vital to understand the importance of combating these two problems! However, this isn't the only contribution a keto diet makes. Ketone molecules themselves are also a major player in many of the benefits experienced.

Ketones act not only as energy molecules, but also as signaling molecules. This means they tell other cells and pathways to do things independently of providing you with energy. Combined, this allows them to promote physiological adaptations that can contribute to many of the proposed health benefits of keto.

Other changes that occur as a result of a ketogenic diet, such as improved hormonal production, better sleep, and an increase in quality nutrient intake, can also contribute to many of the benefits discussed in this chapter and throughout this book.

? HOW LONG WILL IT TAKE TO EXPERIENCE THESE BENEFITS?

> *Short Answer:* The length of time it takes to become adapted to keto is known as the keto-adaptation period and the length of time it takes for this to occur varies for everyone but typically between 2-8 weeks.

The length of time it will take you to see the benefits of keto varies. Some people report seeing improvements within just a couple of days, while others may take a week or longer. Much of this can depend on your individual body and how you were treating it prior to starting the diet.

There is a period of time between starting keto and experiencing its benefits known as the keto-adaptation period. During this period, which we will get into more in Chapter 7, the body is still becoming accustomed to the changes being thrown at it and this can take time. The length of this adaptation period can vary based on factors, such as the degree of insulin resistance or activity level. Someone who is more insulin resistant and less active may take longer to become adapted to burning fat for fuel and producing and utilizing ketones.

The important message here is that keto-adaptation takes time! You will not experience all the benefits of keto right away. In fact, if you look at the side effects of starting keto (also discussed in Chapter 7), you will notice that the exact opposite of the benefits may happen at first. Don't worry, this is normal. Your body is going through a complex series of adaptations. Rome wasn't built in a day, and neither is your body. Be patient and do not give up before you have given your body a chance to adapt and experience the diet's benefits.

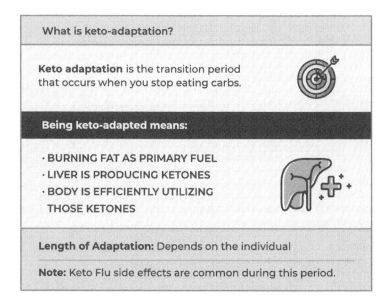

What is keto-adaptation?

Keto adaptation is the transition period that occurs when you stop eating carbs.

Being keto-adapted means:

- BURNING FAT AS PRIMARY FUEL
- LIVER IS PRODUCING KETONES
- BODY IS EFFICIENTLY UTILIZING THOSE KETONES

Length of Adaptation: Depends on the individual

Note: Keto Flu side effects are common during this period.

In Chapter 7, we will talk more about what you can do when you start keto to help get through that keto-adaptation period with ease.

INCREASED ENERGY LEVELS

? WHY ARE MOST PEOPLE'S ENERGY LEVELS SO LOW?

Short Answer: Besides not adequately paying attention to sleep, many people have low energy levels because they consume diets that cause rapid spikes and drops in blood glucose that result in energy swings.

The primary causes for low energy are typically related to problems with sleep, nutrition, hormones, stress, exercise, or a combination of the four. Unless you're just flat out tired from lack of sleep, nutrition is the largest lever to pull here. Within nutrition, the easiest thing to control is the amount of carbohydrates you are consuming.

Consuming carbs leads to an increase in blood sugar (glucose). The good news is that if you aren't extremely metabolically damaged, your body will sense this spike in blood sugar, and your pancreas will secrete insulin to rapidly shuttle glucose into your cells for energy or storage. The bad news is that this leads to a blood sugar crash, a primary driver of your fatigue.

When the blood sugar gets stored or burned, there's no more available substrate for energy. Most people who are "carbohydrate burners" do not possess the ability to easily and effectively transition to burning fat for fuel once they have run out of blood glucose. This means that once their blood sugar crashes, there isn't a whole lot of fuel available to transition to, leading to low energy levels and a need to acquire more energy the only way the body can in this situation—from more food.

Insulin resistance (IR), which we have mentioned numerous times already, can also be a common reason for a decrease in energy levels. Remember, insulin is secreted in response to elevated blood sugar. The purpose of insulin is to communicate with the cells in our body to allow them to take nutrients in for energy use or storage. However, if cells are chronically stimulated by insulin, the line of communication between insulin and our cells can become damaged or in some cases broken. This leads to insulin resistance and the body producing more and more insulin to drive glucose out of the blood and into the cells. This further contributes to the problem. This doesn't just hurt energy levels, it also wreaks havoc on many aspects of your health since IR is considered a precondition to diabetes, heart disease, neurodegenerative disease, and cancer.

If you are insulin resistant but you are still eating a lot of carbs then your body is essentially starving, despite the fact that it has plenty of fuel available. The glucose is in the blood, but it is not efficiently getting into the cell. Furthermore, insulin actually suppresses lipolysis, or fat burning, meaning that someone who has chronically elevated insulin levels is not going to be an efficient fat burner, meaning they are unable to effectively tap into the body's other source of fuel, fat.

? WHAT CAN KETO DO TO IMPROVE ENERGY LEVELS?

One of the primary reasons a keto diet can improve your energy levels is because of its ability to circumvent exactly what we just described. For starters, when you are on a keto diet, you are not eating a lot of carbohydrates, so your blood sugar levels tend to be much more stable. Rather than having sharp increases in blood sugar followed by steep declines, you tend to see consistently level numbers, which can help prevent dips in energy levels.

Once you are adapted to keto, your body can easily tap into stored body fat, which is a much greater, and nearly endless, source of fuel since even the leanest people store plenty of energy in the form of fat. Even better is that fat provides more energy per unit compared to glucose—over double. This means that once you are keto or fat-adapted, you have access to a bigger on-demand fuel tank that is more efficient and produces more energy than blood sugar.

It's not just the burning of fat that contributes to better energy levels on a ketogenic diet. Ketogenesis, or the production of ketones, can also contribute to better energy levels. Ketones are little energy molecules that can be used by nearly all cells in the human body. This is even true for the insulin resistant person, which is why keto is the best option for someone like this.

HUNGER/CRAVINGS

WHY AM I ALWAYS HUNGRY ANYWAY?

Like low energy levels, carbohydrates being your primary source of energy can also stimulate hunger. When your blood sugar crashes after a carbohydrate-based meal and you are unable to tap into fat stores, hunger is stimulated, specifically carbohydrate cravings, to get you to eat and get that blood glucose level back up to provide energy to the body.

Check out this graphic of Anthony's blood sugar after eating an apple:

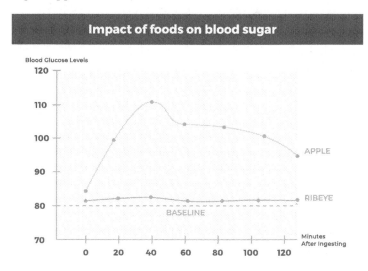

As you can see, his blood sugar looks like a theme park roller coaster. For someone who is following a high-carb diet, especially a high-glycemic, high-carb diet, the hunger stimulations will just lead to another carbohydrate-based meal that starts the cycle over again, leading to a perpetual blood sugar roller coaster. Not only can this eventually cause insulin resistance, it can also cause your hunger and cravings to come on quick and strong.

Appetite is much more complex than most people realize. In addition to unstable blood glucose, appetite signaling also plays an important role in hunger levels. Appetite signaling is regulated by the endocrine system (insulin, amylin, glucagon, pancreatic peptide), the central nervous system (NPY, AGRP, and POMC), and the digestive tract (ghrelin, PYY, somatostatin, secretin, and CCK). Together, all of these signals interact with the brain, particularly the hypothalamus, to regulate food intake.

These various signals are used for both short-term (after a single meal) and long-term (determined by the amount of fat stored in the body) to regulate appetite. In the healthy individual, appetite signaling works well. When there is not a lot of energy available, signals are sent to the brain to stimulate hunger. Conversely, when we have plenty of available energy, signals will be sent to the brain to promote fullness. The problem is that not everyone has proper appetite signaling. In fact, research has found that obese people in particular have impaired appetite signaling; one of the reasons for constant hunger and overeating.[15]

---

15   Jeffrey M. Zigman, Sebastien G. Bouret, and Zane B. Andrews, "Obesity Impairs the Action of the Neuroendocrine Ghrelin System," *Trends in Endocrinology & Metabolism* 27, no. 1 (2016): 54-63.

? HOW IS KETO GOING TO REDUCE MY HUNGER/CRAVINGS?

> *Short Answer:* The keto diet can reduce hunger/cravings by controlling blood sugar, increasing accessible fuel, and altering hunger hormones and signaling.

There have been a lot of studies supporting that a keto diet can suppress appetite, especially when compared to other diets. In fact, one of the most commonly reported benefits of keto is reduced hunger, a great sign of being in ketosis. If you realize you didn't eat for the last 14 hours, still have boundless energy and are not hungry, you are probably in ketosis.

This anecdotal evidence is supported by research like this 2008 study reporting that a keto diet, compared to a moderate-carb diet, led to greater reductions in hunger.[16] This study was very practical because it allowed the subjects to eat as they felt necessary, referred to as ad libitum. Interestingly, the keto diet demonstrated a greater decrease in ad libitum food intake. The subjects on keto actually *chose* to eat less, which supports the reported reductions in hunger.

This is just one of the studies supporting what many keto dieters will report themselves: lack of hunger on keto. The question is, what is driving these reductions in hunger? There are actually several mechanisms at play.

A big mechanism is the stability of blood sugar experienced on a keto diet. Not consuming carbs means not having

---

16 Alexandra M Johnstone, Graham W. Horgan, Sandra D. Murison, David M. Bremner, and Gerald E. Lobley "Effects of a High-protein Ketogenic Diet on Hunger, Appetite, and Weight Loss in Obese Men Feeding ad libitum," *The American Journal of Clinical Nutrition* 87, no. 1 (2008): 44-55.

drastic fluctuations in your blood sugar to stimulate hunger. Furthermore, when adapted to keto, under conditions of low blood sugar your body will transition to burning fat. Since your body has a nearly endless supply of fuel available from fat (the body stores plenty), there is no need for the body to stimulate hunger because it has all of the fuel it needs available. Even further contributing to this effect is ketones since they (and fat) actually provide more energy compared to glucose.[17]

While blood glucose levels have traditionally been thought of as the primary regulator of appetite (the glucostatic theory), research has found that fatty acids can also play a role. Having elevated levels of fatty acids in the blood, like you would on a keto diet, can actually stimulate fullness due to many factors including their impact on insulin and hunger hormone, NPY.[18]

In addition to the fat found inside our body, further contributing to fullness on a ketogenic diet is dietary fat. Fat is more satiating (another term for being full) than carbohydrates, in part due to containing over double the amount of energy compared to carbohydrates. It is also worth mentioning that protein, also consumed on a keto diet, has also been shown to possess satiety-promoting effects.

---

17 Richard L. Veech, "The Therapeutic Implications of Ketone Bodies: The Effects of Ketone Bodies in Pathological Conditions: Ketosis, Ketogenic Diet, Redox States, Insulin Resistance, and Mitochondrial Metabolism," *Prostaglandins, Leukotrienes and Essential Fatty Acids* 70, no. 3 (2004): 309-319.

18 Tanya J. Little, Antonietta Russo, James H. Meyer, Michael Horowitz, Douglas R. Smyth, Max Bellon, Judith M. Wishart, Karen L. Jones, and Christine Feinle–Bisset, "Free Fatty Acids Have More Potent Effects on Gastric Emptying, Gut Hormones, and Appetite than Triacylglycerides," *Gastroenterology* 133, no. 4 (2007): 1124-1131.

Changes in satiety signaling on a keto diet further add to the hunger reducing benefits of the diet. Research has found that being in a state of ketosis can suppress ghrelin, a hormone that is responsible for stimulating appetite.[19] The ketogenic diet has also demonstrated greater production of cholecystokinin (CCK), a hormone produced during fat metabolism, which can further suppress appetite.[20]

Combining all of these mechanisms, we see a pretty impressive recipe for reduced hunger:

How Keto Reduces Hunger

STABLE BLOOD SUGAR

PLENTY OF AVAILABLE FUEL

DIETARY FAT IS SATIATING

PROTEIN IS SATIATING

PRODUCTION OF APPETITE SUPPRESSING HORMONES

Obviously, this is important since constant hunger can lead to overeating, bad relationships with food, and many other

---

19 Antonio Paoli, Gerardo Bosco, Enrico M. Camporesi, and Devanand Mangar, "Ketosis, Ketogenic Diet and Food Intake Control: A Complex Relationship," *Frontiers in Psychology* 6 (2015): 27.

20 P. Sumithran, Luke A. Prendergast, Elizabeth Delbridge, Katrina Purcell, Arthur Shulkes, Adamandia Kriketos, and Joseph Proietto, "Ketosis and Appetite-mediating Nutrients and Hormones after Weight Loss," *European Journal of Clinical Nutrition* 67, no. 7 (2013): 759.

health problems. Additionally, as we will get into in the next chapter, the prevention of increased hunger on a keto diet is one of the reasons why it may be easier to keep off the weight you lose on the diet.

MOOD

? WHY AM I IN A BAD MOOD?

Besides the fact that always having low energy and being hungry is obviously going to cause you to be in a bad mood; the foods you eat also play an important role in your mood, which many people do not want to accept. We used a similar example earlier. If you drank five margaritas and felt like heck the next day, would you blame it on the margaritas? Obviously, yes. But don't forget about the tacos you had with it! Everything you put in your body can affect the way you feel.

Additionally, the neurotransmitters (chemical messengers) that play a role in your mood are produced in your gut and can be impacted by the foods you eat. In fact, many mood disorders, such as depression and anxiety, are rooted in impaired gut function. If you are consuming a diet that is high in pro-inflammatory and highly processed foods, your gut health is being destroyed and this is a huge contributor to poor mood.

Your mood isn't just about what you *do* put in your body. It is also about what you *do not* put in your body. Nutrient deficiencies, such as protein, cholesterol, fat, vitamins, and minerals, and energy availability also play a big role in our mood further emphasizing the importance of diet in our feelings of well-being.

? HOW IS KETO GOING TO IMPROVE MY MOOD?

There is actually growing evidence for the use of the keto-genic diet for mental health disorders, including depression and anxiety, which we will touch on in greater detail later in the book. For now, it is important to know that the combination of improving your energy levels, reducing hunger, improving gut health, minimizing nutrient deficiencies, and improving body image are all ways that a ketogenic diet can improve your mood.

Of course, it is important to note that the quality of your keto diet is important here. As we will get into in the coming chapters, consuming low-quality foods will prevent you from seeing many of the benefits we just discussed.

BRAIN HEALTH AND FUNCTION

? HOW DOES KETO IMPROVE BRAIN HEALTH AND FUNCTION?

Short Answer: Ketones provide more energy to the brain than glucose and do so while producing less oxidative stress, thus causing less inflammation.

The brain has a massive energy demand, around 20-23 percent of the body's total energy demand.[21] This is important because the brain has to utilize the energy that is available to it, and for most people not on a keto diet, this is primarily glucose.

---

21 M. Bélanger, J. Allaman, and P.J. Magistretti, "Brain Energy Metabolism: Focus on Astrocyte-Neuron Metabolic Cooperation," *Cell Metabolism* 14(6) (2011): 724-738.

However, when available, ketones are the preferred fuel source for the brain. In fact, research has shown that the brain's uptake of ketones is proportional to their availability in the blood.[22] What is interesting to note about ketones versus glucose metabolism is the push-pull method that has been so brilliantly explained by one of our favorite keto researchers, Dr. Stephen Cunnane. Dr. Cunnane explains that glucose is pulled into the brain based on the demands of the brain. However, ketones are pushed into the brain based on their availability in the blood. Since ketones provide more energy compared to glucose, this means that ketones possess the ability to provide more energy to the brain to assist in brain function.

It's not just about what ketones are doing, it's also about what they aren't doing. Metabolizing glucose can be oxidative (requires oxygen), meaning it can cause oxidative stress. Over time, that stress can contribute to chronic systemic inflammation, which can damage our cells' mitochondria, the organelles responsible for creating energy. The inflamed brain with damaged mitochondria is an unhealthy, impaired brain.

Ketones are a much "cleaner" source of energy, meaning that when they are burned, they do not promote inflammation. Additionally, since ketones can provide more energy compared to glucose, they are better suited for the brain due to its high energy demands. Ketones are also signaling molecules, and

22 Alexandre Courchesne-Loyer, Etienne Croteau, Christian-Alexandre Castellano, Valerie St-Pierre, Marie Hennebelle, and Stephen C. Cunnane, "Inverse Relationship between Brain Glucose and Ketone Metabolism in Adults during Short-Term Moderate Dietary Ketosis: A Dual Tracer Quantitative Positron Emission Tomography Study," *Journal of Cerebral Blood Flow & Metabolism* 37, no. 7 (2017): 2485-2493.

one thing they are able to signal for is greater antioxidant production—important for anti-aging in general, especially as it relates to the brain.

The health benefits of metabolizing ketones in place of glucose also plays a huge role in brain disease prevention and management, especially since research has found that the brain loses its ability to metabolize glucose as we age.[23] Chronically fueling the brain with glucose is one way to accelerate this. Like all cells in our body, the cells of the brain can become resistant to insulin, causing the brain to struggle to access fuel, thus forcing an energy crisis. A starving brain is also not a healthy brain. In fact, research has shown that insulin resistance is a common driver of neurodegenerative diseases.[24] Alzheimer's has recently been described as Type III diabetes because it is becoming evident that as we age, our brain's ability to metabolize glucose decreases. This can result in a slew of deficiencies that impair cognitive health. This and other indicators suggest that maybe our brain should not be only metabolizing glucose for fuel, especially for extended periods of time—which for many could be their whole life!

Neurodegeneration and other declines in brain health do not have to occur as we age, at least not to the degree that we are currently seeing. Switching to the metabolic state of ketosis can aid in preventing or slowing this. In fact, research in neurodegenerative individuals has demonstrated that keto can

---

23 Mayer B. Davidson, "The Effect of Aging on Carbohydrate Metabolism: A Review of The English Literature And a Practical Approach to the Diagnosis of Diabetes Mellitus in the Elderly," *Metabolism* 28, no. 6 (1979): 688-705.

24 Suzanne Craft and G. Stennis Watson, "Insulin and Neurodegenerative Disease: Shared and Specific Mechanisms," *The Lancet Neurology* 3, no. 3 (2004): 169-178.

improve aspects of brain function such as memory.[25] This is because the insulin resistant brain can still metabolize ketones despite its inability to effectively utilize glucose. This not only solves the energy crisis but also helps reduce neuroinflammation and improve insulin sensitivity, all markers for improving brain health and function.[26]

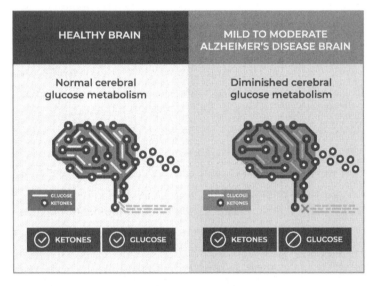

I HEARD THAT OUR BRAIN NEEDS CARBS FOR PROPER FUNCTION?

Short Answer: Your body can make all the glucose it needs for brain function without you eating a single carbohydrate.

25 Maciej Gasior, Michael A. Rogawski, and Adam L. Hartman, "Neuroprotective and Disease-Modifying Effects of the Ketogenic Diet," *Behavioural Pharmacology* 17, no. 5-6. (2006): 431.

26 Robert Krikorian, Marcelle D. Shidler, Krista Dangelo, Sarah C. Couch, Stephen C. Benoit, and Deborah J. Clegg, "Dietary Ketosis Enhances Memory in Mild Cognitive Impairment," *Neurobiology of Aging* 33, no. 2 (2012): 425-e19.

Certain portions of the brain do require some glucose, but this glucose does not have to come from your diet, it can come from a process known as gluconeogenesis, or the production of glucose from non-glucose sources. The rest of your brain can utilize ketones for fuel, and in fact, the brain likely prefers ketones.

Remember, ketones are taken up via the brain in proportion to their availability in the blood. The liver can produce between 100 and 150 grams of ketones per day, which is more than enough to meet the energy demands of the brain. This means that the brain can derive all of the energy it needs from ketones and gluconeogenesis, removing the need for carbohydrate consumption. Combine this with the fact that burning ketones is a lot healthier for the brain, you should trust us in saying "your brain likes the ketones."

It is true that your brain will not immediately start functioning better when you start keto. In fact, the opposite may be true initially. This is due to the keto-adaptation period we mentioned earlier in this chapter, which will be discussed in much greater detail in Chapter 7. For now, it is important to note that you may experience a little brain fog when first starting the diet.

There are several reasons why you may experience this. Once you stop consuming carbs, it takes time before your body is producing a sufficient amount of ketones. This can result in a temporary fuel shortage and thus brain fog. This will quickly subside as your body transitions into ketosis and becomes keto-adapted. Second, dehydration and electrolyte deficiency are very common when starting keto if not properly combatted, and together these two can also be common contributors to brain fog.

In short, brain fog experienced on keto is either a short-term problem or a problem that can be alleviated through proper supplementation, which we will go over in greater detail later in Chapter 7.

First two weeks	Long-term keto dieting
LOW GLUCOSE	LOWER INFLAMMATION
MODERATE AMOUNTS OF KETONES BEING USED FOR FUEL	LOW GLUCOSE
DEHYDRATION	MANY MORE KETONES BEING USED FOR FUEL
ELECTROLYTE DEFICIENCY	GREATER ENERGY PRODUCTION
Brain fog	**Improved brain function**

DISEASE PREVENTION/MANAGEMENT

❓ HOW DOES KETO IMPROVE DISEASE PREVENTION AND MANAGEMENT?

This is an easy one because we have beaten this point home in these first few chapters. Most diseases are rooted in insulin resistance and inflammation. Since keto can target both of these factors, the diet is able to not only improve and manage symptoms of chronic disease, but also reduce the risk of many chronic diseases.

In case you didn't fully pick up on that, the decisions you make in your day-to-day life can reduce your risk of developing chronic disease. Understanding and embracing this concept can be a transformative experience that will allow you to take control of your health and your life.

Besides treating inflammation and insulin resistance, there are other specific mechanisms of various diseases that keto can target. In this book, we are not going to take a deep dive into those mechanisms, but it is important to point out the various conditions in which keto could provide benefits:

- Diabetes
- Cardiovascular Disease
- Cancer
- Epilepsy
- Alzheimer's Disease
- Parkinson's Disease
- Multiple Sclerosis
- ALS
- Traumatic Brain Injury
- Migraines
- Depression
- Anxiety
- Eating Disorders
- PTSD
- Schizophrenia
- Wound Healing
- Lyme Disease
- Inflammatory Bowel Disease
- Hashimoto's
- Lupus

Some of these conditions have more research than others, but regardless, more research is needed so we can fully understand the therapeutic potential of the ketogenic diet.

While many people come to keto for weight loss, which we will discuss in the next chapter, most people stay for the benefits listed in this chapter. When you are eating a diet chock full of processed carbohydrates, sugar, and fake foods, you are slowly poisoning your body. When you make the change to fueling your body with fat and ketones, your body starts to function more efficiently, and you begin to feel better. Ask any keto dieter how they feel if they stuck with the diet for more than just a few weeks. You will hear much of what we discussed in this chapter.

The purpose of going through these benefits first is because of how important we think they are. When you have more energy, less hunger, better brain function, and better mood, you have a recipe for a happy and healthy thriving life. That is what diet should be about. Fuel your body with the nutrients that will allow it to function at a superior level so you can do the same!

CHAPTER 4

BODY COMPOSITION BENEFITS

L osing fat and gaining muscle may be a high priority for you. After all, beach season will come at some point in your future, and everyone wants to look a little better in that bathing suit. However, it is important to stress that body composition goals should not be your sole priority. Being in shape and having a better-looking body does not necessarily mean you are healthy.

When Chris was right out of undergrad, he decided to try a physique competition to prove a colleague that said he couldn't, wrong. After prepping for twelve weeks, Chris was in the best shape of his life, but he wasn't healthy. He wasn't fueling his body with proper nutrients and he was severely calorie restricting while eating a pretty low-fat diet, a recipe for low energy and a metabolic mess.

The point is that six-packs are great, but they do not mean you are healthy. Other diets work for losing weight and improving body composition, but they do not set you up for improvements in health along the way. Going to extreme measures to achieve body composition goals not only sets you up for being unhealthy, but also for failure at maintaining your aesthetic improvements.

As you will see in this chapter, the keto diet is the most robust way to make body composition changes without having to place an immense amount of stress on your body and while providing the body the nutrients it needs to function optimally. A ketogenic diet allows you to experience improvements in your overall health, while still improving the way you look. The gold standard of optimal health!

? HOW DOES A KETO DIET LEAD TO FAT LOSS?

> *Short Answer:* Keto increases the burning of stored body fat, reduces appetite, and improves metabolic function.

When you are following a ketogenic diet, you are putting your body in an optimal fat burning state, the reason why fat loss is so robust on the diet. How does this happen?

When you are no longer providing glucose from carbohydrates, the body must adapt by finding a new fuel source. Fat is this new fuel source and the fat can come from our diet or from our stored body fat. When it comes to burning fat, insulin is of particular importance since this hormone actually inhibits lipolysis or the mobilization of stored fatty acids. However, when glucose levels are low, insulin levels are also low, and the pancreas secretes a hormone known as glucagon instead. Glucagon behaves the opposite of insulin and is able to interact with adipose tissue to stimulate the release of fatty acids into the bloodstream, where they can then be used for energy by various cells in the body and for ketone production.

When you are in ketosis, you literally change your cellular machinery so that it can more effectively burn fat for fuel. Different cell membrane transporters and pathways are activated so your body will more readily use fat instead of sugar for fuel.

Several complementary benefits of a keto diet further contribute to weight loss, such as better energy levels and satiety. Better energy levels tend to lead to an increase in activity, thus greater calorie burning and fat loss. While calorie consumption is not the most important factor for weight loss, which we will get into more soon, keto tends to lead to reduced appetite, which can further contribute to weight loss.

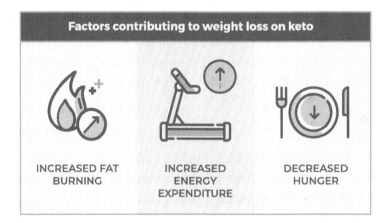

Reduced appetite has its pros and cons. Under-consuming calories for too long is not advantageous to metabolic health, and excessively low protein intake can be damaging to overall health and is counterproductive if you want to preserve or increase muscle mass.

? HOW LONG SHOULD IT TAKE TO START SEEING WEIGHT LOSS?

> *Short answer:* Weight loss can occur within just a couple of days of starting keto; however, the amount of time it takes to see significant *fat* loss depends on the individual and numerous other health and lifestyle factors.

It is important to first differentiate between weight loss and fat loss. It is not uncommon to experience rapid weight loss within the first couple of days of starting keto. In fact, it is not uncommon to report a 7-to-8-pound weight loss in the first week of the diet. Since insulin levels lower when you start keto, fat burning is going to increase to some degree; however, much of this initial weight loss is a result of the body adjusting to a low-carb diet, and not from fat burning alone.

To reiterate: when you first start keto, your blood sugar levels drop, since you are no longer eating a lot of carbohydrates. This forces insulin levels to lower, leading to your body burning more fat but also releasing a lot of stored water. As we will touch on later, this phenomenon is one of the primary reasons hydration is so important on keto, but it is also the reason why we see rapid weight loss initially. Furthermore, during this initiation into keto, your body will burn through much of its carbohydrate stores, known as glycogen. The amount of glycogen burned is not a lot but is a significant contributor to weight loss during the first week of keto.

This rapid weight loss from water and glycogen loss can be experienced almost immediately but will balance itself out as you continue to follow keto. As we will touch on soon, this leads many to think they are experiencing a weight loss plateau, which is usually not the case.

The timeline for experiencing significant *fat* loss is different for everyone. While everyone will be burning more fat from keeping those insulin levels down, the rate at which this occurs can vary depending on your current health status. If you are overweight, have thyroid issues, are insulin resistant, or inflamed, you may experience a slow start to your fat loss. Don't let this discourage you; during these first couple of weeks you will still be burning some fat, and even better is that you will be repairing your body, restoring your metabolism, and setting yourself up for continued robust fat loss.

Activity level will also play a role in when you can expect to start seeing significant progress. We don't need to highlight any studies here to tell you that if you are exercising, you are going to increase fat burning, which could actually accelerate your transition into keto.

It is impossible to determine when you as an individual will start burning significant amounts of body fat, but studies looking at obese individuals, those who may be more likely to experience a slower start, still demonstrate an average fat loss of *at least* 1 pound per week in the first couple of months of the ketogenic diet. In fact, this 8-week study in obese individuals reported nearly 10 pounds of fat loss in just 8 weeks, a weekly average of 1.25 pounds of actual fat loss.[27] While this may not seem like much to a lot of you, consistently losing a pound of actual fat mass each week is pretty substantial.

---

27 Manny Noakes, Paul R. Foster, Jennifer B. Keogh, Anthony P. James, John C. Mamo, and Peter M. Clifton, "Comparison of Isocaloric Very Low Carbohydrate/High Saturated Fat and High Carbohydrate/Low Saturated Fat Diets on Body Composition Aand Cardiovascular Risk," *Nutrition & Metabolism* 3, no. 1 (2006): 7.

? HOW MUCH FAT CAN I EXPECT TO LOSE ON KETO?

Further expanding on the previous question, it is impossible to predict how much weight you will lose on keto since it is so individualized. Depending on your size, we expect weight loss to be between 2-8 pounds in the first week, with a majority of that weight coming from water and glycogen. Bigger individuals will be on the higher side of this initial weight loss due to more water and glycogen to lose. The human body is resistant to drastic shifts in body composition so you cannot expect to lose actual fat mass at the same rate you were dropping water and glycogen in the first week. For this reason, after the first week, weight loss tends to slow down but actual fat burning increases.

The amount you can expect to lose going forward is dependent on many of those same factors we discussed in the previous question, such as your current health status and activity level. Your starting body composition also plays a big role in how much fat you can expect to lose. Despite both having plenty of stored fat to burn, obese and overweight individuals with more body fat to spare will lose more weight compared to leaner individuals with less to spare.

Using that same 8-week study from the previous question, we see obese individuals demonstrating nearly 10 pounds of actual fat loss in the first 8 weeks of keto dieting.[28] However, if we compare to another 8-week study in leaner and healthier individuals, we see only 2.5 pounds of fat loss over the 8 weeks.[29]

28 Manny Noakes, Paul R. Foster, Jennifer B. Keogh, Anthony P. James, John C. Mamo, and Peter M. Clifton,"Comparison of Isocaloric Very Low Carbohydrate/High Saturated Fat and High Carbohydrate/Low Saturated Fat Diets on Body Composition and Cardiovascular Risk," *Nutrition & Metabolism* 3, no. 1 (2006): 7.

29 Salvador Vargas, Ramón Romance, Jorge L. Petro, Diego A. Bonilla,...

While lean individuals still have plenty of stored fat, their total weight loss is going to be less, maybe less than a pound per week. For those with a little more to give, we expect after the first week that you will experience at least 1-2 pounds of total weight loss per week and overtime, that weight loss will slow as you approach your goal weight.

? IS KETO THE BEST DIET FOR FAT LOSS?

> *Short Answer:* Keto allows for greater fat loss, easier fat loss maintenance, and better health improvements compared to other diets.

If you review the literature on comparisons of different diets on fat loss, you will see mixed results. Many studies will show keto as being superior for weight loss compared to other diets while other studies will demonstrate no difference. Here are a few things to consider:

Just because two diets produce the same weight loss does not mean that they have the same impact on the body. Low-calorie diets, while effective at promoting weight loss, have been shown to stimulate hunger, putting you at an increased risk for weight regain following cessation of the diet. As demonstrated in the last chapter, keto can lead to weight loss without stimulating increases in appetite thus making keeping the weight off easier. Another example is low-fat diets, which

---

…Ismael Galancho, Sergio Espinar, Richard B. Kreider, and Javier Benítez-Porres, "Efficacy of Ketogenic Diet on Body Composition during Resistance Training in Trained Men: A Randomized Controlled Trial," *Journal of the International Society of Sports Nutrition* 15, no. 1 (2018): 31.

can produce similar changes in body composition compared to keto, can be harmful to overall health, impair endocrine function, and reduce nutrient absorption. The keto diet can lead to improvements without these deleterious effects.

Many studies show similar *weight loss* between different diets. This is not the same as *fat loss*. As we will discuss later in this chapter, a keto diet tends to lead to a greater preservation of muscle mass. While other diets may show similar weight loss compared to keto, if you break down the composition of the weight loss, you will see keto demonstrating greater actual

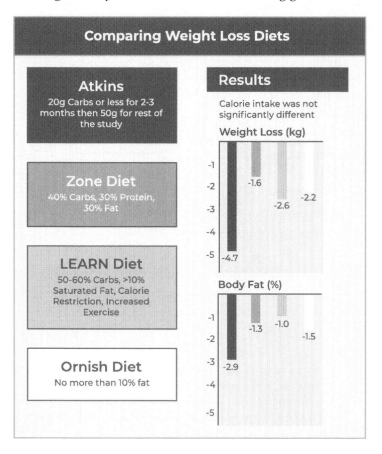

Comparing Weight Loss Diets

Atkins
20g Carbs or less for 2-3 months then 50g for rest of the study

Zone Diet
40% Carbs, 30% Protein, 30% Fat

LEARN Diet
50-60% Carbs, >10% Saturated Fat, Calorie Restriction, Increased Exercise

Ornish Diet
No more than 10% fat

Results
Calorie intake was not significantly different

Weight Loss (kg)
-1.6
-2.6
-2.2
-4.7

Body Fat (%)
-1.3
-1.0
-1.5
-2.9

fat loss and better muscle mass preservation despite total weight loss being very similar.

Individuality is also important to consider when looking at weight loss diets. A prime example of this is insulin resistance. When we look at people who are insulin *sensitive* (meaning they use carbohydrates effectively), there are similarities in the effectiveness of low-carb or high-carb, calorie-restricted diets for weight loss. However, for those who are insulin *resistant*, there appears to be a strong correlation favoring low-carb diets for weight loss. This makes sense. If you are insulin resistant, you do not effectively utilize carbs.

Regardless of the conflicting research, we believe that keto is superior for fat loss. Why? Let's take a look at the research. One study comparing four diets over 12 months in over 300 women found the Atkins Diet to induce the greatest weight loss and *specifically* fat loss.

While the Atkins Diet is not the same as keto, it does offer us insight into the value of carbohydrate restriction and its impact on fat loss, especially since calories were nearly the same in the above study. However, one could still ask, "How can we be sure that carbohydrate restriction was the reason for greater fat loss?" Let's keep digging.

Earlier in the book we presented a study that compared ketone production at varying levels of carb restriction. This study also looked at fat loss and as you can see in the graphic the greater the carbohydrate restriction, the greater the fat loss.[30] This suggests that severe carb restriction, such as

---

30 Charlotte M. Young, Sonia S. Scanlan, Hae Sook Im, and Leo Lutwak, "Effect on Body Composition and Other Parameters in Obese Young Men of Carbohydrate Level of Reduction Diet," *The American Journal of Clinical Nutrition* 24, no. 3 (1971): 290-296.

occurs on a ketogenic diet, may be the superior approach to fat loss.

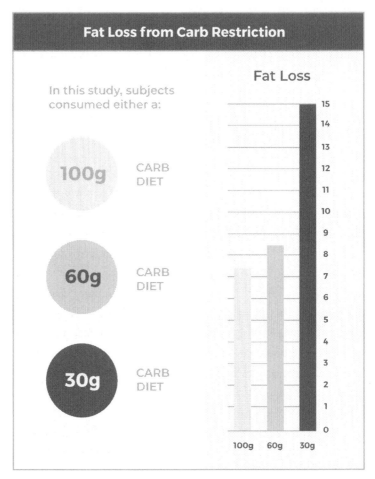

The reduction in insulin and its impact on fat loss is what makes carb restriction so important. When insulin is low, like it would be during carb restriction (and keto dieting), your body is going to be in prime fat-burning mode.

So, how does the keto diet actually stack up when compared to other diets for fat loss? Research looking at the ketogenic diet compared to a low-fat, higher-carb diet has reported "a clear benefit of the VLCK diet (very low-carbohydrate keto-genic) over the LF (low-fat) diet for short-term weight and fat loss, especially in men"[31] concluded "Individuals assigned to a VLCKD achieve a greater weight loss than those assigned to a LFD in the long term; hence, a VLCKD may be an alternative tool against obesity."[32] Given the research and anecdotal evidence, we'd say that's a pretty modest conclusion.

? WOULD I LOSE MORE FAT IF I ATE LOW-FAT AND LOW-CARB?

It seems practical, right? If you stop eating carbs and your body switches to utilizing fat for fuel, maybe not eating as much fat would allow you to burn more body fat. While this does seem intriguing, don't do this to yourself. This approach was why we saw the Atkins Diet fail.

Protein is used for many things in the body, but it is not used well as an energy source for the cells. Thus, a primarily protein-based low-fat/low-carb diet will leave you short of available energy from your diet. Furthermore, the low-calorie nature of low-fat/low-carb diets can cause the body to be

31 Jeff S. Volek, Matthew J. Sharman, Ana L. Gómez, Dan A. Judelson, Martyn R. Rubin, Greig Watson, Bulent Sokmen, Ricardo Silvestre, Duncan N. French, and William J. Kraemer, "Comparison of Energy-Restricted Very Low-Carbohydrate and Low-Fat Diets on Weight Loss And Body Composition in Overweight Men qnd Women," *Nutrition & Metabolism* 1, no. 1 (2004): 13.

32 Nassib Bezerra Bueno, Ingrid Sofia Vieira de Melo, Suzana Lima de Oliveira, and Terezinha da Rocha Ataide,"Very-Low-Carbohydrate Ketogenic Diet v. Low-Fat Diet for Long-Term Weight Loss: A Meta-Analysis of Randomised Controlled Trials," *British Journal of Nutrition* 110, no. 7 (2013): 1178-1187.

reluctant to burn its stored calories leading to weight loss stalls. Finally, going too low-fat can impact numerous aspects of health like hormones, mood, and even long-term brain health. This is not a sustainable or healthy approach to nutrition.

❓ I THOUGHT CALORIES WERE THE ONLY THING THAT MATTERED FOR WEIGHT LOSS?

> *Short Answer:* No, there are numerous other factors impacting weight loss.

The popular explanation for obesity is that we are consuming too many calories. You know what we've been told our entire lives. If you want to lose fat, all you have to do is burn more calories than you are consuming. This is the "calories in vs. calories out" approach to fat loss. We are definitely in the minority in saying this is too simple of a way to look at fat loss. In fact, we think it's pretty easy to debate that theory.

If calories out need to be greater than calories in for weight loss to occur, then why do we see so many people eating 1,000 calories a day, burning 1,500 on the treadmill alone, and still not losing weight—in some cases maybe even continuing to gain weight?

The answer is because fat burning is not just about the caloric load. This is a fallacy of weight loss myths. As nutrition journalist and author Gary Taubes explains, obesity is a disorder of fat accumulation rather than excess calorie consumption. What is causing that fat accumulation? There are many factors, with hormones being one of the biggest, and the composition of our diet plays a big role here.

This should not come as a surprise. To assume that calories are all that matter is to assume that the body handles calories from different macronutrients the same way. This is not the case. For example, we know that consuming carbohydrates stimulates insulin and insulin can hinder fat burning. That macronutrient has a different impact in the body compared to other macronutrients.

Additionally, looking at all calories the same also insinuates that each person handles calories from each macronutrient the same way. As we previously mentioned, for someone who is insulin resistant, consuming a high-carb diet is not going to produce the same results as a keto diet. This is common sense and supported frequently in research.

So, what evidence do we have that calories are not all that matter? The study we previously cited demonstrating greater fat loss on a ketogenic diet compared to a low-fat, high-carb diet should be a good indicator. Especially since the keto dieters in this study ate *more* calories compared to the low-fat diet.[33] That's right, greater fat loss while eating more calories!

Evidence like this favors that there is more to fat loss than just calorie restricting. The research actually demonstrates that carb restriction is a better indicator of weight loss success, especially in those who are obese/overweight and insulin resistant. Again, as we have previously highlighted, the degree of carb restriction also matters. A study from the famous Dr. Eric Westman from Duke University found that a ketogenic diet was superior for not only weight loss but also reducing insulin resistance and improving cholesterol levels compared

---

33 Jeff S. Volek, Matthew J. Sharman, Ana L. Gómez, Dan A. Judelson, Martyn R. Rubin,Greig Watson, Bulent Sokmen, Ricardo Silvestre, Duncan N. French, and William J. Kraemer, "Comparison of Energy-Restricted Very Low-Carbohydrate and Low-Fat Diets on Weight Loss and Body Composition in Overweight Men and Women," *Nutrition & Metabolism* 1, no. 1 (2004): 13.

to a low-glycemic, low-carb diet.[34] Even better, calorie consumption was again higher in the ketogenic group.

Calories matter to some extent, as every food has some impact on insulin, but it appears that on a ketogenic diet, they are a lot less important. Keep insulin secretion low and provide your body with sufficient vitamins, minerals, phytonutrients to do the work of cellular metabolism while relying on fat as a source of energy.

? SO, ALL I HAVE TO DO IS BE IN KETOSIS TO BURN FAT?

To be in ketosis, fat burning has to occur. Restricting carbohydrates is enough to reduce insulin and make you burn more fat, produce ketones, and get into ketosis. However, just because you are in ketosis does not mean that you are optimizing your fat burning.

There are so many additional factors that play a role in fat burning, such as your environment, stress levels, and quality of food. If you are still consuming processed low-carbohydrate foods that can promote inflammation, you will not be an efficient fat burner. If your body is under a lot of stress, it is not going to be an efficient fat burner.

The point is that just because you are in ketosis does not mean that you have optimized your fat burning or your health. As we will get into more in Part III, there is more to keto than just restricting carbohydrates and being in ketosis.

---

34 Eric C. Westman, William S. Yancy, John C. Mavropoulos, Megan Marquart, and Jennifer R. McDuffie, "The Effect of a Low-Carbohydrate, Ketogenic Diet Versus a Low-Glycemic Index Diet on Glycemic Control in Type 2 Diabetes Mellitus," *Nutrition & Metabolism* 5, no. 1 (2008): 36.

❓ DO I HAVE TO WORK OUT TO LOSE FAT?

> *Short Answer:* No, but working out will enhance results and is good for you so we recommend incorporating it into your healthy lifestyle.

There is plenty of research to demonstrate that weight loss can be experienced on keto without the addition of exercise.[35] However, that does not mean that exercise would not lead to more robust benefits. In fact, research looking at a combination of keto and exercise has demonstrated fat loss with simultaneous increases in muscle mass[36] and improved metabolic health.[37]

Exercise pairs well with proper nutrition, no matter if you are following a ketogenic diet or another form of eating. Exercise has numerous benefits, including improving cardiovascular health, maintaining and building lean muscle mass, improving fat loss, improving mood and anxiety, maintaining

---

35 Nassib Bezerra Bueno, Ingrid Sofia Vieira de Melo, Suzana Lima de Oliveira, and Terezinha da Rocha Ataide, "Very-Low-Carbohydrate Ketogenic Diet v. Low-Fat Diet for Long-Term Weight Loss: A Meta-Analysis of Randomised Controlled Trials," *British Journal of Nutrition* 110, no. 7 (2013): 1178-1187.

36 Rachel M. Gregory, H. Hamdan, D. M. Torisky, and J. D. Akers "A Low-Carbohydrate Ketogenic Diet Combined with 6-Weeks of Crossfit Training Improves Body Composition and Performance," *International Journal of Sports and Exerercise Medicine* 3 (2017): 1-10.

37 Matthew J. Sharman, William J. Kraemer, Dawn M. Love, Neva G. Avery, Ana L. Gómez, Timothy P. Scheett, and Jeff S. Volek, "A Ketogenic Diet Favorably Affects Serum Biomarkers for Cardiovascular Disease in Normal-Weight Men," *The Journal of Nutrition* 132, no. 7 (2002): 1879-1885.

and increasing bone density, increasing energy levels, and reducing the risk of chronic disease.[38] [39] [40] [41]

Exercise has also been shown to improve insulin sensitivity, which (as you should know by now) is one of the most important health improvements we can make and is particularly useful at the start of keto, as you are trying to adapt to burning fat for fuel.

Exercising does not have to mean going into the gym every day and killing yourself. It means getting out and moving, doing things you enjoy, such as resistance training, biking, playing a sport, walking, or even just working in your garden. Getting out and moving is important and shouldn't be just a tool for fat loss.

You may not need to add exercise to your keto diet to see progress for fat loss, but doing so certainly can lead to more robust results. Your body is meant to move. You should move it.

38 Wendy M. Kohrt, Susan A. Bloomfield, Kathleen D. Little, Miriam E. Nelson, and Vanessa R. Yingling, "Physical Activity and Bone Health," *Medicine & Science in Sports & Exercise* 36, no. 11 (2004): 1985-1996.

39 Wojtek J. Chodzko-Zajko, David N. Proctor, Maria A. Fiatarone Singh, Christopher T. Minson, Claudio R. Nigg, George J. Salem, and James S. Skinner "Exercise and Physical Activity for Older Adults," *Medicine & Science in Sports & Exercise* 41, no. 7 (2009): 1510-1530.

40 Carol Ewing Garber, Bryan Blissmer, Michael R. Deschenes, Barry A. Franklin, Michael J. Lamonte, I-Min Lee, David C. Nieman, and David P. Swain, "Quantity and Quality of Exercise for Developing and Maintaining Cardiorespiratory, Musculoskeletal, and Neuromotor Fitness in Apparently Healthy Adults: Guidance for Prescribing Exercise," *Medicine & Science in Sports & Exercise* (2011): 1334-1359.

41 Joseph E. Donnelly, Charles H. Hillman, Darla Castelli, Jennifer L. Etnier, Sarah Lee, Phillip Tomporowski, Kate Lambourne, and Amanda N. Szabo-Reed, "Physical Activity, Fitness, Cognitive Function, and Academic Achievement in Children: A Systematic Review," *Medicine & Science in Sports & Exercise* 48, no. 6 (2016): 1197.

? SHOULD I DO KETO IF I AM NOT LOOKING TO LOSE FAT?

> *Short Answer:* Yes, keto provides much greater benefits than just weight loss.

Keto is way more than a trendy fat loss diet. Keto, as we highlighted in Chapter 3, can improve many lifestyle factors, such as energy levels, mood, mental clarity, exercise endurance, and overall health and wellness. As you also know, keto has the unique ability to target two of the most common contributors to many chronic diseases: insulin resistance and inflammation. That means that following this diet not only can improve your overall health but may also help prevent many common diseases.

If you aren't planning on losing weight and you do when you first start keto, don't panic. Remember, some weight loss is inevitable due to increased water and glycogen depletion, a product of low insulin levels. Do not be alarmed by this; it is a physiological occurrence that accompanies carbohydrate restriction and will balance itself out over time.

If you are trying to prevent weight loss, you likely will need to increase your calorie intake. Following keto while maintaining weight will require an even greater individualized approach, so you will have to experiment with calorie intake, see how your body responds, and adjust accordingly. Note that increasing your calories can be challenging on keto, since fullness tends to be a common side effect (or benefit) of ketosis.

❓ HOW DO I MAINTAIN FAT LOSS?

| *Short Answer:* Stay consistent.

Many people discredit keto, since it is not uncommon to experience weight regain when coming off of the diet. While much of that rapid weight regain is retained water, if you go back to eating a poor diet, of course you are going to gain some of the weight back.

If you spent a bunch of time working out, gained a bunch of muscle and then all of a sudden stopped training, would you be surprised if you lost some of the muscle you gained? No. The same can be said for keto.

However, we do see that following a keto diet for an extended period of time impacts our metabolic machinery in a way that can provide long term benefits and be maintained if the right approach is taken. Studies have found that following a low-carb diet after a keto diet can help maintain weight lost on the diet and even allow for continued weight loss.[42]

If you are going to come off of keto (which you shouldn't be thinking about now anyway), you should do so slowly. Rapidly reintroducing carbs, especially after following keto for a while, just preps your metabolic landscape for weight gain. Staying at least low-carb and transitioning to it slowly is the best way to ensure that you maintain the weight you lost.

---

42 Antonio Paoli, Antonino Bianco, Keith Grimaldi, Alessandra Lodi, and Gerardo Bosco, "Long Term Successful Weight Loss with a Combination Biphasic Ketogenic Mediterranean Diet and Mediterranean Diet Maintenance Protocol," *Nutrients* 5, no. 12 (2013): 5205-5217.

(?) I'M FOLLOWING KETO BUT THE NUMBER ON THE SCALE ISN'T MOVING...HELP!

It is very common to experience a slow or stall in your weight loss. This is commonly referred to as a weight loss plateau. You are following the diet just as you have been, but the pounds aren't coming off like they used to. In Chapter 13, we will discuss what to do in the case of an actual weight loss plateau.

For now, it is important to decipher between an actual weight loss plateau and just your body adjusting. If you lose eight pounds the first week of keto and then zero the next week, you are not at a weight loss plateau. Your body is still adjusting to the diet and has not had enough time to reach a weight loss plateau yet.

Additionally, the scale can be deceiving and also make you think you are at a weight loss plateau. As we will get into in the next couple of questions, you can gain muscle and lose fat on a ketogenic diet. If these two things are happening simultaneously, then the scale may not reflect that you have lost weight despite you experiencing improvements in body composition. We will also cover better ways than the scale to measure your body composition in Chapter 13.

(?) WILL I LOSE MUSCLE ON KETO?

Short Answer: If you adjust the diet according to the demands of your body, you should not lose muscle.

Many diets that severely restrict calories can lead to a loss of muscle mass. When our body does not have sufficient fuel coming in and is not adapted to burning fat and producing ketones, it resorts to breaking down muscle proteins, resulting in a loss of muscle mass. However, a ketogenic diet has actually been shown to preserve muscle mass.

You may be able to extrapolate that since on a keto diet you are fat-adapted, you can pull energy from your fat stores, resulting in the preservation of muscle tissue. This theory is supported by the numerous studies we highlighted reporting that while weight loss may be similar on a keto diet compared to other diets, we tend to see a greater percentage of that weight being lost as fat on keto suggesting that more muscle is being preserved on the diet.

A study looking at the infusion of ketone bodies found their ability to spare the breakdown of leucine, the primary muscle protein,[43] demonstrating that it may be ketones that are responsible for the muscle sparing effect of a ketogenic diet.

From an evolutionary perspective, this makes perfect sense. If access to food is limited, especially for a long duration, it would be advantageous to be able to produce and use a fuel source that prevented breaking down precious muscle.

Research has also demonstrated that ketones may be able to stimulate protein synthesis or the biological production of muscle proteins.[44] Since maintaining an appropriate balance of protein synthesis to degradation is important for maintaining muscle mass. This is another mechanism that can allow us to refer to a keto diet as a muscle-preserving diet.

---

43 K. Sreekumaran Nair, Stephen L. Welle, David Halliday, and Robert G. Campbell, "Effect Of Beta-Hydroxybutyrate on Whole-Body Leucine Kinetics and Fractional Mixed Skeletal Muscle Protein Synthesis in Humans," *The Journal of Clinical Investigation* 82, no. 1 (1988): 198-205.

44 Tijs Vandoorne, Stefan De Smet, Monique Ramaekers, Ruud Van Thienen, Katrien De Bock, Kieran Clarke, and Peter Hespel, "Intake of a Ketone Ester Drink During Recovery from Exercise Promotes Mtorc1 Signaling but not Glycogen Resynthesis in Human Muscle," *Frontiers in Physiology* 8 (2017): 310.

However, like any diet, muscle loss can certainly occur on keto if appropriate measures are not taken. This is something that we see in research and anecdotally. There are a couple of reasons why this can occur.

As we will discuss in greater detail in Part III, there is no one-size-fits-all approach for our macronutrient intake. Despite this, many have made an attempt to make one. You may have heard of the common keto macronutrient recommendations of 75 percent fat, 20 percent protein, and 5 percent carbohydrates. While this approach may work for some, especially in certain therapeutic models, it is still too general and too low for most; especially for those who are exercising and have greater protein demands.

Besides too general of macronutrient recommendations, eating too little protein on keto also occurs from the fear of gluconeogenesis, or the production of glucose from non-carbohydrate sources like protein. However, this is a natural process that is activated to meet the demands of the body. It has not been supported in the literature that consuming a higher protein diet will impair your state of ketosis. In fact, it may actually lead to better results for some.

The amount of protein you need is very individualized and depends on various factors, such as activity level, your diet in its entirety, and even your gender. A 2019 study published found that a keto diet including 20 percent of calories from protein led to muscle loss in men, but not women.[45] These men

---

45 Nina Mohorko, Maša Černelič-Bizjak, Tamara Poklar-Vatovec, Gašper Grom, Saša Kenig,Ana Petelin, and Zala Jenko-Pražnikar, "Weight Loss, Improved Physical Performance, Cognitive Function, Eating Behavior, and Metabolic Profile in a 12-Week Ketogenic Diet in Obese Adults," *Nutrition Research* 62 (2019): 64-77.

were not even exercising that hard, which tells us that current protein recommendations on keto seem to be suboptimal. We will get into that more in Part III.

Eating too few calories, a result of the fullness effect of keto, is another common cause of muscle loss on keto. A calorie deficit on a keto diet is safe, due to the availability of stored fat and the presence of ketones; however, too large a calorie deficit for too long could still cause your body to break down muscle for fuel. If you have a rampant metabolism, you are exercising, or you have a very low body fat percentage, you may need more calories to contribute to muscle preservation.

Muscle loss does occur on a ketogenic diet if not properly combatted against. While there is a focus on carbohydrate restriction, we want to make sure we are still fueling our body with nutrients through protein and fat to function optimally.

? CAN I GAIN MUSCLE ON KETO?

| *Short Answer:* Yes, muscle can be built on a ketogenic diet.

Carbohydrates can help with muscle gain, but they are not required. Remember, ketones offer a unique ability to prevent the breakdown of muscle, and they also have an ability to stimulate protein synthesis, offering up a combination that could lead to muscle gain.

There is not a ton of evidence in the research of increased muscle mass on keto. This is because the diets used in research are not set up to promote muscle gain. Here are three factors to help muscle gain on keto. As you will see, they are an extension of how not to lose muscle as well.

1. Eat adequate protein: This will range depending on your bio-individuality but should be between .8 grams to 1.2 grams per pound of lean body mass.
2. Eat enough calories: To effectively gain lean muscle mass you may need to eat more calories. If you are losing muscle mass or not gaining it, increasing calories will help.
3. Create the appropriate stimulus: Exercising is important for muscle growth. This is no different on a ketogenic diet. Keto scientist Dr. Jeff Volek has demonstrated that the combination of resistance training and keto leads to muscle growth[46] which has also been supported in other studies, including keto and CrossFit.[47]

It is absolutely possible to increase muscle mass on a ketogenic diet, but it is also possible to lose it if the diet is not tailored correctly. We will get more into the specifics of tailoring your diet for your specific goal in Part III.

When it comes to the numerous benefits of a ketogenic diet, changes in body composition may be the most robust. This is due to the unique metabolic characteristics of the diet and their impact on the human body. While body composition is not the most important health factor, it does play a major

---

46 Jeff S. Volek, Matthew J. Sharman, Dawn M. Love, Neva G. Avery, Timothy P. Scheett, and William J. Kraemer, "Body Composition and Hormonal Responses to a Carbohydrate-Restricted Diet," *Metabolism-Clinical and Experimental* 51, no. 7 (2002): 864-870.

47 Rachel M. Gregory, H. Hamdan, D. M. Torisky, and J. D. Akers. "A Low-Carbohydrate Ketogenic Diet Combined with 6-Weeks of Crossfit Training Improves Body Composition and Performance," *International Journal of Sports and Exerercise Medicine* 3 (2017): 1-10.

role in the prevalence of chronic disease. If you are overweight, improving your body composition is a huge first step toward improving your health.

Another benefit that accompanies improved body composition and health from a ketogenic diet is improved physical performance, which is next on our list of keto benefits.

CHAPTER 5

PERFORMANCE BENEFITS

The topic of keto and physical performance is controversial, despite there being a lot of anecdotal evidence, and a fair amount of research supporting its use. Outdated beliefs and poorly designed research have again skewed our understanding.

While we do have research supporting the diet's use for physical performance, there is plenty of research indicating that keto will impair exercise performance. Why the variability between studies?

Many studies that demonstrate keto leading to decrements in physical performance metrics, like endurance capacity and strength, are very short studies. As we know, adapting to a ketogenic diet takes time. If a study is less than four weeks, of course we would expect to see some decrements in exercise performance. The body is still adapting to the diet. Anyone who has tried keto will tell you, physical performance is not optimal in the first couple of days or even weeks of the diet.

However, when we take a look at longer keto studies, we see different results. Thankfully, several scientists have provided us with valuable insight by conducting studies of long enough duration to induce keto-adaptation. Or in the case of Dr. Jeff Volek of Ohio State University, have studied the impact keto has on performance in long-term keto-adapted athletes. Let's dive in.

? ARE CARBS ESSENTIAL FOR EXERCISE PERFORMANCE?

Short Answer: The body can perform exercise just fine without the use of carbohydrates.

A hint to the answer can be found in a story of a two-year Arctic expedition that began in 1878. A group of explorers— four Caucasians, three Inuit families, and 44 dogs pulling sleds—set out from the west side of Canada's Hudson Bay in search of the HMS *Franklin*, a British Royal Navy ship lost in the Arctic.[48]

The group set out with a month's supply of food that consisted almost entirely of walrus blubber. After they ate that, they lived off the land and sea, eating what they hunted. In other words, for the duration of a two-year, 3,000-mile foot journey through the Arctic, they ate primarily meat and fat.

Every man and dog returned safe and sound, leaner and healthier than ever. This is a great example of the human capacity to perform exceptional physical feats on very few carbohydrates.

---

48 Charles Francis Hall, *Narrative of the Second Arctic Expedition Made* (Cambridge University Press, 2014).

Nevertheless, conventional wisdom among the fitness and nutrition community is that carbohydrates must make up a high portion of your diet in order to maintain physical performance. If you had asked someone ten-to-fifteen years ago, they would have said you were crazy for thinking you could improve exercise without carbohydrates, especially endurance exercise. These beliefs mostly stem from studies in the last hundred years looking at muscle glycogen and its relationship to exercise performance.

Muscle glycogen is the stored form of carbohydrates found in our muscles that serves as an energy reserve tank. It is traditionally thought that having full glycogen stores is important to ensure enough energy is available to fuel the body for optimal physical performance. It is this understanding that has led to carb loading being the most popular strategy for improving physical performance. The problem is that research has not supported that carb loading before exercise actually improves performance.

Furthermore, the fuel you rely on during exercise differs based on your diet. If you are following a high-carbohydrate diet, then yes carbohydrates will be fueling your physical performance. Don't let this understanding lead to you thinking that carbohydrates are the best fuel source or that it is particularly good to have exercise primarily fueled by them.

As you know, on a ketogenic diet, the body is running on a different fuel source; fat and ketones. Later in the chapter, we will demonstrate the benefits of this as it relates to exercise performance. A couple worth highlighting here have been found by Dr. Volek.

In a study conducted on highly trained endurance athletes who were either keto or carb adapted, it was discovered that keto dieters burn a similar amount of glycogen during exercise and possess a unique ability to replenish glycogen at rates similar to carb-adapted athletes.[49] All this despite consuming no significant amount of carbohydrates.

This tells us that when someone is adapted to a ketogenic diet, the role of glycogen may be diminished and the need for dietary carbohydrates to support glycogen levels may not be required. Thus, carbohydrates are not, in all circumstances, essential for physical performance.

You may be wondering if the type of exercise matters. Conventional wisdom holds that carbs provide more fuel for the body to perform at higher intensities and fat is what provides more energy during exercise at lower intensities. Again, the fuel you rely on during exercise differs based on your diet. In Volek's study, it was demonstrated that the athletes following a ketogenic diet burned mostly fat during exercise at up to 70 percent of their max intensity, while the high-carb athletes burned fat up to 55 percent of their max intensity[49]. In other words, the fat-adapted athletes in this study demonstrate that the demand for carbs as fuel during greater exercise intensities can change under different dietary conditions. Thus, carbohydrates are not, in all circumstances, essential for physical performance.

However, it is true that carbohydrates may provide an ergogenic effect, meaning they can improve physical performance. Additionally, some elite athletes may require energy more quickly than the rate at which they can get it from fat, so more research is needed on this subject to fully understand

---

49 Jeff S. Volek, Daniel J. Freidenreich, Catherine Saenz, Laura J. Kunces, Brent C. Creighton, Jenna M. Bartley, Patrick M. Davitt, et al., "Metabolic Characteristics of Keto-adapted Ultra-endurance Runners," *Metabolism* 65, no. 3 (2016): 100-110.

the details. Regardless, none of these possibilities mean that carbohydrates are a superior energy source for exercise. Furthermore, the goal of optimizing physical performance likely only applies to elite athletes. The majority of us are not elite athletes and perhaps achieving the most optimal exercise performance shouldn't be the primary focus. Instead, the focus should be on health, which when improved, can still contribute to greater exercise performance.

CARB MOUTH RINSE

There is actually research demonstrating that simply swooshing carbohydrates around in your mouth can produce an ergogenic effect, without the need to actually consume the carbs. This phenomenon is known as the "Carb Rinse," which could potentially have implications for keto athletes or athletes in competition who may experience upset stomach from carb intake.

? DO I NEED CARBS FOR EXERCISE RECOVERY?

As we briefly touched on earlier, there is a commonly held belief that carbohydrates are essential for exercise recovery due to the need to replenish glycogen after exercise. However, as you now know, under different dietary conditions, the bodies need for carbohydrates to provide fuel and replenish glycogen, is reduced. This debunks much of the perceived benefits supporting the use of carbohydrates during recovery from exercise.

Additionally, remember that consuming carbohydrates following a workout will increase blood glucose levels, thus stimulating insulin production to drive that blood glucose down.

This can lead to lethargy, carb cravings, and brain fog during exercise recovery. Insulin can also halt fat burning and may even reduce the improvements in insulin sensitivity generated by exercise.

Finally, when the body is burning carbs, there is more oxidative stress and inflammation. This would be counterproductive for recovery. So maybe smashing tons of carbs post-exercise isn't the absolute best approach.

❓ HOW DOES KETO IMPACT ENDURANCE EXERCISE PERFORMANCE?

> *Short Answer:* Being keto allows athletes to tap into stored fat, a much larger fuel source, to provide energy to support endurance exercise.

There are two primary fuel reserves in the body: muscle glycogen and stored fat (stored in adipose tissue). What is the difference in these two different fuel reservoirs? Skeletal muscle and your liver can store up to 2,000 calories from carbs in the form of glycogen. Yet even the leanest of athletes can store 20,000 calories as fat in their adipose tissue.

You hear that you should load up on carbs prior to exercise to give you energy. However, when you run out of carbs, if you are not fat-adapted, your body cannot readily switch to burning your stored fat fuel supply. That means that despite the fact that you have a way larger stored fuel source available in stored fat, your body has to resort to burning glycogen for energy.

What happens when the carb-adapted athlete runs out of glycogen? They may start burning muscle and begin to experience fatigue. If they continue exercising, they "bonk"—their central nervous system, a.k.a. the brain, shuts down because there is not enough available energy. The common prescription to preventing this is continuing to refuel on carbohydrates to meet the energy demands of the body during exercise.

Is eating more carbs the best approach though? Or should we realize that carbs are inhibiting the use of fat during exercise and that the real reason why we suffer from fatigue during exercise is reduced carb availability combined with an inability to utilize a huge, latent fuel source in adipose tissue? If we looked at it like that, then we would understand that maybe finding a way to tap into this huge supply of fuel is the best strategy for improving exercise endurance.

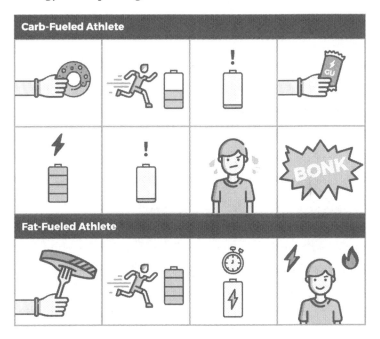

Insert the ketogenic diet. Becoming keto-adapted means becoming an efficient fat burner, and fat burning during exercise is no exception. The study by Dr. Volek also found that athletes who were keto-adapted demonstrated the ability to burn up to 2.3 times more fat than the high-carb group during a three-hour run.

We have mentioned a lot of data from Dr. Volek. Putting it all together, he has demonstrated that when adapted to a keto, the body can access a much greater fuel supply, burn more fat, and replenish glycogen at similar rates as carb-adapted athletes.

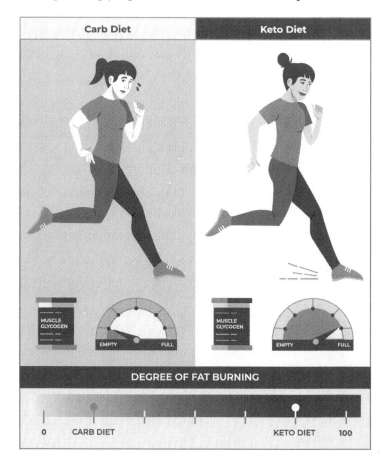

If that is not enough to get you on board with keto for endurance performance, then what if we told you that fat provides over twice the amount of energy compared to glucose, *and*

ketones can fuel the brain to prevent bonking or any other kind of central nervous system fatigue that could limit performance?

Furthermore, becoming keto-adapted allows the body to sustainably provide fuel to our muscles without all of the added inflammatory side effects of eating carbohydrates. This could have huge implications on endurance performance and recovery.

Here is a summary of the several ways in which a keto diet can help you improve exercise without the need for carbs:

- Preventing fatigue when doing longer bouts of exercise
- Improving performance on low-to-moderate intensity levels of exercise when keto-adapted
- Improving health and losing more fat through regular exercise and low-carb eating
- Maintaining stable blood glucose during exercise
- Adapting the body to burning more fat, which might be able to help the body preserve glycogen in the muscles during exercise

Being able to list why a keto diet is better for endurance exercise is one thing. What does the actual research say on endurance performance while on a ketogenic diet? Those who do not have a lot of experience in endurance training can expect to see improvements in performance once adapted to the diet. A six-week study in untrained obese subjects found a 155 percent increase in treadmill duration time.[50] However, when it comes to those who are

---

50 Stephen D. Phinney, Edward S. Horton, Ethan AH Sims, John S. Hanson, Elliot Danforth, and Betty M. Lagrange, "Capacity For Moderate Exercise in Obese Subjects after Adaptation to a Hypocaloric, Ketogenic Diet," *The Journal of Clinical Investigation* 66, no. 5 (1980): 1152-1161.

more experienced in endurance exercise, the results are a little more mixed. A four-week study in endurance athletes found that keto did not impact aerobic performance,[51] while another four-week study demonstrated a significant increase in markers of endurance performance and a decrease in markers of fatigue.[52]

Based on these findings, it seems like there are many factors that may impact whether or not improvements in performance will be experienced by well-trained endurance athletes. A couple worth mentioning are the training stimulus, whether or not electrolytes are sufficiently replenished, and the adaptation time an individual requires

Regardless, we do not see many studies demonstrating that if sufficient time to adapt is allowed for, that endurance performance is impaired on keto. It is either staying the same or improving. Couple this with the greater benefits of a ketogenic diet and you have an ideal diet for endurance exercise, which is why more and more athletes are choosing the ketogenic lifestyle.

? HOW DOES KETO IMPACT STRENGTH?

Short Answer: During keto-adaptation, strength will often be impaired but usually returns or improves once the body is given enough time to properly adapt to the diet.

51 Stephen D. Phinney, Bruce R. Bistrian, W. J. Evans, E. Gervino, and G. L. Blackburn, "The Human Metabolic Response to Chronic Ketosis without Caloric Restriction: Preservation of Submaximal Exercise Capability with Reduced Carbohydrate Oxidation," *Metabolism* 32, no. 8 (1983): 769-776.

52 Adam Zajac, Stanisław Poprzecki, Adam Maszczyk, Miłosz Czuba, Małgorzata Michalczyk, and Grzegorz Zydek, "The Effects of a Ketogenic Diet on Exercise Metabolism and Physical Performance in Off-Road Cyclists," *Nutrients* 6, no. 7 (2014): 2493-2508.

Strength and power-related movements work from different energy systems compared to endurance exercise, but we aren't going to go into that here. The task of optimizing the use of certain energy systems to maximally optimize performance is for highly trained professional athletes, not for the average Joe. What is important for people like us is the ability to effectively exercise at a high enough intensity to stimulate improvements in health.

One of the studies we highlighted in the previous chapter found subjects following a ketogenic diet for six weeks while training CrossFit four times per week demonstrated improvements in strength to go along with improvements in body composition.[53] We like this study because it is a very practical study using normal individuals, putting them on a keto diet and a training program, and seeing what happens.

However, not all research demonstrates improvements in strength. A 2012 study from keto researcher Antonio Paoli found that elite gymnasts put on a keto diet for twelve weeks did not demonstrate improvements in strength.[54] However, they did not experience decreases in strength either. The point here is that even in highly trained athletes, keto will not impair strength if enough time to adapt is allotted for.

Our take on keto for strength is that it depends on your training status. If you are a well-trained athlete, you will see

53 Rachel M. Gregory, H. Hamdan, D. M. Torisky, and J. D. Akers. "A Low-Carbohydrate Ketogenic Diet Combined with 6-Weeks of Crossfit Training Improves Body Composition and Performance," *International Journal of Sports and Exercise Medicine* 3, (2017): 1-10.

54 Antonio Paoli, Keith Grimaldi, Dominic D'Agostino, Lorenzo Cenci, Tatiana Moro, Antonino Bianco, and Antonio Palma, "Ketogenic Diet does not Affect Strength Performance in Elite Artistic Gymnasts," *Journal of the International Society of Sports Nutrition* 9, no. 1 (2012): 34.

decreases in strength at first, followed by a return to baseline strength and maybe improvements later. If you are an untrained or lightly trained person, the novel stimulus of exercise alone will lead to improvements in strength measures irrespective of diet.

Do not become discouraged if you lose strength initially; give your body time to learn to depend on its new source of fuel and you will find that your strength returns and, in some cases, even improves.

? WHAT SPORTS WOULD KETO BE BEST FOR?

There are many sports where a keto diet could provide a lot of benefit. Before we dig into them, it is important to point out that you should not adapt to keto in season or too close to an event. As we highlighted earlier, your performance may dip during keto-adaptation so make sure you have enough time to adapt prior to competition. We recommend at least eight weeks.

Here is a short list of sports keto could be good for, and why:

ENDURANCE SPORTS (I.E., RUNNING, CYCLING)
The ability to tap into a much larger fuel supply make keto a superior diet for endurance sports where having sustainable fuel availability is important.

STRENGTH ENDURANCE SPORTS
(I.E., SOCCER, BASKETBALL, CROSSFIT)
Long-term keto-adaptation can lead to maintenance of strength (if not improvement) and improvements in endurance. Furthermore, the anti-inflammatory component of keto would provide additional benefits toward recovery.

CONTACT SPORTS (FOOTBALL, FIGHTING)

The benefits of strength endurance apply for these sports as well; however, keto has also been shown to provide benefit following head trauma, making a strong case for keto in these sports.

WEIGHT CLASS SPORTS (I.E., FIGHTING, WRESTLING, BODYBUILDING, PHYSIQUE)

Keto could be particularly beneficial in sports where meeting a weight class is a requirement. Most of these sports require drastic action to be taken that can be harmful to both overall health and performance. A keto diet is a better choice because it can lead to rapid weight loss, retain muscle, and (given enough time) can lead to at least strength performance maintenance.

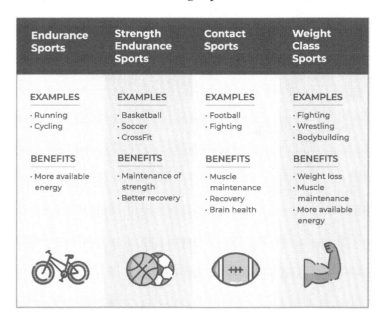

Endurance Sports	Strength Endurance Sports	Contact Sports	Weight Class Sports
EXAMPLES	EXAMPLES	EXAMPLES	EXAMPLES
· Running · Cycling	· Basketball · Soccer · CrossFit	· Football · Fighting	· Fighting · Wrestling · Bodybuilding
BENEFITS	BENEFITS	BENEFITS	BENEFITS
· More available energy	· Maintenance of strength · Better recovery	· Muscle maintenance · Recovery · Brain health	· Weight loss · Muscle maintenance · More available energy

Of course, some of the ability of keto to improve physical performance is a result of improvements in body composition. However, as you should be able to tell from this chapter, keto can also improve performance through mechanisms unrelated to body composition.

As we have highlighted numerous times throughout this chapter: if physical performance is measured within the first couple of days or even couple of weeks of keto, expect to experience decrements in performance. This is inevitable for most people because your body has to adapt. Furthermore, the motivation to exercise on keto may be lower when first starting. We recommend finding a way to exercise in some capacity regardless.

There are a few things you can do to help improve exercise performance while on keto, such as supplementing with electrolytes, staying hydrated, consuming enough calories (especially protein), and even using exogenous ketones, which we will get more into in Chapter 8.

PART 3

KETOSIS AND YOU

Now that we have debunked a lot of nutrition myths and you have a better understanding of the basic science behind a ketogenic diet, why you should follow it, and what benefits you can expect to experience, we hope that you have discovered your why.

Discovering your why is an important aspect of dietary adherence. Most people can discipline themselves enough to start a diet but sticking to it is a different story. Establishing why you are following a particular diet will help with this. If you have discovered your why, then it is time to take the next step and learn how you can start a successful ketogenic diet.

The title of this section of the book is "Ketosis and You," because as you should have realized by now, there is no one-size-fits-all approach to nutrition. Taking control of your health means learning what works best for you as an individual. This may seem like a tall task, but helping you get there is the point of this section!

We do not view keto as just some diet that you follow for thirty days before returning to your previous lifestyle or trying the next fad diet. We see keto as a lifestyle, one that you adopt long term to build and maintain optimal health. The goal is to teach you what the best foods to eat are, different ways to alter the diet to meet your needs, how to supplement for success, how to adopt the diet as a lifestyle, and how to be a scientist with your own nutrition if that is something you are into.

This section is about practical application. As you are going through the next couple of chapters, start thinking more about how the practices that we are teaching can be applied to your lifestyle. By the end, you will be ready to start your own journey.

CHAPTER 6

KETO FOODS

The first step to getting yourself started on a ketogenic diet is understanding which foods you can eat. While most people think that any foods that are "low-carb" are fair game on a ketogenic diet, we recommend something different.

If you recall from earlier in the book, we mentioned that we have a slightly different approach, what we refer to as Keto+. The purpose of Keto+ is to make sure that you are optimizing your nutrition by focusing on nutrient intake. This will mean not just eating low-carb foods but the right low-carb foods that will help you get the most out of your diet.

Let's get you started already!

? WHAT FOODS SHOULD I EAT?

In this chapter we are going to go into much more detail on each food category; however, here is a simple list of healthy food options for you to start with, in case you were getting tired of waiting.

Not everyone should consume every food on this list. Certain individuals may have intolerances to various keto-friendly foods, while others may be able to tolerate almost anything. In the self-experimentation chapter, we will get into the specifics of how to find out what foods are most optimal for you.

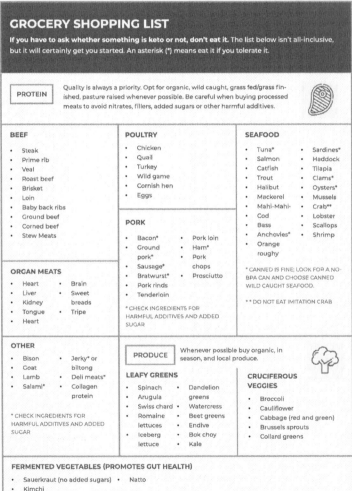

GROCERY SHOPPING LIST

If you have to ask whether something is keto or not, don't eat it. The list below isn't all-inclusive, but it will certainly get you started. An asterisk (*) means eat it if you tolerate it.

PROTEIN

Quality is always a priority. Opt for organic, wild caught, grass fed/grass finished, pasture raised whenever possible. Be careful when buying processed meats to avoid nitrates, fillers, added sugars or other harmful additives.

BEEF
- Steak
- Prime rib
- Veal
- Roast beef
- Brisket
- Loin
- Baby back ribs
- Ground beef
- Corned beef
- Stew Meats

ORGAN MEATS
- Heart
- Liver
- Kidney
- Tongue
- Heart
- Brain
- Sweet breads
- Tripe

POULTRY
- Chicken
- Quail
- Turkey
- Wild game
- Cornish hen
- Eggs

PORK
- Bacon*
- Ground pork*
- Sausage*
- Bratwurst*
- Pork rinds
- Tenderloin
- Pork loin
- Ham*
- Pork chops
- Prosciutto

* CHECK INGREDIENTS FOR HARMFUL ADDITIVES AND ADDED SUGAR

SEAFOOD
- Tuna*
- Salmon
- Catfish
- Trout
- Halibut
- Mackerel
- Mahi-Mahi·
- Cod
- Bass
- Anchovies*
- Orange roughy
- Sardines*
- Haddock
- Tilapia
- Clams*
- Oysters*
- Mussels
- Crab**
- Lobster
- Scallops
- Shrimp

* CANNED IS FINE; LOOK FOR A NO-BPA CAN AND CHOOSE CANNED WILD CAUGHT SEAFOOD.

** DO NOT EAT IMITATION CRAB

OTHER
- Bison
- Goat
- Lamb
- Salami*
- Jerky* or biltong
- Deli meats*
- Collagen protein

* CHECK INGREDIENTS FOR HARMFUL ADDITIVES AND ADDED SUGAR

PRODUCE

Whenever possible buy organic, in season, and local produce.

LEAFY GREENS
- Spinach
- Arugula
- Swiss chard
- Romaine lettuces
- Iceberg lettuce
- Dandelion greens
- Watercress
- Beet greens
- Endive
- Bok choy
- Kale

CRUCIFEROUS VEGGIES
- Broccoli
- Cauliflower
- Cabbage (red and green)
- Brussels sprouts
- Collard greens

FERMENTED VEGETABLES (PROMOTES GUT HEALTH)
- Sauerkraut (no added sugars)
- Kimchi
- Natto

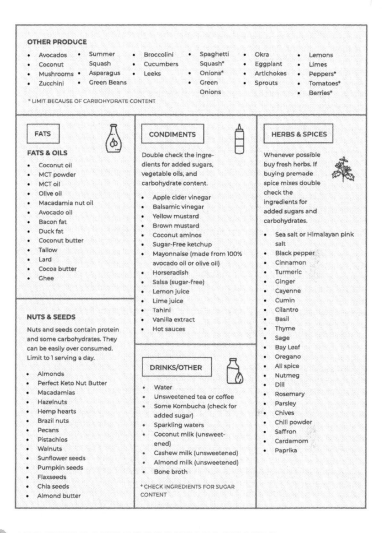

OTHER PRODUCE

- Avocados
- Coconut
- Mushrooms
- Zucchini
- Summer Squash
- Asparagus
- Green Beans
- Broccolini
- Cucumbers
- Leeks
- Spaghetti Squash*
- Onions*
- Green Onions
- Okra
- Eggplant
- Artichokes
- Sprouts
- Lemons
- Limes
- Peppers*
- Tomatoes*
- Berries*

* LIMIT BECAUSE OF CARBOHYDRATE CONTENT

FATS

FATS & OILS

- Coconut oil
- MCT powder
- MCT oil
- Olive oil
- Macadamia nut oil
- Avocado oil
- Bacon fat
- Duck fat
- Coconut butter
- Tallow
- Lard
- Cocoa butter
- Ghee

NUTS & SEEDS

Nuts and seeds contain protein and some carbohydrates. They can be easily over consumed. Limit to 1 serving a day.

- Almonds
- Perfect Keto Nut Butter
- Macadamias
- Hazelnuts
- Hemp hearts
- Brazil nuts
- Pecans
- Pistachios
- Walnuts
- Sunflower seeds
- Pumpkin seeds
- Flaxseeds
- Chia seeds
- Almond butter

CONDIMENTS

Double check the ingredients for added sugars, vegetable oils, and carbohydrate content.

- Apple cider vinegar
- Balsamic vinegar
- Yellow mustard
- Brown mustard
- Coconut aminos
- Sugar-Free ketchup
- Mayonnaise (made from 100% avocado oil or olive oil)
- Horseradish
- Salsa (sugar-free)
- Lemon juice
- Lime juice
- Tahini
- Vanilla extract
- Hot sauces

DRINKS/OTHER

- Water
- Unsweetened tea or coffee
- Some Kombucha (check for added sugar)
- Sparkling waters
- Coconut milk (unsweetened)
- Cashew milk (unsweetened)
- Almond milk (unsweetened)
- Bone broth

* CHECK INGREDIENTS FOR SUGAR CONTENT

HERBS & SPICES

Whenever possible buy fresh herbs. If buying premade spice mixes double check the ingredients for added sugars and carbohydrates.

- Sea salt or Himalayan pink salt
- Black pepper
- Cinnamon
- Turmeric
- Ginger
- Cayenne
- Cumin
- Cilantro
- Basil
- Thyme
- Sage
- Bay Leaf
- Oregano
- All spice
- Nutmeg
- Dill
- Rosemary
- Parsley
- Chives
- Chili powder
- Saffron
- Cardamom
- Paprika

ARE THERE ANY FOODS THAT I SHOULD LIMIT OR AVOID ON KETO?

Obviously, anything that contains a significant amount of carbohydrates, especially sugar, is out. As a good rule of thumb, most foods that contain more than 5 g of net carbs are out (hint: they give you this on nutrition fact panels).

However, Keto+ is about a lot more than just cutting out carb-containing foods. It is about consuming quality keto-friendly foods that help you produce ketones, as well as provide your body with the nutrients it needs for optimal health. Here are a few foods that would appear to be keto-friendly that you may need to limit or, in some cases, avoid:

- **Dairy:** Not everyone tolerates dairy well. Later in this book, we'll get into the specifics on how to approach dairy to see if it works for you.
- **Nuts:** These do not have to be avoided but should be limited, since they contain a decent amount of carbs and are *very* easy to overeat!
- **Peanut Butter:** Peanuts are actually not a nut, they are a legume. Besides containing a lot of carbs, they are pro-inflammatory and typically manufactured with the addition of pro-inflammatory hydrogenated oils.
- **Lunch Meat:** While lunch meat is technically keto-friendly, most lunch meats are low-quality and contain a lot of preservatives. In a pinch they may make a good option, but in general should be limited.
- **Vegetable Oils:** Don't even get us started! Vegetable oils are going to get their own section, but for now note that these oils are extremely pro-inflammatory and should be limited at all costs. This includes sunflower oil, canola oil, corn oil, peanut oil, safflower oil, soybean oil, and any other partially hydrogenated oils (check the labels!).
- **Processed and Prepackaged Foods:** Avoid any foods that are highly processed or manufactured using poor practices. If it is packaged and has a long ingredient label, it probably falls into this category.

- **Soy:** Soy contains phytoestrogens, which can be problematic for your hormone levels. Additionally, many people react poorly to soy.

? HOW IMPORTANT IS FOOD QUALITY?

Short Answer: You can see progress without emphasizing food quality but to take better control of your health, food quality is important.

Not many people in keto world want to talk about this, but food quality is just as important as cutting carbs out of the diet. Bold statement, right? Let's take a look at why.

Ignoring food quality while following a keto diet is "dirty keto." A dirty keto diet is one in which the focus is on keeping carbs low, fat high, with no attention paid to the quality of the foods you are putting in your body. A dirty keto dieter may eat a lot of keto treats, pork rinds, processed meat, cream cheese, bacon, and not even pay attention to anything that spoils. This is not the keto diet that we are recommending.

Sure, regardless of what types of foods you put in your body, cutting your carbohydrate intake can lead to improvements in our overall health, especially in the short term and particularly if you already have metabolic damage. However, long term health is determined by the quality of foods you eat. Higher quality foods contain more nutrients that your body needs to function optimally.

Imagine someone rummaging around a junkyard and collecting a bunch of scraps to build an airplane. Would you climb in and take off with them? I doubt it. You wouldn't build an airplane out of scrap metal and expect it to fly very far, so why would you build your body with garbage?

Your biological human body is made of cells. We all know that fact at some "I remember middle school" level, but do you stop and think about what that implies? The cells in your body exist to carry out very complex biological processes and their ability to exist and function properly is predicated on how you fuel your body.

The food you eat is responsible for your cells, your hormones, your gut microbiome, every muscle, every blood vessel, every nerve. Yes, the body is adaptable and can break things down to some usable parts, but this is not the most optimal approach to maximizing our health, especially in the long term. You are *literally* what you eat. If you want to be the best version of you, or even just a non-ill and normally healthy human being, you must start with the right materials first.

There's no arguing that eating real, high-quality food is a great idea and a constant that shouldn't really change. This is no different on a keto diet.

Why do we see so many differences between individuals or subjects in studies following a keto diet? We believe that's because of food quality. One person may be following a keto diet consisting of grass-fed, grass-finished beef and organically grown/pesticide-free/micronutrient dense produce. Another person may be eating a very similar looking diet but is consuming low quality processed meat cooked with vegetable oil and topped with a slice of neon-colored "cheese." The point here is that while both of these diets would appear to be "keto," they can lead to drastically different health outcomes.

To give you a real-world example of how this could make a difference, let's take another look at LDL cholesterol levels, which we have already touched on a bit. Remember that LDL, typically considered to be bad cholesterol, serves a purpose in the body. Due to its function, it can become elevated on a keto diet, but is only a problem if other markers are also elevated—like inflammation. If LDL is elevated in conjunction with elevated inflammatory markers, then health may be impaired. No worries for keto since keto reduces inflammation, right? This is true for a keto diet rich in high-quality foods, but what about that keto diet rich in low quality beef being fried in pro-inflammatory vegetable oils? That *can* cause inflammation.

Now do you see what we are saying? Food quality is extremely important and taking shortcuts in this area is not advisable. Yes, higher-quality foods are more expensive, we understand that, but your health is an investment, not an expense.

❓ HOW DO I ENSURE THAT I AM GETTING THE HIGHEST QUALITY FOODS?

Eating higher quality foods means improving the way you shop to ensure you are buying food that is grown, raised, and produced properly because all of these factors affect the makeup and nutritional value of the food. One great way to ensure that you are eating the highest quality foods is by shopping at local farmers markets. Here, you can speak directly to the source of the food. You can ask questions about how animals are fed or if there are any pesticides used on the produce. This is a huge advantage; however, not everyone has access to quality farmers markets so learning how to shop at grocery stores for the best food becomes more important.

If you have ever tried looking for higher quality foods at any commercial grocery store, chances are you came up empty handed and frustrated. Our massive population, as well as the obesity epidemic for that matter, has led the food industry to take steps to increase food production. These steps have led to lower quality, nutrient deficient, and potentially harmful foods. Furthermore, food industry labeling has made things even more confusing.

It is easy to be tricked into thinking that anything "organic" and "non-GMO" is healthy, but that's just not true. You can end up spending tons of unnecessary money and still not get healthy quality foods. Furthermore, many processed foods that appear to be healthy are filled with hidden carbs, sugars, and additives. Learning to decipher claims and labels will prevent you from falling prey to the food industry.

A good rule of thumb: don't eat foods with ingredients that you can't pronounce or don't know what they are. While ideally you will eat mostly real unprocessed foods, here is a list of some of the most common ingredients to avoid:

- Vegetable oils (soybean, canola, corn, grapeseed, peanut, sesame, sunflower, safflower)
- Carrageenan
- Citric acid
- Potassium sorbate
- Monosodium glutamate (MSG)
- All syrups (high-fructose corn syrup, maple syrup, malt syrup, rice syrup, etc.)
- Cane juice
- Corn starch
- All types of sugar (brown sugar, coconut sugar, cane sugar, beet sugar, etc.)
- Most sugar alcohols (maltitol, xylitol, glycerol, etc.)
- Artificial sweeteners (aspartame, sucralose, saccharin)
- Other names used for sugar (dextrose, maltodextrin, maltose, lactose, fructose, monosaccharide, glucose, disaccharide, polysaccharide, etc.)
- Agave

- Molasses
- Honey
- Dates
- Fruit juice

Now that you know about some of the ingredients on food labels to look out for, we are going to talk specifically about oils, meats, eggs, and produce individually so you can learn how to choose the best quality foods in these categories.

NUTS/OILS

? WHAT ARE THE BEST OILS?

Not all fats are created equally, and this is especially true for oils. In general, the best and most beneficial oils are:

- Coconut oil
- MCT oil
- Palm oil

- Avocado oil
- Macadamia nut oil
- Olive oil

What makes these fats healthier is their unique fatty acid profiles, which allow them to contribute to a healthy and well-functioning metabolism. While these oils are healthy, if you treat these oils the wrong way, they can actually become unhealthy. To avoid this, understand the concept of "smoke point." Smoke point is the temperature at which an oil begins quite literally to smoke. When you are cooking, you never want to cross this point, as the fats become very oxidized and thus damaging to your health.

Lower smoke point oils are also a little less stable than other fats. Interestingly, lower smoke point oils don't just become damaged through surpassing their smoke point; they can also oxidize by becoming rancid in storage.

So, basic tip: If you're not cooking with an oil, don't worry about the smoke point. If you are cooking with an oil, choose one that has a higher smoke point. Here are common keto cooking oils, ordered from highest to lowest smoke point:

- Coconut oil
- Palm oil
- Avocado oil
- Olive oil

Olive oil is one of the most ubiquitous oils in the kitchen. Everyone knows this is a healthy addition to any meal and a "heart healthy" fat. But with that comes caveats.

Olive oil can turn rancid a little quicker than other oils. Olive oil should be stored in amber or green glass (or tin) and out of sunlight. Many of the main brands of olive oil aren't olive oil. They use blends of other oils that are inflammatory and oxidized. The good stuff should be a light green in appearance and almost fruity and nutty in taste. Once you use high-quality olive oil, you'll notice all the garbage that most people call olive oil.

? ARE THERE ANY OILS TO AVOID?

After cutting sugar, if you were to make one giant change that would impact your health radically, it would be cutting out vegetable oils. Frighteningly enough, these are the oils we have been guzzling for decades in the Western world. These include:

- Canola oil
- Soybean oil
- Corn oil
- Peanut oil
- Vegetable oil
- Sunflower oil
- Safflower oil

Vegetable oils may be just as harmful to your health as refined and processed carbohydrates. Despite this, many people think that vegetable oils are healthy. When we demonized animal fat, we opened up a market in which an oil called "vegetable oil" could thrive. We have seen a sharp increase in the use of vegetable oils since the low-fat diet recommendations were made. This increase in vegetable oil usage correlates with our increased prevalence of many different diseases.

Another reason why vegetable oils are used so often is they are cheap. These oils come from agricultural wastes and the methods of extracting the oil are inexpensive and damaging to the oil. Think about this for a second. Where does the oil come from in corn? Or a soybean? There is hardly any oil in corn or soy, right? Producers use high heat extraction methods that result in an oxidized, pro-inflammatory oil—a recipe for disaster for your health.

Now you can see why the widespread and commonly accepted use of these vegetable oils is a problem. Vegetable oils are everywhere. They can be found in salad dressings, in roasted nuts, and in other packaged foods at the store. In some cases, these packaged foods can't even differentiate between which oil they are actually using.

Ingredients: Almonds, Expeller-Pressed Sunflower Oil and/or Expeller-Pressed Peanut Oil, and Sea Salt. **CONTAINS ALMOND INGREDIENTS.**

Allergy Information: *This product is produced on equipment that makes other products containing peanuts and other tree nuts.*

A general rule of thumb on which oils to avoid is to ask if the source of the oil is a naturally fatty source. Avocados, coconut, and olives are juicy and fatty, you can literally squeeze the fat out of them. What is a safflower? Or a canola? Try taking sunflower seeds, soybeans, or corn kernels and squeezing them to get fat out. Good luck.

Since these oils are so cheap, they are also used by many restaurants, even the highest end hipster hotspot. Vegetable oils are used to sauté virtually everything, to fry foods, and they will absolutely be in any sauce and condiment you order.

This leaves you with two options when eating out. You can either choose things that you know don't have any sauces or oils in them, or you can ask if they can use olive oil or butter instead.

? WHICH NUTS CAN I EAT ON A KETO DIET?

Nuts can be a great snack on a keto diet, but they do contain carbs and since they are very easy to overeat, the amount consumed should be monitored. Nuts are often roasted in vegetable oil or a combination of vegetable oils, so opt for raw or dry roasted nuts whenever possible.

Here is a list of approved nuts/seeds on a keto diet:

- Almonds
- Macadamias
- Hazelnuts
- Hemp hearts
- Brazil nuts
- Pecans
- Pistachios
- Walnuts
- Sunflower seeds
- Pumpkin seeds
- Flaxseeds
- Chia seeds
- Almond butter

? WHAT ABOUT NUT BUTTER?

Nut butter can also make for a great keto snack, and we offer the same precaution as nuts. Nut butters have carbs and they taste good, so be careful. Again, check the ingredient label on nut butters, since many of them contain hydrogenated or partially hydrogenated oils. Additionally, some nut butters may actually be a blend of a specific nut combined with peanuts. You will want to avoid this as well.

What's wrong with peanuts and peanut butter? They are not a nut and are quite pro-inflammatory. Peanuts also have a higher carb content compared to other nuts. If you are going to be indulging in nut butters, avoid peanut butter and opt for choices such as:

- Almond butter
- Macadamia nut butter
- Walnut butter
- Brazil nut butter
- Coconut butter

PRODUCE

? WHAT ARE THE BEST KETO VEGETABLES?

As we mentioned earlier, the best veggies on keto are leafy greens. However, other vegetables and even some fruits may be acceptable in moderation. Here is the list again.

Reminder: Whenever possible buy organic, in season, and local produce.

- Leafy Greens
- Spinach
- Arugula
- Swiss chard
- Romaine lettuce
- Iceberg lettuce

- Dandelion greens
- Watercress
- Beet greens
- Endive
- Bok choy
- Cruciferous Veggies
- Broccoli
- Cauliflower
- Cabbage (red and green)
- Brussels sprouts
- Collard greens
- Other Produce
- Avocados
- Coconut
- Mushrooms
- Zucchini
- Summer squash
- Asparagus
- Green beans
- Broccolini
- Cucumbers
- Leeks
- Spaghetti squash*
- Onions*
- Green Onions
- Okra
- Eggplant
- Artichokes
- Sprouts
- Lemons
- Limes
- Peppers*
- Tomatoes*
- Berries*
- Fermented Vegetables (promotes gut health)
- Sauerkraut (no added sugars)
- Kimchi
- Natto

Limit because of carbohydrate content

❓ HOW DO I SELECT THE HIGHEST QUALITY PRODUCE?

Short Answer: Learning how to read labels and where to shop is the best way to select the highest quality produce.

When it comes to actually selecting your produce, think about colors. If you think you are eating healthy by eating a single plant, think again. Different colors essentially mean different nutrients. Mix it up and mix your colors up.

Don't be surprised that we are going to also drive home food quality as it relates to produce. One of the first things you can do to ensure higher quality produce is to check the source.

Much of the soil in this country, especially on farms that mass produce vegetables and fruits, is depleted of minerals and the necessary compounds for plants to achieve their highest levels of nutrition. Pesticides and herbicides also destroy the natural eco-system in the soil upon which the plants depend. A farmer who wants to maintain truly healthy soil rotates his crops, planting different species over the years. He also introduces animals to the land. Their presence helps till the soil, mix in manure, bring bugs to the surface, increase the overall mineral composition, and improve the overall health of the soil. Healthy soil makes for healthy plants. Healthy plants make for healthier humans.

What is the takeaway here? Shop locally. Go to the farmer's markets in your area. Ask questions. Ask if they rotate crops. Ask if they use fertilizers. Ask if they use pesticides and herbicides. The more they know, typically the more you can trust their methods.

Another reason why shopping locally is important is transport time. The second you pull a plant out of the ground, off a stem, or from the tree, it starts oxidizing and losing flavor. This means the longer it takes to get to you, the less healthy and flavorful the plant is going to be. There is an inverse relationship between the transportation time of plants and how many micronutrients are left in them:

Short transportation time = more micronutrients
Long transportation time = fewer micronutrients

You can taste the difference in carrots you pull out of the ground versus the ones in a giant twenty-pound bag from

Costco. They actually taste like something. Sweet. Crunchy. This is no coincidence.

The loss of flavor corresponds to a loss of nutrients. To eat the most nutritious plants, you have to get those plants cultivated closer to you. This means going to the farmer's market and eating what is local and in season. If you're eating pineapple in Alaska in the middle of winter, chances are you're not getting a very fresh fruit. Eat seasonally—that is, eat what is in season in your region. Some areas may be trickier than others, but when you eat seasonally, you are going to get the healthier vegetables and fruits by default. Another perk of eating with the seasons is nutrient variety. Your body likes to shift from one thing to another to avoid processing the same nutrients constantly, so tweaking your diet according to the seasons will help you achieve this.

If you do not have access to a farmer's market, understanding labeling on produce will be crucial to ensuring proper food quality. Here is an explanation of many of the common claims you will likely encounter at a store or market.

NON-GMO

Genetically modified organisms (GMOs) are foods that have their genetic code manipulated to give us a desired trait. Many people think that these plants are just modified to be tastier; however, some modifications make plants genetically resistant to pesticides. This allows farmers to overspray crops with pesticides and herbicides—chemicals that are designed to kill things that live. You are alive. So, it's probably not a great idea to eat these things in any amount. But pesticides can arguably be washed off, cooked down, and removed from the plant. Or so we thought.

Some GMO foods are manipulated to actually produce their own toxins that kill living things. Yes, that's right. The plants themselves are making the pesticides, such as the common bacillus thuringiensis (Bt) toxin. If plants are genetically manipulated to produce compounds to kill living things, and you're a living thing, do you think you should be eating those plants? This is insanely frightening for reasons beyond what you can even imagine.

Looking for foods labeled as Non-GMO will ensure that these foods have not undergone any of these modifications.

ALL NATURAL

Foods containing the label "natural" customarily contains no artificial ingredients or preservatives *but may still contain antibiotics, growth hormones, chemical preservatives, and GMOs.* Safe to say, "all natural" is not the gold standard for produce quality.

CERTIFIED ORGANIC

Certified Organic means that foods are grown without antibiotic, growth hormones, pesticides, fungicides, herbicides, or food additives. Certified organic foods must meet the standards and regulations of the National Organic Program (NOP) and be non-GMO.

Certified organic is among the healthiest food you can choose. But not everyone can afford or have access to organic, non-GMO produce. If you can't, then prioritize. Every year, the Environmental Working Group puts out two lists to help consumers make smart food choices: The Dirty Dozen and Clean Fifteen. They research these lists and rank foods based on levels of toxin and pesticide contamination. Here are the 2018 results:

The twelve *most* contaminated and pesticide-ridden produce items as of 2018 are:

- Strawberries
- Spinach
- Nectarines*
- Apples*
- Grapes*
- Peaches*

- Cherries
- Pears*
- Tomatoes

- Celery
- White Potatoes*
- Sweet Bell Peppers

The fifteen *least* contaminated produce items are as of 2018:

- Avocado
- Sweet Corn*
- Pineapple*
- Cabbage
- Onion
- Frozen Sweet Peas*
- Papaya*
- Asparagus

- Mango*
- Eggplant
- Honeydew Melons*
- Kiwi*
- Cantaloupe*
- Cauliflower
- Broccoli

Not keto!

CERTIFIED NATURALLY GROWN (CNG)

Certified Naturally Grown is a third-party certification program utilized by small scale farmers who choose not to obtain the Certified Organic label, typically due to cost. CNG standards meet or exceed the standards for Certified Organic.

Once you have the produce, you are not out of the woods yet! The way you store your produce is important to their micronutrient profile. When exposed to oxygen, the micronutrients oxidize, reducing nutritional benefit.

How do we minimize this? Keeping produce in your crisper drawers is a great idea, but even better is opting for more airtight solutions. Glass Tupperware works well if you want a fresh vegetable or fruit to keep nutrients as long as possible. There are also microperforated bags that do a great job.

❓ CAN I HAVE FRUIT ON KETO?

Fruit contains a lot of sugar, specifically fructose. Fructose is not only harmful to ketosis but can actually promote inflammation. For this reason, avoid most fruits to properly follow a ketogenic diet.

However, some fruits have a lower glycemic index and can fit into a ketogenic diet in moderation. As you will see most berries are good to go. Berries contain a lot of antioxidants and polyphenols while being relatively low in carbs. While some non-keto fruits may be dense in various micronutrients, these micronutrients can be acquired through more keto-friendly foods. For example, avocados contain much more potassium than a banana.

As with all foods, check the nutrition label or your nutrition tracking app to see the carb content on fruit before choosing which ones to consume. If you do opt to eat fruit, stick to moderate quantities of these fruits:

- Avocados
- Coconuts
- Strawberries
- Blueberries
- Blackberries

- Raspberries
- Cherries
- Cranberries
- Mulberries

❓ WHAT ARE FERMENTED FOODS?

Several of the foods on the list we provided are classified as fermented foods. Fermented foods are created when natural sugars from the food interact with various microbes and bacteria, leading to not only a chemically different food but also a more bioavailable food. Fermented foods are very dense in probiotics that can help populate your gut with good bacteria. A healthy gut is at the foundation of a healthy body.

In addition to improved gut function, fermented foods can also improve the immune system and even improve cognitive function! The most popular fermented foods are:

- Kefir
- Kombucha
- Sauerkraut
- Pickles

- Kimchi
- Raw cheese
- Yogurt
- Natto

These products naturally contain sugar and different brands will have varying carbohydrate amounts, so check your food labels when making choices. Two very popular fermented foods not mentioned here are Miso and Tempeh which we have excluded due to their soy content.

MEAT

? WHAT ARE THE BEST MEAT CHOICES ON KETO?

Making the best meat choices on keto is all about variety and sourcing. You should eat a combination of beef, pork, poultry, game meat, and seafood to ensure that you are obtaining enough diversity in your protein selection. Different proteins have different fatty acid profiles. Different meats contain different amounts of omega-3 and omega-6 fats, and as we will discuss later in this chapter, a balanced omega-6 to omega-3 fat ratio may be important for keeping inflammation low.

Different protein sources also contain drastically different micronutrient profiles. For example, salmon is extremely rich in B vitamins while grass-fed ground beef is high in CLA.

Diversity in your meat consumption will better ensure that you are getting as many quality nutrients into your body as possible.

? WHICH CUTS OF BEEF SHOULD I EAT ON KETO?

There are many different cuts of beef and as long as quality is maintained, all make great keto options.

- Beef
- Steak (ribeye, sirloin, T-bone, etc.)
- Prime rib
- Veal
- Roast beef
- Brisket
- Loin
- Beef ribs
- Ground beef
- Corned beef
- Stew meats

Choosing the right cut of beef depends on your goal. If you are looking to get more fat in your diet, a ribeye is a great option. However, if you are looking to get more protein in your diet, choosing a cut like a New York strip may be a better choice. Later in the book, we will get more into making choices based on your goal.

? HOW DO I CHOOSE THE HIGHEST QUALITY BEEF?

When choosing the best beef, it is important to ensure that the animals have been fed a diet that most closely resembles what they would have been eating in the wild.

Ruminants are a classification of animals that include cows, lamb, goats, and bison. Rumination is not just about thinking! It actually refers to the process of chewing up, partially digesting, regurgitating, then rechewing a plant-based diet to aid in the animal's digestion. Interestingly, it is this process that allows ruminant animals to obtain nutrients from plants that we as humans cannot absorb.

Just as in humans, grain-fed, carb-eating animals have an extremely high amount of inflammation. This inflammation leads to a high amount of inflammatory omega-6 fats in the tissues of the animals, and these fats are transferred to us when we eat them. When animals eat the things they are supposed to, like grass, clovers, shrubs and other colorful things (how many colorful animal feed troughs can you think of?), they end up with a much higher density of nutrients.

These include beneficial omega-3 fatty acids, conjugated linoleic acid (good for brain function, weight loss and cancer prevention), beta-carotene (good for eyes) and essential fat-soluble vitamins (good for many things), all of which make achieving ketosis and being healthy so much easier. The ratio of omega-6 to omega-3 fatty acids is 6:1 in grain-fed cows and closer to 1:1 in grass-fed cows. This is important since omega-6 fatty acids can promote inflammation if consumed in excess. The average American eats a 20:1 ratio of omega-6 to omega-3 fatty acids, a recipe for increased inflammation. Don't be the average American.

Odd how when animals eat what they're supposed to, the nutrition we get from them is what we actually need. To help you shop, these are the three types of meat you will find at the supermarket or butcher shop:

GRAIN-FED (CAFO)

The majority of beef you will find will be from concentrated animal feeding operations (CAFOs), although the marketing will never tell you that, because it's not the sort of thing advertisers want to draw attention to. A large number of these operations aren't only feeding these animals inflammatory grains, corn, and soy-based products, but also candy. Yes, candy. And plastic. Oh, and also the ground-up by-products of the sick animals that die in the feedlot. That, too.

CAFO animals are also commonly fed antibiotics and growth hormones. Why is this necessary? Because the animals are kept in such close quarters and fed such an awful diet that they get sick very easily (just like humans). They are malnourished and they don't grow as large, so they're given growth hormones. These chemical compounds can be stored in the meat and passed down to the consumer.

Chances are, if your label doesn't say where the meat came from, this is what you're getting. These are *not* healthy meats and are even more inflammatory if high in fat content.

GRASS-FED, GRAIN-FINISHED

This is one of many examples of sneaky marketing in the food business. A good portion of grass-fed meat is actually not worth the extra price. This is because the animal is grass-fed, then "finished" on grain, spending 30-60 days in a CAFO. When you buy red meat that is grain finished, you're getting a runaround for your money. Most of these cows are stuffed with grains to plump them up. This plumping-up not only drastically increases the inflammatory omega-6 fatty acids, but can also destroy the previously high levels of omega-3, fat-soluble vitamins, and conjugated linoleic acid.

Whether at a farmer's market or a grocery store, if are you unsure about whether meat is grain- or grass-finished, just ask. At farmers' markets you will very easily get your answer and usually the staff at Whole Foods and other similar stores will know where they get their meat and how the cows ate during their last few weeks.

The extra cost for grass-fed meat is not justified if the beef is grain-finished, as you're likely getting close to what CAFO animals have in terms of reduced nutrition.

100 PERCENT GRASS-FED

To get this label, the cow (or other animal) must be fed a natural grass diet up until the day they are slaughtered. When buying red meat that is 100 percent grass-fed you are getting the highest nutrient concentration possible, and definitely healthy meats. This is also known as grass-fed/finished.

Stress on the animal plays a huge role in the formation of inflammatory fats. The stress hormone cortisol persists in cows just as it does in humans. This stress hormone leads to fat gain and chronic inflammation. In general, most grass-fed cows graze on pastures until they are slaughtered, leading to a reduction in cortisol, thus a reduction in harmful fats.

The fat in grass-fed beef is also sometimes darker and more colorful (yellow to orange) than in their CAFO counterparts. This is a result of increased colors in their diet and resultant increased levels of beta-carotene (you want this) in the animal's fat.

There is a caveat with grass-fed, however. Unlike with chickens, there is no regulation regarding whether grass-fed or pastured animals can be injected with growth hormones, antibiotics or fed a bunch of GMO feed. This is another reason why asking questions about how the animals are raised is important

If you can't afford the higher price at farmers markets, Whole Foods, or other specialty stores, there are plenty of other options for beef, lamb, bison, goat, etc. Use Google to find cow-share programs in your area. Find local sources through resources like EatWild.com and LocalHarvest.com that feature local farms in your area that are easily accessible. Check Craigslist. Seriously. There are plenty of very small-scale farmers offering their cows on Craigslist. These farmers often allow you to visit the farm and ask further questions about how the animals are raised.

Can't fit a whole cow in your freezer? Find a few friends, co-workers, people at your gym, whatever, to split a whole, half or quarter of a cow. When you purchase meat this way, all of the cuts average out to $4-5/lb. This includes organ meats (you should be eating these), ground beef, New York strip, tenderloins, rib eyes, rib roasts—all of it! This quickly becomes exceedingly affordable, and usually much more so than even your general grocery store CAFO-based animal products.

ORGANIC

This is a strict term highly regulated by the USDA. Even though grass-fed meat is fantastic, the responsible thing would be to make sure the animals aren't pumped full of antibiotics and hormones and given potentially dangerous GMO crops to graze on.

Is there organic, grass-fed beef? Yes. More often than not, these two things go together. When farmers take the time and care to raise their animals on fully organic standards, they are not going to ruin their insides with grains, corn, and soy-based products.

Keep in mind the absence of an organic label doesn't always mean the meat is not organic. Some of the smaller family farms you may purchase from simply can't afford to be officially designated as organic (it's quite an expensive and time-consuming process). They may follow organic rules and regulations but lack the designation and overview from the USDA to certify their animals as organic. In that case, you can again talk to the source about how they raise their cattle.

Organic is worth purchasing to avoid any additives to the animals. Most of the toxins and inflammation concentrate in the fat of animals. This means if you can't afford the 100 percent grass-fed, organic beef, go for the leanest cuts possible and at least look for antibiotic- and hormone-free. If you are able to purchase organic, grass-fed meats, spring for the fattier cuts.

BEEF SUMMARY

- Go 100 percent grass-fed and organic if at all possible
- If CAFO, buy lean meats and get fats from other sources to avoid toxins
- If grass-fed, buy fattier cuts
- Visit local farms and buy direct if possible

? WHAT IS UP WITH ORGAN MEAT?

You may have noticed that we have organ meats on the food list. This is not a mistake. If you ask your grandparents, chances are they used to eat organ meat, especially if they grew up on a farm. Times were tough and food couldn't go to waste. What your grandparents may not have realized is that these meats are extremely nutrient dense! Even better is that the nutrients in these organs are more bioavailable, meaning they are more readily absorbed by the body. This makes organ meat like a natural meat version of a multivitamin. This is one of the reasons someone can follow an all meat diet without having to suffer from nutrient deficiencies. We will get more into that later but for now know that organ meat, while it may take some getting used to, is a great food to include in an optimized ketogenic diet.

If you were to rank all foods on a spectrum of nutrient density, organ meats sit unchallenged at the top. Yes, far above kale. Organ meats do not have to just come from cows, they can also come from pigs, lambs, goats, chickens, and ducks. Organs commonly consumed are:

- Liver
- Tongue
- Heart
- Kidneys

- Brain
- Sweet Breads
- Tripe

When it comes to actually eating organ meat, it is all about preparation. If overcooked, organ meat can produce a pungent taste that may require you to hold your nose to get down. However, if you season organ meat and cook it slow and low, just enough to cook the outside of the meat, you will notice little to no taste or maybe even a taste you prefer.

WHICH PORK OPTIONS ARE THE BEST TO EAT?

Pork is one of the most popular meat sources on keto. Think bacon. One of the problems with pork is that many sources contain a lot of additives or added sugar. This and source of your pork is just as important as it is with beef. Since pigs will eat nearly anything, the food typically fed to these animals is suboptimal and worth considering when sourcing pork. Again, asking questions from the source can help here.

Here are some of the pork options you may elect for:

- Bacon*
- Ground pork*
- Sausage*
- Bratwurst*
- Pork rinds
- Tenderloin

- Pork loin
- Pork shoulder
- Ham*
- Pork chops
- Prosciutto

*Check ingredients for harmful additives and added sugar.

Note that while pork rinds may make for a great crunchy snack on keto, they contain hardly any nutrients and are often fried in vegetable oils. They are a low-carb food but not a health food.

? BUT REALLY, IS BACON HEALTHY?

We think bacon is fine…in moderation. The problem with bacon is that it is typically highly processed, contains a lot of additives, and does not have much of a nutritional profile. Since most people have been under the impression that bacon is bad for them, finding out they can have it on keto makes them go hog wild (see what we did there?).

But overall, there aren't many nutrients in bacon, so you're just not getting a big bang for your buck. We like to choose the foods that have the highest nutrient density as possible. Like organ meats. Moral of the story, don't let bacon be a primary meat source in your diet.

? WHAT SEAFOOD SHOULD I EAT ON KETO?

Adding seafood to your keto diet helps bring variety to your diet, which also increases variety in your nutrient intake. Leaner fish like tuna tend to have a lower nutrient profile compared to fattier fish like salmon.

Here is a list of seafood options:

- Tuna*
- Salmon
- Catfish
- Trout
- Halibut
- Mackerel
- Mahi-Mahi
- Cod
- Bass
- Anchovies*

- Sardines*
- Haddock
- Tilapia
- Clams*
- Oysters*

- Mussels
- Crab**
- Lobster
- Scallops
- Shrimp

Canned is fine; look for a no-BPA can and choose canned wild caught seafood.
** Do not eat imitation crab.*

? WHY IS EATING SEAFOOD ON KETO IMPORTANT?

Many people know about the benefits of eating fish—the oil, right? That's one reason fish oil is one of the most popular supplements. Fish and fish oil contain omega-3 fats, particularly EPA and DHA. These two fats have been shown not only to help combat inflammation but also improve brain development and function.

As we alluded to earlier, getting enough omega-3 fats in your diet is extremely important for maintaining an appropriate omega-6 to omega-3 fatty acid ratio. Consuming low-quality red meat containing a lot of omega-6, and not consuming seafood, is a recipe for a high omega-6 to 3 ratio and thus inflammation.

The benefits of seafood go much further than healthy omega-3s and a quality protein. Antioxidants, such as astaxanthin found in seafood, can aid many different bodily processes and can protect the brain. Micronutrients like magnesium, potassium, selenium, zinc and B vitamins are also often found in fish.

? HOW DO I CHOOSE THE BEST QUALITY SEAFOOD?

With beef and poultry, it is fairly easy to lump animals into better and worse categories. Grass-fed or pastured? Good choice. Grain fed/CAFO? Not a great choice. Unfortunately, categorizing seafood is not as simple. The same rules do not apply. Wild-caught sea creatures aren't always the best option and farmed is not always a problem.

While the benefits of fish are pretty robust, pollution is cause for concern in several large populations of fish. It is much less problematic with river and stream fish, but wild ocean fish can accumulate substantial levels of heavy metals such as mercury. Unfortunately, just as we are what we eat, so are fish, so the larger fish near the top of the food chain concentrate mercury and other toxins from the smaller fish they eat and the mercury (or any other metal) in the fish is passed along to the human who eats the fish.

Farmed fish can sometimes be just as polluted, if not more. Artificial feeding is a problem for some fish, but not for others. It can be hard to know, so here is a breakdown for what to look for when buying seafood at your local market.

SALMON

Salmon is one of the best sources of omega-3 from an animal product. However, farmed salmon is akin to farmed chicken or beef. In the past, these fish were fed pellets of fish meal. But that's far too expensive for modern farms, where fish are often fed pellets of corn and soy. Sounds like a familiar way to get fat and sick, right?

Farmed salmon get so sick that up to a third of them die in the farms. They are so devoid of nutrients that their flesh is gray, and the salmon are fed coloring pellets to make their flesh a more recognizable pink color. The tanks are loaded with various chemicals like PCBs and flame retardants to keep them running smoothly. No thanks.

Stick with wild-caught Alaska, California, or Oregon salmon. These fish are going to be a much deeper pink, will have lower levels of toxins, and a higher concentration of omega-3 than most any other healthy fish you can find.

TUNA

Tuna is a very large fish that lives in deep waters and eat many smaller fish. This means the tuna have concentrated the mercury and heavy metals contained in all of the fish they've consumed into their own flesh.

If you are going to eat tuna, try to avoid long-line-caught tuna, which tend to be very large. Pole-caught tuna are smaller fish, thus typically less contaminated with heavy metals and a better option for your body. If you are buying tuna and can't determine any of this, it's probably not a good sign.

TILAPIA

Tilapia is the real chicken of the sea. Similar to chicken breast, tilapia is a good source of protein, but not much else. It is a relatively lean fish, but because of what farmed tilapia are fed, the omega-6 to 3 ratio is high. Additionally, it is relatively tasteless and ends up mostly as a plate of mush when you cook it.

Tilapia are vegetarians. This means they love all of the corn and soy that gets thrown at them during farm feeding. They also enjoy all of the other garbage that other fish don't eat. Skip tilapia if you're trying to eat fatty fish and have healthy seafood be part of your diet. It was probably fed an awful diet and you're not getting much of that healthy fish fat from it anyway.

CRAB AND LOBSTER

Who doesn't love crab and lobster? Especially when dipped in some ghee or grass-fed butter, crab or lobster can be one of the best-tasting seafood options. Lucky for us, these creatures are like rats of the ocean.

This means there is no reason to farm them, so the crabs or lobsters you buy in the grocery store are wild. What's more, these little sea monsters have organs called hepatopancreas that filters out and concentrates toxins and heavy metals, leaving the meat untainted. They are rich in magnesium, zinc, and antioxidants. Go crazy here if you can afford it.

COD

Cod is rarely farmed. However, cod fishing is destroying habitats and has placed them onto endangered species lists. Cod is similar to tilapia in the form of the flesh, meaning you're getting mostly protein out of the fish. There are certain cod that are a little better, like wild black cod, but fishing for them is still a disruptive practice.

If you'd like some cod, go for it. If you're interested in sustainability and not screwing up marine habitats, probably best to skip this one.

ANCHOVIES, SARDINES, AND MACKEREL

Sardines are one of the best budget meals on a ketogenic diet. You can buy these fish fresh or canned, but canned is a great way to get tons of fatty delicious fish, usually soaked in olive oil. These tiny fish have very short lifespans, meaning they have very little time to concentrate any sort of heavy metals or toxins. They also rank exceedingly high in omega-3s, making them the common source for very high-end fish oils.

SHELLFISH (MUSSELS, CLAMS, SCALLOPS, OYSTERS)

Shellfish are the king of healthy seafood. You can't force-feed it any garbage. Farming is just fine for this group. You can throw all the corn and soy in the water you want, and shellfish will filter it out and take only the nutrients out of the water that they need. Shellfish don't concentrate anything in the water, passing what can't be used. Furthermore, shellfish are extremely high in magnesium, selenium, zinc, iron, B12, and have very high amounts of omega-3 fats, about a 15:1 omega-3-to-6 ratio.

Go crazy on these shellfish no matter the source, as they are highly nutritious and extremely low in contaminants. Canned oysters are another way to provide a lot of bang for your buck on a ketogenic diet.

SHRIMP

Shrimp are a pretty complicated seafood to purchase. Shrimp are the most-consumed sea creatures in America, by a long shot. There are plenty of varieties from many countries, making it tricky to choose the right shrimp, and they aren't all that nutritious to begin with. They have some B vitamins and a little protein, but you're really not gaining that much by eating them. They aren't full of micronutrients like other shellfish, and don't have a lot of omega-3s like salmon or sardines.

You can get shrimp from four different sources:

1. **Internationally Farmed.** Nearly 90 percent of the shrimp consumed in this country come from Asian or Latin American farms. These farms are entirely disruptive to ocean ecosystems and are chock-full of antibiotics and chemicals. The shrimp marinate in these chemicals and concentrate them pretty heavily. If the shrimp aren't marked as being from some other source at the supermarket, assume that this is what you're getting.
2. **Generic Wild Caught.** Generic wild-caught shrimp are no better. They are caught by a technique called trawling that bulldozes the ocean floor. Think of this

as pulverizing underwater rain forests. "Bycatch" is the term for the wasted and unusable animals that get caught by this method. It is estimated that up to 20-30 sea creatures die for each shrimp caught. While this doesn't necessarily affect the nutrient profile, it is not a sustainable method and is harmful to the environment.

3. **Domestic Wild Caught.** Domestically-caught wild shrimp are generally caught by trap, which is far less destructive and produces far fewer bycatch deaths. These are smaller shrimp, like bay shrimp and cocktail shrimp. These are better options.

4. **Domestically Farmed.** Domestically farmed shrimp are regulated; farmers can't use the antibiotics and chemicals that foreign farms are getting away with. This makes both domestic wild and farmed shrimp an okay choice.

The Gulf of Mexico is technically considered "domestic," but because of the little oil spill BP had not too long ago, we would recommend staying clear of shrimp from these waters for a while. The cleanup efforts are still underway years later.

If you're a shrimp fanatic, go for US farmed shrimp, or domestic wild bay shrimp, cocktail shrimp or trap-caught shrimp. Avoid imported farmed or wild and Gulf of Mexico shrimp.

Those are the most common types of fish that you'll see at the supermarket. Remember, general rules don't always apply here, so do some research (www.seafoodwatch.org is a good resource) before you go buying seafood in massive quantities. If there are two different types of the same fish, there's probably a reason one is more expensive. Unless you're dealing with some local surplus, stay away from extremely cheap seafood and pay higher prices for the fattier stuff.

FISH SUMMARY

- Quality matters; pay attention to the source
- Watch out for fish that concentrate metals
- Wild-caught salmon, shellfish, crab, lobster, sardines, anchovies, and mackerel are great seafood options

---

WHICH POULTRY IS BEST ON KETO?

While poultry is a great source of protein, it is typically pretty low in fat and does not contain a ton of additional nutrients. For this reason, we do not recommend poultry being your primary source of protein.

Eggs, on the other hand, are a completely different ball game. Eggs are rich in protein, fat, and a wide variety of nutrients. The problem with eggs is sourcing, but we will get into that in a second.

Here are some of the best poultry sources on a keto diet:

- Chicken
- Quail
- Turkey

- Wild Game
- Cornish Hen
- Eggs

HOW DO I CHOOSE THE BEST POULTRY/EGGS?

Buying healthy chicken and eggs can be quite the headache. Poultry products typically have some of the most poorly marketed and deceptive labels of any animal products. Let's first break down the different products and terms that you're likely to see when buying chicken and eggs.

CONCENTRATED ANIMAL FEEDING OPERATION (CAFO)

Similar to beef, you're not going to find much label information on these items. These are the average $1 per dozen eggs or run-of-the-mill economy-size package of chicken parts at your local grocery stores. You know all of those disgusting videos you see of sick animals crammed into large cages or warehouses being sprayed with antibiotics and covered in each other's feces? Their unused parts get chopped up and turned into some bizarre slime and fed back to the animals or to young children as tasty little nuggets. Yes, that's what you're eating here.

The animals' living conditions matter not only in relation to what the animal ate (never mind the ethics of it all) but also because, remember, stressed animals have higher levels of cortisol. Like beef, this high-stress environment and shift in hormones leads to a higher percentage of chronic inflammation and omega-6 fatty acids, just as it does in humans. The low nutrient diets of these animals leads to meat and eggs that are also low in nutrients, and the practices of raising these animals is sickening. These are not healthy chickens. Steer clear if at all possible.

CAGE-FREE

Believe it or not, this term actually has no formal regulation or definition. Essentially, cage-free means that the animals are not confined in small cages smashed next to each other. They can still be (and likely are) in a gigantic warehouse smashed next to each other. Since this term is clearly misleading, several different groups are pushing for renaming this high-density floor confinement. Again, not healthy chickens. Don't worry about paying extra for anything cage-free, you're wasting your money and still supporting the awful plants that execute animal production this way.

FREE RANGE

This term can also be misleading; the USDA defines free range as allowing animals short access to the outdoors—for a full *five* minutes per day. While this sounds like a luxurious lifestyle for the chickens, it usually means no more than a concrete slab with access through a tiny door. The whole point of being outside is so they can peck away at their natural diet of insects. Simply another marketing ploy to add $2 a dozen to the price of eggs. Despite these being the most expensive eggs, you will find at most commercial grocers, the increase in price is not worth the five minutes of play time. They are not given any access to eat a real diet and are still crammed in a giant and disgusting warehouse.

HORMONE FREE

We laugh when I see labels claiming that a producer's hens were never given any hormones. US law prohibits any hormone administration to poultry, so these manufacturers are simply abiding by the law. This label is like a water bottling company advertising no hormones in their new brand of water. Ridiculous and means nothing. Do not pay extra for this.

OMEGA-3 ENRICHED

"Our hens were fed a diet rich with omega-3 fortified flax, grains, etc." Sounds fantastic, doesn't it? Sure, until you realize that the chicken isn't eating what it is supposed to be eating. Given that there is also no regulation as to how much of the percentage of feed given to the chickens is actually fortified with omega-3, who knows if it is even a high enough concentration to trickle down to the consumer? If it says the percentage of omega-3 diet on the label (some do), and it is fairly high, this is a better bet than CAFO, but still far from optimal. The chickens are still given feed, which is not what you want.

100 PERCENT VEGETARIAN FED

This also sounds good—except healthy chickens are not vegetarians. They omnivorously eat insects, bugs, worms and other crawling things for a good portion of their nutrients. What this implies, however, as in the case of the omega-3 enriched diet, is that the chickens were intentionally fed something other than what they would naturally eat. This defeats the whole purpose of a proper and natural diet. Many times, this 100 percent vegetarian feed is also nearly 100 percent GMO grains and full of chemical fertilizers.

On the positive side, some CAFO animals are known to be fed ground up feces and parts of other animals that have perished in the lot. So, not using that as feed is a plus. If you want insurance that the chicken wasn't fed animal by-products and you're going to spring for the extra price on 100 percent vegetarian fed, make sure it is also 100 percent organic.

ORGANIC

Organic eggs and chickens are not all that they are cracked up to be (ha-ha, we couldn't help ourselves!). Organic here means that the chickens are being given feed that is 100 percent organic, non-GMO, and free of any pesticides, herbicides, or other chemical fertilizers. While this is better than other options, the chickens are still being given feed that is different from what they should be eating. This makes organic eggs and meat less nutritious compared to chickens that are eating their natural diet.

The good news here is that there are a few hoops to jump through to get chickens and eggs labeled organic. An outdoor play period is required for organic designation, but there are no requirements on time (like the five-minute free-range minimum) or accessibility. An organic designation usually means that the birds are raised better, but more and more companies are catching on to marketing under the organic label, so they are just tossing a ton of "organic" feed into big pens.

PASTURE RAISED

This is essentially what free range should mean. This is truly naturally raised healthy chickens on a farm, roaming around on grass, pecking away at bugs and insects. When compared to commercially raised eggs, pastured eggs contain a much higher level of omega-3 fatty acids, lower level of inflammatory omega-6, 36 percent more vitamin A, 100 percent more vitamin E and 260 percent more beta carotene.

These eggs have been hard to find even at places like Whole Foods, but the demand has made this a much more common staple at the store. Your best bet is to find local farmers and ask them how they raise their chickens. Chances are, the product will be more expensive, as is usually the case with quality food. We know, no one wants to pay extra for eggs but just as handmade furniture made of real wood is more expensive than comparable furniture made of flimsy press board at IKEA, you get what you pay for in terms of nutrition with chickens (and all things). And this isn't just your living room, this is your body and your health we are talking about here. Maybe forego a Starbucks run to compensate?

FIND THE BEST EGGS

Open the carton. If the eggs are all different shapes, size, and color, chances are you are getting them from a good source. Crack an egg—if the yolks are a deep yellow/orange and different colors, this is a great sign of nutrient density in the yolks. The difference in shape, size, and color across the spectrum is indicative of a varying diet of the animals, the way it should be.

If you can find fully pastured chickens and eggs, you should be eating everything. Eat the skin, eat the fat, eat the yolks. This is packed with nutrients as well as fats that your body will be burning through on a ketogenic diet. Use the bones and cartilage left over to make bone broth to get even more out of the chicken. No waste.

Most of the harmful chemical fertilizer by-products, inflammatory fats, and other negative ramifications from mass-produced animals are concentrated as toxins in the fats. What does this mean for you? If you are buying chickens and eggs on a budget and only get CAFO animals, spring for the whitest and leanest meats and gravitate away from the fat and skin. These would not be healthy chickens, but at least you are not eating all of the bad stuff.

POULTRY SUMMARY

- Try to find poultry and eggs from a farm, not from a commercial grocer
- Go for pastured if you can and eat every part of the animal
- Free range and cage free mean nothing, skip these poultry products
- If you can't afford pastured, eat lean meat and egg whites

DAIRY

? CAN I HAVE DAIRY ON KETO?

This is a loaded question and the answer is, it depends. Dairy does contain sugar, particularly lactose, and this sugar when consumed in high amounts can be harmful not only to your state of ketosis but your health as a whole. At the very least we can say that dairy should be consumed in moderation and choices that are higher in sugar, like most commercial yogurts and milk, should be avoided.

As for dairy choices that are lower in carbohydrates, the answer is less clear and depends on your ability to tolerate dairy. There are two potential reasons why some people are sensitive to dairy: intolerance to either the sugar (lactose) or to one of the proteins (casein) normally found in dairy. Simply put, some people don't have the enzymes needed to properly break down these proteins and sugars, while others do. If you are unable to break down these components, you may experience some very unpleasant and serious side-effects like fatigue, metabolism issues, skin problems, and/or digestive problems.

There are a few things to consider before assuming you are lactose intolerant. If you have to run to the bathroom fifteen minutes after consuming "dairy," it doesn't necessarily mean you are sensitive or allergic to dairy. In fact, the likelihood that you are getting the real food version of dairy is low. Ninety-nine percent of commercially available dairy is "franken food." The majority of dairy most people consume is weird, watery, over-processed made-up foods—nothing like what comes out of an animal.

Real foods spoil. Real foods are consumed close to how they are found. Is this how you are getting your dairy? All people, tolerant or not of dairy, should avoid ingesting milk and dairy that is highly pasteurized, homogenized, and/or processed.

Pasteurization typically kills all of the beneficial bacteria and enzymes that help you digest dairy. Moreover, homogenization forces fat through a tiny little screen, which breaks the fat particles into smaller damaging and oxidized versions of otherwise stable and beneficial saturated fats. Processing of dairy is hard to miss. Think of the super bright orange shredded cheese found in groceries, or the cheese that comes in brick form that won't be growing mold any time soon. These cheeses last approximately three years. Alert: they are not good for you.

In our upcoming chapter on self-experimentation, we will go over in greater detail how to test and see if you are intolerant to dairy.

? DOES DAIRY OFFER ANY HEALTH BENEFITS?

For those who can tolerate dairy, it can be an excellent nutrient dense food if properly sourced. Dairy is packed with fat soluble vitamins like A, D, and K2. These nutrients not only play key roles in your body, they are also pretty tough to get if you're not eating a lot of organ meats or fermented soy. Can I get a raise of hands of those who regularly consume organ meats and fermented soy?

Dairy also contains high levels of calcium. Now, the vegans may say, "Yeah, but you can also get calcium from leafy greens!" Ah, touché! However, vitamins A, D, and K2 (the ones found in dairy, remember?) can lower your need for calcium, so you may be able to obtain all the calcium you need without those leafy greens.

Dairy also contains short chain fatty acids like butyrate that are excellent for gut energy. Conjugated linoleic acid is another type of fat found in dairy that can aid in fat burning. Some dairy also includes medium chain triglycerides, which are highly ketogenic fatty acids. This and the associated saturated fats in dairy can make it an excellent ketogenic food.

In addition, certain fermented dairy foods have high probiotic densities (i.e., yogurt, kefir, and cheese) that can help populate your gut with good bacteria—bacteria that is tremendously good for your overall health. For many people, fermented dairy products like whole-fat yogurt are more palatable sources of probiotics than raw sauerkraut (my personal favorite), kimchi, or other fermented foods.

? HOW DO I CHOOSE THE BEST DAIRY?

As you can see, if you are consuming dairy, choosing the right type is important. Let's take a look at some of the common claims you will see on nutrition labels.

HOMOGENIZED

Dairy should not be homogenous. There should be a cream top layer to milk that separates from the more liquid solution. Many people find this gross or inconvenient, so we invented a machine to spray milk through a very fine screen. This process chops up the fat, so it stays suspended in the milk, eliminating the cream layer on top and creating "whole milk."

The fat that was chopped up in the screen is no longer made up of the same molecular strands; it is fragmented. What does that mean? Just as you wouldn't recognize the milk fats and proteins under a microscope, your body isn't going to recognize them either. This leads to inferior quality liquid that your body doesn't know what to do with. It is not advantageous to your health when your body doesn't know what to do with things that are inside it. High-quality fat is a must.

What does this mean for the ever so popular skim, 1 percent, and 2 percent milk? Well, it means that the fats and proteins are fragmented and destroyed. If you don't like the taste of whole milk, go for non-homogenized and skim off the top cream layer! Homemade skim milk! But that isn't really keto and you're throwing away tons of beneficial nutrients and fat here. So, don't be silly—eat the fat.

PASTEURIZATION

Dairy was consumed raw for thousands of years on farms and ranches. Then things changed. People started living in dense cities without refrigeration. Buying dairy was difficult. Transportation time increased and dairy wasn't kept cold, so bacteria grew. People got sick from consuming that bacteria. We can all agree that wasn't a good thing.

So, what happened? A French man named Louis Pasteur invented a process to heat dairy up to a certain temperature to kill all of the bacteria. Great! No one got sick anymore! But all of the beneficial bacteria and natural enzymes were destroyed along with the dangerous bacteria. Some of the fats and milk proteins were destroyed as well. What were we left with? Some liquid mysterious to our bodies. The same milk proteins remained, but all of the helpful enzymes and fats that assisted our bodies in breaking them down in our digestive system did not.

Unfortunately, raw milk is outlawed in some states. Some farmers are, unbelievably, being raided by law enforcement for producing raw milk. If you are lucky enough to be able to purchase raw in your state, then spring for this much more nutritious form. Google your way to finding if you can locate raw, local dairy close to your area to support your farmers and get the most nutrient dense, tolerable form of dairy.

ORGANIC

Organic is better than conventional, but not always optimal. What does organic mean for dairy? It ensures that the animal ate organic and wasn't given any hormones. However, you will likely still be consuming mystery dairy that has been processed and heated beyond repair. When buying dairy, if you're for some reason not going to go with raw, non-homogenized, then we fully suggest at least springing for a jug of organic.

GRASS-FED DAIRY

Why is buying dairy that is grass fed important? Just like beef, it increases the beneficial omega-3 fats and balances out the ratio of omega-3 to omega-6 fats. Grass-fed leads to much higher levels of fat soluble vitamins and important compounds like CLA that help burn fat and provide usable energy. Grass-fed is a crucial step if you can afford it.

When it comes to butter, especially don't waste your time with traditional butters. They are devoid of nutrients and good fats. However, when butter comes from grass-fed animals, it is full of usable and healthy fats, vitamins, and fat burning compounds. There are a lot of local brands, depending on where you live, and some commercial brands that produce butter and other dairy products from grass-fed cows. Sometimes this is branded as "European Style" butters. Check the labels to make sure.

> ## DAIRY SUMMARY
>
> - Skip skim, 1 percent or 2 percent dairy—go full fat
> - Get non-homogenized dairy
> - Get non-pasteurized (raw) dairy if possible
> - Look for "grass-fed" when possible
> - Try to eat what is local

? WHY DO PEOPLE SAY THAT DAIRY IS BAD?

There is a lot of misinformation about dairy in this day and age, especially in the paleo community. Usually when people are extremely divided on a topic like this, both sides are right. Some people can thrive on dairy products and some people will destroy themselves on dairy. It is clear that some people have the enzyme to break down milk proteins and others do not. What is less clear is whether dairy is inflammatory to a particular individual. Even if you can digest healthy dairy, you may not be getting it from the proper source, increasing the likelihood that you'll have an inflammatory response.

Some people who follow a paleo diet think dairy can't be consumed because they believe that humans haven't had the evolutionary time to adapt genetically to process dairy. They argue that we are unable to break down dairy, thus consuming dairy leads to a host of inflammatory conditions.

Although these are common reasons for adopting a limited-food paleo or primal diet, they don't hold up in this case. In fact, it has been proven several times that the Northern European regional humans experienced genetic shifts that helped them successfully process dairy. Even if you did not descend from this region, that doesn't mean that dairy won't work for you, too.

Another argument we hear is that humans are the only animals to drink other animals' milk, and that it is not proper. This is true—we are the only animals who do this. We're also the only animal to cook food. No other animal does that, not even those super-smart dolphins. Nor do other species domesticate other animals, have any system of agriculture, develop complex societies with millions of members, build shelters from the elements that contain down blankets, pillows, and thermostats, have running water, or use the internet. So, consider this: Would you give up any of those things just because other animals don't have access to them? No, of course not. We should use whatever we can, not just to survive, but to thrive.

SNACKS/OTHER

DO I HAVE TO PUT BUTTER IN MY COFFEE?

No, you do not, and putting butter in your coffee does not make you keto. This phenomenon of butter in your coffee was made famous by the company Bulletproof, which promotes the sale of their proprietary coffee beans which they encourage drinking with butter. We simply call it fatty coffee.

Putting fat in your coffee can be a great way to increase your consumption of beneficial fats and keep you feeling full during the day. However, it can also drastically increase your calorie consumption and destroy your fat loss goals.

Butter in your coffee isn't going to kill you, but it isn't necessary either. However, if it helps you get through the day and adds focus to your life, feel free to use it as a tool if that works for you! Just don't complain if you're drinking 750 calories of fat and not losing fat.

MCTs can be used to get way more of the benefit without having to jack fat intake. We will chat about this more in our fasting chapter.

? WHAT SNACKS CAN I HAVE ON KETO?

You may find that not snacking between meals will lead to better results on keto. However, with the concept of following the diet as a lifestyle, you may find yourself at times in need of a snack between meals. Here are some of the best options:

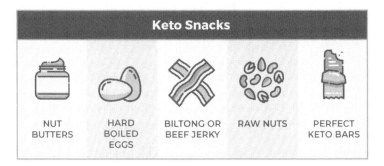

Keto Snacks				
NUT BUTTERS	HARD BOILED EGGS	BILTONG OR BEEF JERKY	RAW NUTS	PERFECT KETO BARS

If you find yourself constantly in need of a snack, try to add additional calories from fat or protein to your meals to keep you satiated between meals. Generally speaking, eating real meals and not snacking frequently is the best approach for optimizing health and being productive.

As we mentioned at the beginning of the chapter, learning what to fuel your body with on a keto diet is the first big step toward starting this lifestyle. Taking control of your health isn't just about what not to put in your body. It is also about what foods you can put in your body to help it function better and improve your health.

We understand that not everyone is going to want to take the extra steps to understand where your food is coming from or how it is being made. However, we think this is important to not only your health but also to help discourage current popular food manufacturing practices. Use your dollars to vote for higher quality health food made the right way—your body will thank you!

CHAPTER 7

STARTING KETO

A t this point you should have a pretty good grasp on which foods to eat and which foods you should stay away from on keto. Again, this is the first big step toward setting yourself up for success on keto. However, you probably have numerous other questions before you are ready to jump in to the diet. The goal of this chapter is to address these questions.

Starting keto is simple—just cut the carbs, right? Actually, it's much more complex than that, but that is the first step. Many times, people who flirt with the idea of keto think a better approach is slowly lowering carbs or transitioning to a low-carb diet before going full blown keto. While this approach may seem plausible, all it will do is delay the time it's going to take you to get adapted to the ketogenic diet. There are some side effects of starting keto and you are going to have to endure at least a few of these whether you do a low-carb transition or just jump right into keto. So why wait?

Once you have decided to make the jump to full blown keto, the next step is educating yourself. If you have been reading this book from the start then great job, you have already done that and are ready to start!

Education is important because when you know why you are eating or not eating certain foods, you are more likely to stick to a diet. For example, if you understand that a diet chock-full of processed carbs leads to inflammation and insulin resistance, then you would understand why cutting them out is important. Education is a powerful tool for taking control of your health and wellness and adhering to that control.

⊘ HOW DO I START KETO?

Once you have acquired a basic understanding of keto, the next step is to start. Starting doesn't have to be as challenging as many people think. Remember, keto meals consist of moderate portions of meat, seafood, or eggs, nutrient dense, low-carbohydrate vegetables, additional sources of healthy fats, and herbs and spices. Simply switching to consuming only foods from the approved list in the previous chapter is enough to get you started on the right track!

To begin, you will have to complete your first keto trip to the grocery store. To help yourself be a more efficient shopper, try planning your meals for your first week before heading to the grocery store. This will ensure that you get enough for the week but not too much. Your productivity and wallet will appreciate this. To plan your meals, use the grocery shopping list and follow the simple steps listed here. Visually speaking, your plate should look something like:

STEP 1	STEP 2	STEP 3
Pick a high quality protein	Pair your protein with nutrient-dense, low-carbohydrate produce	Cook with healthy fat or add healthy fat/oil *

* SOME PROTEIN SOURCES CONTAIN ENOUGH FAT AND WON'T NEED ADDITIONAL FAT ADDED TO THE MEAL

TIP : Eat enough at each meal to satisfy your hunger and prevent cravings in between meals.

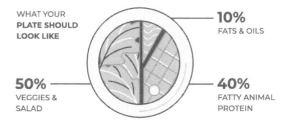

WHAT YOUR **PLATE SHOULD LOOK LIKE**

10% FATS & OILS

50% VEGGIES & SALAD

40% FATTY ANIMAL PROTEIN

STEP 1: PICK A HIGH-QUALITY SOURCE OF PROTEIN

Pick grass fed/finished meat, wild caught seafood, or a pasture raised poultry source. Portion size should be around a fist to two fist sizes, depending on your size. Which source of protein you choose will determine the amount of additional fat you will add in Step 3. Leaner protein sources will require a little additional fat while fattier cuts of meat will not. Below we have classified meats based on their amount of fat.

- **Least Fat:** Skinless chicken breast, skinless turkey breast, pork tenderloin, pork chop, 93 percent lean ground beef, 95 percent lean ground turkey, bone broth, deli turkey/ham/beef, crab, lobster, shrimp, prawns, mussels, scallops, tuna in water, white fish.
- **Moderate Fat:** Whole eggs, skinless chicken thighs,

turkey bacon, bison, flank steak, beef shank, lean sausage, beef jerky, salmon, canned sardines, lamb chop, lamb leg, pork sirloin, leg ham, organ meat (liver, heart, kidney).

- **Highest Fat:** Ribeye steak, top sirloin, porterhouse steak, New York steak, T-bone steak, filet mignon, beef/pork/lamb ribs, beef tri-tip, bacon, pork belly, pork spare ribs, chicken with skin, sausage/chorizo, salami, 80 percent lean ground beef, salmon fillet with skin, canned fish in oil, lamb shank, hot dogs, any meat with lots of untrimmed fat or skin.

STEP 2: PAIR PROTEIN CHOICE WITH NUTRIENT DENSE LOW-CARBOHYDRATE PRODUCE

Choose organic, local, and in season nutrient dense vegetables whenever possible. Vegetables should fill about half of your plate for each meal. While the nutrients in vegetables are not best absorbed by humans, vegetables can still provide additional benefits such as helping you feel full as you are transitioning to a ketogenic diet.

STEP 3: COOK WITH HEALTHY FAT OR DRESS IN HEALTHY FAT/OIL

Choosing the right types of fat to formulate your diet is extremely important. We emphasize eliminating all processed and refined vegetable oils and most seed oils. These types of oils are found in almost all store-bought dressings, condiments, and other processed foods and are linked to a long list of unwanted metabolic and inflammatory conditions. Replace canola, corn, soybean, sunflower, margarine, butter spread, with healthy fats and oils such as coconut oil, avocado oil, ghee or olive oil. Think if that food is naturally fatty or not. Avocados have fat. Canolas have…what's a canola?

The amount of fat you add for each meal will be determined by your protein choice. If your protein source is coming from the high-fat list, no or minimal additional fat is needed for the meal. If your protein source is coming from the moderate list, add 1-2 thumb-sized servings of a healthy fat source. If your protein source is coming from the lean list, add 2-3 servings of a healthy fat source. Here are examples of fats you can add to proteins found on the moderate or lean protein list.

Moderate Protein + Fat Examples:
- ½ avocado
- ½ handful of nuts
- 1-2 tablespoons healthy salad dressing
- 1-2 tablespoons ghee
- ¼-½ cup full fat coconut milk

Lean Protein + Fat Examples:
- 1 avocado
- 1 handful of nuts
- 2 tablespoons healthy salad dressing
- 2-4 tablespoons ghee
- ½-¾ cup full fat coconut milk

Once you have planned out your meals, go to the grocery store and get the foods you need for the week. Remember the tips we taught you in the previous chapter to ensure you are purchasing high-quality food. Focus on eating 100 percent real, unprocessed foods without a long ingredients list, or at least a very short ingredient list that consists of ingredients that you know and can pronounce.

In addition to becoming educated, planning, and getting your shopping done, you can use other strategies to ensure starting off on the right foot. One great way to ensure you stick to keto and avoid eating unapproved foods is to clean your pantry out before starting. Getting the temptations out of the house will set you up for success. Throw out or donate the foods you won't be eating. If others in your household are not participating in keto, clean off a separate shelf in the fridge and pantry for all of your keto-approved foods. You don't want to have to push behind the cookies to reach your macadamia nuts.

❓ HOW LONG DOES IT TAKE TO GET INTO KETOSIS?

Some people say that it takes a couple of days, or a couple of weeks, or even a couple months. To answer this question, we think it is important to differentiate between three different words: ketogenesis, ketosis, and keto adaptation.

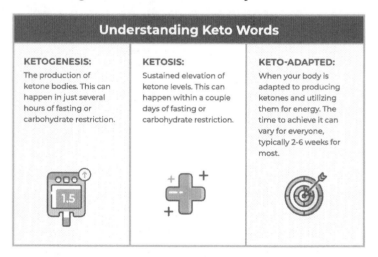

Understanding Keto Words		
KETOGENESIS:	**KETOSIS:**	**KETO-ADAPTED:**
The production of ketone bodies. This can happen in just several hours of fasting or carbohydrate restriction.	Sustained elevation of ketone levels. This can happen within a couple days of fasting or carbohydrate restriction.	When your body is adapted to producing ketones and utilizing them for energy. The time to achieve it can vary for everyone, typically 2-6 weeks for most.

Ketogenesis is the production of ketone bodies. This can happen in just several hours of fasting or carbohydrate restriction.

As ketogenesis ramps up, you start to see a more sustained elevation of ketone levels. This is ketosis and can happen within a couple of days of fasting or carbohydrate restriction. Once you are in ketosis, you will start to experience some of the benefits of keto, but your body is still becoming adapted to producing the ketones and utilizing them for energy. This is called the keto-adaptation period, and the time to achieve it can vary for everyone, typically 2-6 weeks for most.

Most times when people ask the question, "How long does it take to get into ketosis?" they are asking how long it takes to become keto-adapted—or for your cells actually using the ketones for energy.

WHAT IS KETO ADAPTATION?

Keto adaptation is a state that occurs when your body has become efficient at producing and utilizing ketones for energy and primarily relying on fat for fuel.

As we noted earlier, just being in ketosis does not mean that you are keto-adapted. Your body has not used fat and ketones for fuel for a long time—for most people, not since they were babies. For this reason, the cells in your body must upregulate the processes necessary to take in ketones and use them as fuel. Typically, this takes a little longer than it does to start producing ketones. This is why you may see a lag time between when you start producing ketones and when you actually start to feel some of the benefits of ketosis.

During this time, our cells are upregulating monocarboxylate transporters or MCTs (not the same as the fat you put in your coffee). These transporters are necessary for opening the door for ketones to come into the cell to be utilized for energy. Since prior to starting keto, more people are using carbohydrates as their primary fuel and glucose uses a different transporter, a family of GLUT transporters, it takes the body some time to "wake up" the MCTs in our cells to allow those ketones we are producing to be burned more efficiently.

As you start to become more efficient at utilizing ketones, you will start to experience the more noticeable benefits of keto, such as increased energy and better exercise performance.

❓ WHAT ARE THE SIDE EFFECTS OF KETO ADAPTATION?

Since it takes time to become keto adapted, it is not uncommon to experience a few side effects while the body is transitioning. These side effects are typically referred to as the keto flu.

There are several contributors to the keto flu. The first is that you are no longer providing your body with its expected fuel source in glucose, but the body is still adapting to burning fat, producing, and utilizing ketones (remember keto-adaptation), so there may be a degree of energy deficit in the body that can come with some side effects.

The second, and more common, is dehydration and electrolyte deficiencies. Remember, when you stop eating carbs, your pancreas responds by secreting less insulin. Lower insulin levels cause your kidneys to release more water. This leads to dehydration and a loss of electrolytes. Electrolyte deficiency can lead to many of the side effects experienced when starting keto. These side effects can include the symptoms listed on the graphic opposite.

Of the symptoms listed, brain fog tends to be one of the most commonly reported. This is for the same reasons listed above: fuel shortage and electrolyte deficiencies. The brain cannot use fat for fuel—it can only use ketones and glucose.

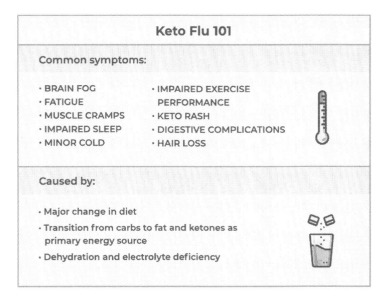

When glucose is cut out, but the body is still adjusting to producing and utilizing ketones, impaired brain function can be expected. Additionally, the electrolyte deficiencies, especially salt, can be a major contributor to brain fog. This symptom will quickly subside as your body transitions into ketosis and becomes keto-adapted.

Not everyone will experience all of the side effects mentioned here, and some people may hardly experience any. Regardless, there are many strategies to manage your keto flu symptoms or even avoid them altogether.

? IS IT NORMAL TO HAVE HEADACHES ON KETO?

It is not uncommon to experience headaches when you first start keto or at any point on a ketogenic diet, since low-carb dieting can lead to an increase in water excretion and electrolyte loss. Headaches on keto are commonly due to dehydration and electrolyte deficiencies and can be alleviated through proper hydration and electrolyte replenishment.

Headaches when first starting keto can also be due to the insufficient energy availability for the brain that we just mentioned. This side effect will take care of itself over time and exogenous ketones, which we will talk more about in Chapter 8, can be a great way to alleviate headaches.

? IS IT NORMAL TO FEEL TIRED WHEN FIRST STARTING KETO?

Fatigue is a common symptom during the onset of a ketogenic diet and is one of the symptoms of the keto flu. Fatigue on keto can again be a result of your body not having its common energy source in glucose and not yet being fully adapted to burning fat and producing and utilizing ketones for energy. Stick with it; this is something that takes time!

Like headaches, fatigue also can be a result of dehydration and electrolyte deficiency, which can be managed through proper hydration techniques and replenishing electrolytes.

If you have been following keto for a while and experience fatigue, chances are you may need to make some adjustments to your diet, since on keto you should be full of energy! In this case, give some of the following strategies a go:

- **Improve your sleep:** if you are not getting quality sleep, your energy levels will suffer.
- **Exogenous ketones:** These supplements can help provide a rapid source of energy to the brain and body.
- **MCTs:** These unique fats can be rapidly digested and used for energy or to produce ketones for additional energy.

- **Increase your calories:** If your caloric intake is too low for too long, fatigue can be expected. Track your calories, and if they seem to be too low, try increasing them. Adjusting caloric intake is especially important for people who are exercising or have just started exercising.

Tips for Battling Fatigue

IMPROVE SLEEP QUALITY AND QUANTITY

SUPPLEMENT WITH EXOGENOUS KETONES

ADD MCTS

INCREASE YOUR CALORIES

? HOW DO I AVOID KETO FLU SYMPTOMS?

One of the best ways to limit or prevent symptoms is to stay hydrated and replenish electrolytes. This will take attention to detail. Staying hydrated on keto can be a challenge, especially when you first start. Ensure that you are drinking enough water; signs of thirst are already indicative of the onset of dehydration. Our best practices for staying hydrated are:

- Drink a glass of water upon waking

- Keep a bottle of water available at all times
- Avoid thirst
- Finish at least a shaker bottle full of water during exercise
- Finish another shaker bottle full of water after exercise
- Adjust water intake based on activity level

Avoiding keto flu symptoms will also require replenishing electrolytes. Electrolytes are electrically charged minerals that help support numerous functions in the body. Just to name a few:

- Balance water levels
- Balance pH
- Support muscular contractions
- Help build new tissue
- Transmit nerve signals

Imbalances in your electrolytes can lead to many of the keto flu symptoms listed. The most common electrolytes as it relates to keto are:

- Sodium
- Potassium
- Magnesium
- Calcium
- Phosphorus

There are two ways in which electrolytes can be replenished:

- Whole food sources
- Electrolyte supplements

The best whole food sources of electrolytes are:

- Salting your foods
- Mixed nuts
- Avocados
- Salmon
- Leafy green vegetables

While you can find a decent quantity of electrolytes in several whole food sources, it is likely that you will still need to support your electrolyte replenishment efforts with supplementation, which you can refer to Chapter 8 for details on how to do so.

In addition to staying hydrated and replenishing electrolytes, another way to help combat the keto flu is by getting keto-adapted faster.

? IS THERE ANYTHING I CAN DO TO GET KETO ADAPTED FASTER?

This is a challenging question, because the length of time it takes to become keto-adapted varies from person to person, and there isn't really an objective way to measure keto adaptation since it is more of a subjective measurement, which we will get into more in a bit. So, this will be pretty theoretical.

Remember being keto-adapted means you're an effective fat burner, ketone producer, and ketone utilizer. The latter of the three is dependent on the upregulation of those monocarboxylate transporters we mentioned earlier. These transporters become upregulated via exposure to increased blood ketone levels. Thus, we theorize that taking strategies to increase and sustain that increase in ketone levels will promote a faster keto-adaptation period.

❓ HOW DO I GET MY KETONE LEVELS HIGHER?

Before we dig into this, we want to point out that current research does not support a reason for the general population to chase higher ketone levels. As we discussed in the previous chapters, just because you have high ketone levels does not mean that you are burning more fat, are healthier, or are having a more successful ketogenic diet. However, there could be a case for higher ketone levels for certain therapeutic cases, for improving brain function and energy levels, or for quicker adaptation to keto.

When you are first starting keto, getting those ketone levels up will be important to induce ketosis, push toward keto-adaptation, and reduce keto flu symptoms. There are several strategies that can be taken to increase ketone levels:

FASTING

Fasting, the restriction of food, is a great way to further stimulate the body to produce ketones. When no food is provided to the body, there is an even greater dependence on ketones for energy. Note that this strategy may not be the best for every beginner since fasting and keto together can be a pretty drastic change at one time. Refer to Chapter 9 for more on fasting.

MCTS

MCTs or medium chain triglycerides are unique fats that are more rapidly digested compared to other fats and can contribute to natural ketone production. Refer to Chapter 8 for more on MCTs.

EXOGENOUS KETONES

Exogenous ketones do not stimulate the production of ketones in the body, but they can provide you with short term ketosis, an energy boost, and reduced keto flu symptoms to allow you to stick to carbohydrate restriction and help your body to get in ketosis. Exogenous ketone salts also contain a blend of electrolytes, which gives them another benefit on a keto diet, especially during keto-adaptation. Refer to Chapter 9 for more on exogenous ketones.

EXERCISE

Exercise is a great way to stimulate fat burning and thus ketone production. In addition, exercise can help drive blood glucose down and increase ketone uptake into our cells. High-intensity exercise may be the best for stimulating ketone production, making it a preferred exercise type to push keto-adaptation.

Using these strategies can be effective for ensuring that you are elevating your ketone levels, promoting keto-adaptation, and possibly managing or improving some of your keto flu symptoms. With all diets, keto included, there is a constant question of what is optimal and what is sustainable.

IF WE WERE TO PRESCRIBE HOW TO GET ADAPTED TO KETO AS QUICKLY AS POSSIBLE, IT WOULD LOOK LIKE THIS:

- Commit to 60 days of high-quality keto-approved foods only
- Start with a 24-hour fast, followed by intermittent fasting
- Use MCTs in the late morning
- Use exogenous ketones in the afternoon
- Exercise daily, with an emphasis on exercise intensity

While this approach may be the most effective for getting you keto-adapted, it may not be the most sustainable. For instance, fasting may be very difficult for someone who is just starting keto, thus making the diet harder mentally and physically. Additionally, others may not have the capacity to do much exercise when they first start keto. For this reason, the most important item on that list is number one: stick to keto. Even if it takes you a little longer to adapt, that's okay. At the bare minimum, stick to the commitment to eat higher quality, keto-approved foods, and you will become keto-adapted in no time.

? HOW DO I KNOW IF I AM IN KETOSIS?

The most common way to see if you are in ketosis is by testing your ketone levels. In Chapter 13, we discuss testing for ketosis in greater detail. A few things to note about testing ketones is that there are several different ways to test ketone levels; each method has pros and cons; it is unclear what the optimal level of ketones in the blood is; and there are many factors that can impact your results.

Regardless, measuring your ketone levels will only help you determine that you are in ketosis; it will not help you determine if you are actually keto-adapted. For these reasons, another way to determine if you are in ketosis and keto-adapted is to listen to your body. Here are a few subjective measures you can use. These are not accurate enough to know your blood ketone level but can be a good gauge of how quickly you are adapting to the diet.

- **Mental Clarity:** Your brain constantly uses a significant amount of energy. When you are eating carbs you experience energy swings, and therefore mental performance swings. When you are keto-adapted, your brain will rapidly use ketones for fuel and there will be a marked mental state of ketosis that is different. When you're in it, you know.

- **Weight Loss:** If you are losing weight, especially consistently, then it is likely that you are keto-adapted.
- **Sustained Energy:** Approximately 90-120 minutes after you eat carbohydrates your body runs out of readily available energy produced from the mitochondria in your cells, so you start "crashing," or lowering your energy. When you are in ketosis and keto-adapted, your body can run off your body fat, which is an essentially limitless source of fuel. This prevents any crash in energy.
- **Hunger Control:** Being able to tap into stored fat means your body has such a constant supply of energy, it doesn't crave food the way it would if your energy depended on carbohydrates. If you experience reduced hunger pangs throughout the day, that could be a good sign that you are keto-adapted. Realized you didn't eat for the last fourteen hours, still have boundless energy and not hungry? Probably in ketosis.
- **Increased Thirst, Dry Tissues:** When you're adapting to a ketogenic diet, your body will use up excess glycogen and increase urine production. This typically leads to dehydration, which will cause thirst and lead to drier tissues in the short term. This can be a good sign of ketosis but should subside, if planned against, once keto-adapted.
- **Not Breath, but Mouthfeel:** You may have read that if your breath is fruity smelling, this is a good indication you are in ketosis. This is not accurate. Fruity breath is more of an indication of ketoacidosis, which is *not*

to be confused with nutritional ketosis and is typically associated with out-of-control diabetes. Acetone levels in the breath under nutritional ketosis should not be high enough to cause a detectable scent. However, when you wake up in the morning, a lot of times you'll have a distinctive mouth feel when in ketosis. There's almost a film-like feeling. You'll know.

? HOW MANY MEALS A DAY SHOULD I EAT ON KETO?

However, many meals you require to be satisfied. We eat when we are hungry, and don't eat when we're not. This changes when we are intentionally fasting, but that isn't the majority of the time like most people think is necessary.

The real answer is based on preference and necessity. Traditional meal frequency recommendations are based around carbohydrate-rich diets in which blood glucose levels are more prone to fluctuations which increases the need for meal frequency to ensure a source of energy is available.

On a ketogenic diet, you will not experience drastic fluctuations in blood sugar, meaning you may not require meals as frequently. However, you want to make sure you are sufficiently satisfying the calorie demands of your goals and lifestyle. This is different for everyone. For example, someone who is very active will want to make sure not to chronically under-consume calories due to reduced hunger. Learning how much to eat on keto can be an intuitive process. Over time, you will gain the skills to listen and learn from your body. A couple of ways to know if you are undereating calories on keto are:

- Extreme hunger
- Fatigue

- Impaired recovery
- Poor sleep
- Impaired exercise performance

These seem similar to keto flu symptoms, right? Keto flu symptoms can be triggered by the same caloric shortage. You may notice that your calorie demands decrease the longer you follow keto, but again this is very dependent on the individual.

? SHOULD I TRACK CALORIES ON KETO?

If there is one thing we've learned by working with countless patients, it is that humans are pretty awful at guessing how much food they eat.

In general, tracking calories is beneficial with any large dietary change. For example, if you moved and are eating an entirely different set of foods; or if you are changing your foods to lose weight instead of reduce inflammation; or if you are starting a new workout program. All of these are factors that could change your calorie intake and understanding how many calories you are consuming can be beneficial.

Anthony recommends that his patients track their food for the first week or two of keto to make sure that they are not over or undereating calories. If you invest a little bit of time into tracking for a week or two, you will have a pretty good template that you can use to eyeball food for the next couple of months, or even years.

Weighing out food is important when it comes to tracking calories and, in the beginning, can be a pain—we get it. But within a week or two, you'll realize you don't really vary the food you eat that much anyway. You'll look at a piece of steak and say, "Oh yeah, that's probably four ounces," and be able to nail it. Measuring for yourself for a while is the best way to learn how to do this. Once you get good at eyeballing foods, this becomes a much easier task to hammer out.

There are many ways to track your food, but by far the easiest is using your smartphone and an app that does a lot of the heavy lifting for you. Our preferred app is Cronometer. It lets you search by barcode (not that you should be eating that much packaged food anyway!), type of food, how it is prepared, etc. What makes Cronometer so great is its ability to break down the nutritional content of a meal. If you're trying to shore up nutritional deficiencies or see how balanced your general nutritional intake is, this is the app to go with.

Use whatever app is easiest and most intuitive for you, because the most important thing is to actually use it, at least while you are getting started. Once you learn what to eat to get into and stay in ketosis, you can pull back from tracking your food.

As discussed in Chapter 4, we do not believe that calories are as important as many think, especially on a ketogenic diet. Calories play a role but not as big of a role as the composition of those calories. However, calorie tracking through food tracking apps can provide you with this more useful information as well.

? WHAT ARE MACRONUTRIENTS?

Macronutrients are energy-containing molecules found in the foods we eat. The energy in macronutrients is what makes up the calories of our food and provides energy to our bodies. There are technically four primary macronutrients: carbohydrates, proteins, fats, and fiber. The food and diet industry have done an admirable job at making these words commonplace, but many people still couldn't identify what these macros actually are and what they do.

While counting calories is a great way to determine the energy content of your diet, counting macros allows you to determine the composition of those calories. As you know from the last few chapters, all calories are not the same, so this is important.

Macronutrients are essentially structures made out of different types of building blocks—think LEGOs. Carbohydrates are built from sugars, protein from amino acids, and fats from fatty acids.

Since the effectiveness of a ketogenic diet does relate to the composition of macronutrients in your diet, it is important that we discuss them in greater detail. Let's dive a little deeper into each macronutrient.

CARBOHYDRATES

Different types of carbohydrates are essentially different buildings made from different sugars (LEGO pieces). This means that not all carbohydrates are created equally. Specifically:

Monosaccharides are a type of carbohydrate that is just one sugar molecule. This is sugar in its most simple form. *Examples: glucose and fructose.*

Disaccharides are a carbohydrate of two sugar molecules. *Example: Table sugar.*

Polysaccharides are more complex sugars build up from multiple sugar molecules. *Example: Starches.*

All carbohydrates are not evil. The problem with carbohydrates is that many of the most commonly consumed carbs are processed and consumed in unnatural amounts that can wreak havoc on our health. It is worth noting that carbohydrates are also non-essential, meaning that the body does not require consuming them for survival. You can make all of the carbs you need endogenously or inside the body (remember gluconeogenesis). If you are going to consume carbs on a keto diet, get carbs contained within a cell wall of a plant. What do we mean? Get them from eating plants.

PROTEIN

Protein is the easiest macronutrient for most people to visualize. Think of protein and you usually think of meat, the staple of the American diet—alongside a massive whack of carbohydrates, of course (meat and potatoes, anyone?).

Think of protein as building blocks for all of your tissues. Protein is the LEGO set that makes up the structure of you. Protein, in other words, creates the scaffolding and support that we need to be an organized mass of energy. Protein's building blocks are called amino acids.

Protein can also come from plant sources, but these sources are not complete proteins, meaning they do not contain all of the essential amino acids. For this reason, protein from animal origin is superior.

Now, we always focus on quality, right? (*Yes! Yes, we do!*) With protein, the way you prepare it determines the net quality and bioavailability you'll be getting out of it. Proteins are folded structures of amino acids that become unfolded and then combined into different tissues for different reasons. When a protein is degraded, it is "denatured." Overcooking meat can lead to denatured protein that is voided of much nutritional benefit. Generally, proteins do better when they are closer to raw forms, as they exist in nature. Cooking meat is entirely fine if done in a reasonable fashion. Typically, the lower and slower you cook it, the easier it is for your body to break down the amino acids into better building blocks.

FAT

You shouldn't need a biochemistry background to read this book, and the structure of fat molecules is relatively unimportant, so we are just going to highlight the basics here. A common theme you will see when it comes to fat is that the source of the fat matters. Dietary fat comes in three primary forms:

Unsaturated Fat

These fats have traditionally been considered the "good fats." The problem is that these fats are found in both good *and* bad sources. There are two primary fats that make up this category; monounsaturated and polyunsaturated fats. Monounsaturated fats (MUFAs) are found in foods like avocados, nuts, and seeds; however, they are also found in some pro-inflammatory oils like peanut and canola oils. Polyunsaturated fats (PUFAs) are found in healthy sources like walnuts and fish but are also found in high concentrations in vegetable oils like soybean and safflower oil.

The saturation of these fats is important because it impacts oxidation. When oxidation to a fat occurs, the fat can become pro-inflammatory and dangerous. Unsaturated fats contain double carbon bonds. The more double carbon bonds a fat has, the more prone it is to oxidation. Polyunsaturated fats contain multiple double carbon bonds, making them especially prone to oxidation. This is why vegetable oils are so dangerous. They are made up primarily of PUFAs and are obtained through high heat extraction methods, turning these fats into firecrackers inside our bodies. Not a good thing. That is not to say that PUFAs are bad. It depends on how they are treated.

Within the classification of polyunsaturated fat, there are both omega-3 and omega-6 fats. Typically, omega-3 fats, found in foods like fish, seeds, and nuts, are considered to be the "good fats" for their ability to combat inflammation. Omega-6 fats, which can be found in nuts but also those pro-inflammatory vegetable oils, are considered to be "bad fats" due to their ability to promote inflammation.

Like most of our understandings of dietary fat, this is also too simple of an outlook. Not only does the source matter here but also the ratio between omega-3 and omega-6 fats. The Standard American Diet tends to have a much higher ratio of omega-6 to omega-3 fats than what is recommended. As we will get into throughout this book, much of this can be combated through a keto diet, increasing your consumption of fish, supplementing with omega-3 supplements, and lowering your intake of foods high in omega-6 fats.

Saturated Fat

The most demonized of fats, saturated fat is found not only in foods like dairy, meat, and coconut oil but also in processed desserts, pizza, and other unhealthy foods. A fat is saturated when it has predominantly single carbon bonds, making it a solid at room temperature. The single carbon bonds of saturated fat are important because it makes the fat more stable and less prone to oxidation. This is essential to not only the quality of the fat but also its effect on the body.

Of course, the source matters and this is one of the reasons why there is much confusion behind the safety of this fat. Refer back to Chapter 2, to learn more about why saturated fat is falsely blamed for poor health. To date, there has been no research to support that saturated fat is a contributor to poor health and on a keto diet, saturated fat can provide numerous benefits to the body.

Trans Fat

Nearly everyone knows that trans fats are the worst of the worst, and this is almost true. The problem is again that there are some good sources of trans fat. CLA, found in grass-fed meat is technically a trans fat and can provide numerous health benefits.

However, most of the trans fats people are getting in their diet are industrially produced trans fats created through hydrogenation. Hydrogenation is a process that changes the chemical configuration of unsaturated fats to give them more desirable physical properties for use in packaged foods. Hydrogenation results in the production of a type of trans fat that is not naturally occurring. These artificial fats are extremely pro-inflammatory and can cause many health problems.

Minus that naturally occurring CLA found in high-quality meat, trans fats should be avoided at all cost. Additionally, anything that says hydrogenated or partially hydrogenated on the label should also be avoided.

FIBER

We included fiber last here because, despite it technically being a macronutrient, it does not supply a significant amount of energy. Fiber, by definition, is the portion of a plant that is not able to be fully broken down by digestive enzymes. Fiber isn't food for your body, but food for the colony of microbes that live inside your gastrointestinal tract.

Most of us have been trained to understand that fiber is important because a lack of adequate dietary fiber is commonly associated with many health-related issues such as colon cancer. However, as you should be fully aware of now, just because something is associated with something does not mean that it is the cause. One important aspect to consider is that your nutrient needs change based on the diet you are following.

Many people consuming 0-carb diets with no fiber experience little or no digestive problems.

While research has not clearly demonstrated that fiber is essential, it can add volume to your diet to help you feel full, and most fiber-rich foods are dense in other micronutrients. For this reason, fiber coming from vegetable origin are acceptable on a ketogenic diet.

? SHOULD I COUNT MACROS?

> *Short answer:* For new ketogenic dieters, counting macros may not be essential but for those who are trying to push through a plateau or want to take greater control of their diet, tracking macros can help.

For many people, macronutrients are their first introduction to a ketogenic diet (remember those 70 percent fat, 25 percent protein, 5 percent carb recommendations?). This makes sense: many people need guidelines to follow and we know that macronutrient ratios do play a role in inducing ketosis. The problem is that the macronutrient approach to nutrition in general has led many to decide that foods are just made up of macronutrients, and that is all that matters. This is the "macro" camp. These people also apply the heavy use of the social media hashtag #IIFYM, which stands for "if it fits your macros." (Search for pictures of buff people eating Pop-Tarts to see what we mean.) The rationale here is that as long as you are eating the correct ratio of protein to fat to carbohydrate, you will be healthy. Donuts, soda, and pizza are all gravy IIFYM, bro!

But fuel is only one part of the equation. Your car uses fuel, but it is made up of hundreds of components made from different materials. It needs continual maintenance, or you won't have a car anymore. Parts wear out and must be replaced. Things break and must be repaired. Different fluids keep everything running smoothly. Think of macronutrients (protein, fat, and carbs) as the fuel that drives you forward. But if you want to actually be healthy, you need much more than just macronutrients. You constantly need the materials to sustain every component and maintain all the systems in your body or it's going to crash and burn way quicker than you want it to. This is why macros should not be the primary focus of your ketogenic diet.

Looking at your macros and your overall "fuel" system is a quantity-based perspective on food. You should have a quality-based perspective. We hit on this concept a lot (have you noticed already?), but quality is always better than quantity when it comes to nutrition. The right quality and the right quantity is a winning combination not just to survive as a human, but to thrive with optimal health.

The point here is that keto is about so much more than just tracking macronutrients and as we will get into in the next question, our understanding of the most optimal macronutrient intake is limited.

Furthermore, tracking your calories and macros is much more stressful and less sustainable. If you can learn to eat intuitively, keep your calories under control, and more importantly, keep your carbohydrate intake in check, then don't worry about the stresses of tracking macros. Instead, keep the focus on eating a variety of high quality, keto-approved foods and let your body handle the rest.

However, if you are someone who is wanting to take a more personalized approach to your nutrition, then tracking macros will allow you to know exactly what you are putting in your body, so that you can make adjustments later based on how you are feeling or if you are shifting to a new goal.

Note that for some people, tracking just carbs or calories could be enough. If you find that you are having a hard time adapting to keto or you aren't seeing progress, tracking your carbs and calories to make sure that they are in check may be just what you need.

If you are going to be tracking macronutrients, your next question is probably what those macronutrients should be at.

? WHAT ARE THE BEST KETO MACRONUTRIENTS?

Typically, you will see the best macronutrients for keto listed at or around 70 percent of your calories coming from fat, 25 percent from protein, and 5 percent from carbohydrates. Despite what anyone else might tell you, there is no macronutrient ratio that is most optimal for everyone. The current commonly recommended macronutrients were made in the '20s to help children suffering from drug-resistant epilepsy. To think that everyone, regardless of goal, should also be following these same macronutrient recommendations seems far too simplistic.

To be brutally honest, we can't make a general macronutrient recommendation because everyone is too different. Anyone who thinks they can is wrong. However, we know this isn't the answer you are looking for so we are going to try our best here to make as general of a macronutrient recommendation as we can.

The above-listed macronutrient ratio (70 percent fat, 25 percent protein, 5 percent carbs) will allow you to induce a state of ketosis, meaning that for the general population who is new to keto, this is a great starting point. This higher fat approach to keto is also a great way to ensure that you are consuming enough energy to fuel the body as you are adapting to the keto diet.

These macronutrients will not meet the demands of everyone, especially not permanently. After becoming keto-adapted, the next priority will be adjusting these macronutrients based on your individual needs as well as goals. For example, if you find that your training and recovery from training is suffering, you may benefit from increasing your protein. If you find that you are not losing weight, your body may respond better to lowering your fat intake a bit. The point is to experiment and see what works best for you! In Chapter 13 we will talk more about how to make adjustments to your macronutrients based on your goals.

❓ WHAT ARE MICRONUTRIENTS?

Micronutrients are non-energy containing substances that are required to support the body's growth, development, and function.

Notice that we said *required*. Micronutrients are extremely important and often overlooked when it comes to our nutrition despite the fact that without them, our bodies cannot function properly. Many micronutrients act as coenzymes or cofactors for enzymes in our bodies, meaning they are essential to the function of enzymes in the body.

Micronutrients can come from the foods you eat, synthesis in the body, and supplementation. When we refer to micronutrients, we are referring to compounds like:

- Vitamins as coenzymes
- Minerals as cofactors
- Phytonutrients
- Antioxidants

Unfortunately, micronutrient intake is also personalized so there are not general recommendations we can make on which and how much you require. However, doing your research and understanding common symptoms of specific micronutrient deficiencies can be a great way to determine which foods you should be incorporating more often in your diet and which supplements would be beneficial to add to your diet. In general, a great way to prevent micronutrient deficiencies is by eating high quality, whole foods, especially meat.

? HOW DO I MEASURE MACROS AND MICROS ON WHOLE FOODS THAT DON'T HAVE LABELS?

If you are consuming whole foods that do not have nutrition labels, logging your calories, macros, and micros may be a little more challenging.

In general, the majority of whole foods are going to be similar in macronutrients, so using apps like Cronometer or MyFitnessPal can give you a pretty accurate measurement for whole food macronutrients.

Micronutrients can be more varied from food source to source, so you may not be able to get the most accurate prediction of micronutrients in whole foods that do not have nutrition labels. Do your best to choose options on these apps that most closely resemble the food you are eating.

? HOW MANY CARBS CAN I EAT?

As with macros, there is no optimal carb range for everyone and for every goal. Under 30 grams of total carbs is a good place to start, since this is typically enough to ensure that ketosis occurs.

Adjust your carbs and see how your body responds. Many people may find that lowering their carbs even as low as 0-20 grams may lead to better results and benefits on keto.

Additionally, some people may find that having a few extra carbs helps them perform better with exercise. This is also something that can be tested.

As a general rule of thumb, if you are a starter, you should stick to less than 30 grams of total carbs. In Chapter 13 we will tell you more on how to self-experiment to determine your optimal carbohydrate range.

? WHAT ARE NET CARBS?

You will often hear people refer to net carbs when talking about keto. Net carbs refer to the carbohydrates you have left when you subtract fiber and sugar alcohols from the total carb count.

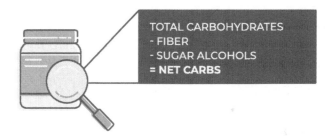

TOTAL CARBOHYDRATES
- FIBER
- SUGAR ALCOHOLS
= **NET CARBS**

Since many people think that fiber and sugar alcohols do not have any impact on blood sugar, the thought is that net carbs are most important to keep track of. This approach may not be best for everyone.

? SHOULD I COUNT TOTAL OR NET CARBS?

In principle, tracking just net carbs seems like a great approach. The problem with counting net carbs is that it can lead to a higher total carb intake and a higher sugar intake, which could inhibit ketosis. If you are trying to keep your carbs below 30 but you are tracking net carbs, that could mean 30 grams of sugar and 50+ grams of total carbohydrates. While some keto dieters may be able to tolerate this, many can't.

Making things more difficult, many companies take advantage of our understanding of net carbs by loading products up with sugar alcohols and fibers, which in high amounts, may stimulate a glucose response. Don't fall victim to this.

Our recommendation is if you are new to keto, stick to tracking total carbs to ensure that you are not going overboard on total carbs and sugar.

If you have been following keto for a while, you may be able to transition to tracking net carbs, but you should take time to test your tolerance and make sure that you are not overconsuming carbs from taking this approach. If you notice a dip in energy levels, increase in hunger, stall in progress, or lower ketone levels, chances are you are overdoing it with your carbs. In Chapter 13 we will get more into how to experiment with different carbohydrate amounts.

? WHAT ARE HIDDEN CARBS?

Hidden carbs are the carbs found in foods you would least expect and in some cases are hidden on nutrition labels. Processed foods and packaged foods are especially guilty of this. Hidden carbs are important to watch out for.

The problem with hidden carbs is that while they may seem minimal, they can add up. Several grams of carbs from this dressing, several from that cheese, a few from that packaged meat, and next thing you know, you have hidden carbs making a pretty big contribution to your total carb intake. This is why reading nutrition labels is so important.

Additionally, knowing what foods to be suspicious of for hidden carbs is important when you can't read nutrition labels, like when dining out. In this case, sauces and dressings are the biggest culprits. Here is a short run-through on hidden carbs and some tips for avoiding them.

SEASONING AND SAUCES

You should already know to steer clear of sweet sauces, but other flavorings, no matter how healthy (and delicious!), add up to your carb count daily and may be the source of uncalculated carbs. Here's a tally of carbs in seasonings, sauces, herbs, and spices (in 1 tablespoon):

- Ground Cumin 2.75 g
- Garlic Powder 6 g
- Onion Powder 5.4 g
- Chili Powder 4.1 g
- Oregano 3.3 g
- Cayenne 3 g
- Paprika 3.3 g

Dried/ground, less than 1 g per tsp:

- Tarragon, Mint, Basil, Cinnamon, Ginger
- Cloves, Black pepper, Coriander

Blended spices, 1 g per tsp:

- Curry powder
- Chinese 5-spice
- Garam masala
- Pie spice

For all other blended spices, read the label carefully. Look at huge tubs in Target or Costco if smaller containers/shakers don't have sufficient information.

FRESH

- Ginger root, 1 g/tbsp
- Garlic, 1 large clove/1tsp minced, 1 g
- Lemon/lime juice, 1 g/tbsp
- Lemon/lime rind, 1 g/tsp

VINEGAR, SOY SAUCE, HOT SAUCES

- White, cider and wine vinegar are zero carb
- Balsamic vinegar 2 g/tbsp
- Balsamic oil: plain has 3 g of carbs and processed has 9-12 g in 2 tbsps
- Soy sauce, 0.5 g/tsp
- Tabasco and Red Hot (zero carb). Read the label carefully for Cajun, Trinidad, Jamaican
- Flavor concentrates/extracts (almond, vanilla, orange, etc.), 0.5 g/tsp
- Bouillon cubes and powders, 1 g per 1/2 cube

MUSTARD AND MAYO

- Plain, Dijon, less than 0.5 g/tsp
- Real mayonnaise, 0.5 g/tbsp

PROCESSED MEATS

Deli meats, loaves, ham, sausages, corned beef and hot dogs all have starch and sugar (and the more processed they are, the worse they get—these are the meats that may actually contribute to health risks). If you are eating, read the label for the carb count. Some genuinely healthy, all-natural options have 1 gram or less per serving, but some of the lesser quality meats could reach 10 times that! Canned fish in any sauce may also have starch and sugar added.

MEAT AND EGGS

Beef, poultry, pork cuts, lamb, goat—the top recommended meats in the ketogenic diet—have zero carbs. Other protein sources have the following carb content:

- Liver 4 oz: veal/calf liver: 3.1 g, chicken liver 1.0 g
- Kidney 4 oz: 1.1 g
- Eggs: 0.6 g per one large egg, egg substitutes 1 g/1/4 cup
- Shellfish 4 oz: Oysters: 8 g, Scallops: 2.5 g, Shrimp: 1 g, Natural crab: 1 g, Imitation/Surimi crabmeat: 12-15 g, mussels: 8.4 g

DAIRY

All dairy products contain some carbs. Full-fat dairy is better because of its high-fat and lower-carb content. Lower fat dairy, such as 1 percent, 2 percent, low-fat and nonfat varieties replace the fat with carbohydrates, leading to a much higher total carb count. Here is a breakdown of the carbs found in dairy:

- Greek yogurt, 6 g to 7 g from the naturally-occurring sugars
- Natural butter, zero carbs
- Heavy cream, 0.8 g in 2 tbsp
- Sour cream, 1 g/oz
- Cheese, 1-8 grams depending on type of cheese and how processed it is

VEGGIES

While vegetables are typically very low in carbs, they do still contain carbs, some more than others. A hundred grams of kale has 9 grams of carbs, 100 grams of spinach has 3.6 grams, and 100 grams of lettuce has 2.9 grams. While the majority of these carbs come from fiber, meaning that vegetables have a low amount of net carbs, be cognizant of how much you are getting. Even if you are not kicked out of ketosis, too much fiber can cause other health-related problems.

"SUGAR-FREE" "FOODS"

Hidden carbs also lurk in "healthy" options, like sugar-free foods (which we don't think of as real foods). Sugar alcohols, also called "the polyols," are in everything labeled "sugar-free" and even "carb-free." They're not zero-carb and some of them are associated with insulin spikes and increased blood sugar levels. These include:

- Xylitol
- Sorbitol
- Maltitol
- Splenda
- Honey
- Agave
- Molasses

If you are looking to use sugar replacements, which shouldn't be done too frequently, opt for stevia or monk fruit, since these actually provide some benefit and have a much more minimal, if any, impact on glucose levels.

? ARE THERE ANY TIPS FOR STAYING FULL ON KETO?

Not everyone will experience satiety on a keto diet, especially not at first. For these individuals, strategies for promoting fullness may be beneficial. On a ketogenic diet you consume the majority of your calories from fat. One gram of fat has more than double the caloric value of one gram of carb or protein. Fat also has the ability to signal for fullness. If you are experiencing a lot of hunger on keto, adding in fat can be a great way to help solve this.

The other macronutrients can also contribute to reduced hunger. Protein also has a bit of satiating effect so making sure you get adequate protein to meet the demands of your body is also important. Carbs in the form of fiber from leafy green vegetables can also contribute to fullness and can be added in response to hunger without having much of an impact on blood glucose or caloric intake.

If you are frequently hungry on keto, you may need to increase your water intake. Lots of people confuse thirst for hunger. Drinking water will ensure you are hydrated and can help you feel fuller for longer. Lastly, supplementing with ketones and MCTs will boost ketone levels in your blood, which has been shown to suppress appetite.

HOW DO I KNOW IF I AM EATING ENOUGH FAT?

Since keto is a high-fat diet, many people wonder what exactly high-fat means and how to know if they are getting enough. The answer is also very individualized and dependent on many factors. We have seen numerous people benefit by increasing their fat intake, and others benefit by decreasing it.

When you start a keto diet there are different demands for dietary fat, and those demands may change the longer you follow a keto diet. In Chapter 13, we will explain how to manipulate your macronutrients to better align with your individual needs. For the moment, learn the common signs of eating insufficient dietary fat. The most obvious is hunger. Fat is very calorie dense, denser than protein and carbs combined. If your fat intake is too low, you may be heavily restricting your calories, resulting in increases in hunger. Other signs of not getting enough fat could be low energy levels, hormone imbalances, altered mood.

However, undereating fat is not as common of a problem as most people think, especially if you are eating the fattier cuts of meat we recommended earlier in this chapter.

HOW MUCH PROTEIN SHOULD I HAVE ON A KETO DIET?

As with all macros, there is no set-in-stone, optimal protein range for everyone. It will take self-experimentation to find what works best for you based on your individual needs and goals.

For a beginner, starting at 25 percent of total calories or 0.8-1.2 grams per lb. of lean body mass is a minimal starting point for most people. Going much lower than this, unless for certain therapeutic applications, could result in adverse side effects. From here, adjust your protein intake based on how you are feeling.

Do not be afraid to increase your protein intake. The body can produce glucose from excess amino acids from protein, a process known as gluconeogenesis; however, the body will only activate this process to the degree needed to meet the demands of the body. It has not been supported in the literature that consuming a higher protein diet will impair your state of ketosis. In fact, it may actually lead to better results for some.

? WHAT ARE SOME OF THE COMMON MISTAKES MADE ON KETO?

A ketogenic diet is tough for many people to implement. It requires a little more attention to detail than other nutritional approaches, leading to many mistakes. These mistakes lead to a lack of results, making these people want to quit. The best path we've found for success is to address all the mistakes you could make; then provide solutions before you've even begun a keto diet. Here are the top six mistakes I've seen on a ketogenic diet and how you can prevent or fix them.

1. **Not tracking protein intake.** A couple of years ago we would have been much more concerned with making sure you are not eating too much protein; now we feel like the majority of people are not eating enough. The high-fat nature of a keto diet has led many to focus only on fat and less on protein. This is a mistake, since protein demands vary depending on the individual and the goal. If you feel like something is off with your keto diet, this would be a good time to track your protein and experiment with making adjustments.

2. **Overeating carbs a.k.a. The Carb Creep.** Keeping your total carbohydrate intake low is essential to success on a keto diet; however, carbs can easily sneak into your diet without you even knowing it.

   Not only do vegetables contain some carbohydrates, but so do a lot of sauces and seasonings, which can easily lead to the overconsumption of carbohydrates. We can't tell you how many times someone has asked us why they aren't seeing success on a keto diet, yet when we ask them to track their carbs, we find they are eating closer to 50 grams a day when they thought they were eating less than 30 grams. This is the carb creep and it can happen very easily.

3. **Eating the wrong amount of fat.** If you take away one of the big three macronutrients, you need to increase another source. This is where dietary fat comes in. It is sometimes hard mentally to eat enough fat since we have been told our whole lives that it's bad for us. There are also a lot of people who eat too much fat—this is also a mistake. The easiest way to make sure you're getting enough is to be aware of it. Look at the food you are eating. Read the labels. Look up macros every once in a while. This will help you understand where your fat is at and determine how to adjust it.

4. **Not eating high-quality fats.** Just because you are in ketosis doesn't mean you should sacrifice quality. A huge mistake on most ketogenic diets is the absence of high-quality fats. Yes, you can get into ketosis by eating a very low-carb diet that's high in low-quality foods. No, that type of ketosis is not healthy. Garbage in equals garbage out.

Fats are the backbone for making new cells, brain tissue, neurotransmitters, hormones, and most bodily functions. Since keto is centered around dietary fat, focusing on getting the highest quality fat possible is even more important.

Think of whole, non-processed food choices. This means grass-fed meats, wild fish, cold pressed oils, avocado, nuts, etc.; not Frankenfood fats that come in super bright packages like low quality processed fluorescent cheese and other non-food dairy products.

5. **Not eating enough calories.** When you cut carbs, many changes occur that can promote under eating calories. While this can be effective for reducing body fat in the short term, it can be detrimental to hormonal processes in the long term. When you eat fat, you are fuller, which makes it easy to eat fewer calories, but that doesn't mean you should. When Anthony first ate a true ketogenic diet, it was difficult for him to get more than about 1,600 calories. He's a lean 175 lb. male who works out and needs about 2,600 kcal a day. You see the problem here.

When your body has fewer calories than it needs, it goes into starvation mode. It thinks the trend will continue, so it hoards precious resources (stored body fat, substrates to make hormones and neurotransmitters), and doesn't try to thrive. Most of the metabolic and thyroid problems people claim are caused by a ketogenic diet are just a low-calorie problem (this especially applies to women).

Start the ketogenic diet by trying to get a maintenance level of calories. A good way to do this is by tracking what your diet has been and noting the number of calories your body has been eating lately. That is a good place to start your calories at and over time, adjust accordingly.

6. **Not getting enough micronutrients.** Since bunless burgers and bacon are approved on a keto diet, many people tend to overeat foods like these that while they

may be keto-friendly, can contain fewer micronutrients. This can lead to micronutrient deficiencies that can be difficult to pinpoint.

Consuming vegetables is one way to increase micronutrient intake, but remember that these micronutrients tend to be less bioavailable or not absorbed as well. Therefore, another strategy that can be taken to increase micronutrient intake is through higher consumption of high-quality meats. Remember that when the quality of the meat is emphasized, the micronutrient quantity is higher, and these micronutrients are more bioavailable to humans.

A final way to increase micronutrient intake is by consuming organ meats like liver and heart since they are some of the most micronutrient-dense foods on the planet.

Starting a ketogenic diet does not have to be overcomplicated. While everyone requires a personalized approach with their nutrition, starting keto is similar for everyone. Stick to the approved food list from Chapter 6, try to consume a variety of high-quality keto-approved foods, listen to your body, and adjust accordingly.

At this point, you have all of the information you need to at least get started on a ketogenic diet, so get to it. But don't stop here. While starting the diet is similar for most people, how you need to adjust your diet as you progress will be very individualized. Keep reading to learn more on how to tailor the diet to your specific needs. This will be essential to dietary adherence as well as continuous success on keto.

CHAPTER 8

USING SUPPLEMENTS AND KETO

Thus far, we have put the emphasis on the foods to eat and not to eat on keto. Real food should certainly be the foundation of your nutrition but depending on your food preferences or even your goals, supplements can be a great way to fill in some of the nutritional gaps not met by your diet. Supplements are named correctly. They are not replacements and should never be viewed as such. You should eat an adequate amount of nutrient dense real foods first, then add in supplements to, well, *supplement* your food intake. Not replace it.

We believe certain supplements are essential for a human to thrive in the modern world. Eating a nutrient dense and diverse representation of meat and plants isn't always enough to provide the necessary levels of phytonutrients, vitamins, and minerals for a modern human to thrive. The need for supplementation may have increased over the years due to our food system, which has modified plants to be less nutritious and have higher sugar contents, while mono-cropping and destructive farming practices have led to nutrient-depleted soil, meaning nutrient-depleted produce. Supplements can help fill some of these voids as well as help you progress toward various goals that you may be chasing.

Full disclaimer: Anthony is the founder and CEO of Perfect Keto and Equip Foods, and Chris is heading up keto education for Perfect Keto. It will come as no surprise that many of the supplements that we recommend in this chapter are products that we sell. We are not making these recommendations because we have these products; we have these products based on these recommendations. You do not have to buy from us—that is not the goal here. The purpose of this chapter will be to introduce which supplements may be beneficial on keto and why.

? ARE THERE ANY SUPPLEMENTS I SHOULD BE USING ON KETO?

Even the most well-rounded ketogenic diet can be optimized through appropriate supplementation. Here is the list of supplements that we think are important to discuss for keto:

- Electrolytes
- MCT oil
- Vitamin D
- Vitamin K2
- Protein powders
- Greens powders
- Organ meat capsules
- Omega-3 supplements
- Exogenous ketones
- Insulin sensitizing agents
- Nootropics
- Probiotics
- Prebiotics
- Digestive enzymes
- Adaptogens

During this chapter, we will break down each supplement, what it does, why you need it, and how to take it. Note that, depending on your diet, you will not require every supplement in this chapter. Learning how to optimize your ketogenic lifestyle includes finding which supplements you require as an individual.

ELECTROLYTES

(?) WHAT ARE ELECTROLYTES?

> *Short answer:* Electrolytes are minerals that play a vital role in numerous bodily processes. Replenishing electrolytes is very important on low-carb diets.

Electrolytes are a class of minerals primarily found in our cells (intracellular) and in our organs and tissues with a small percentage located in our bloodstream. Electrolytes work together to help regulate fluid balance and play a key role in many bodily processes, including:

- Muscle contractions
- Heartbeat regulation
- Body temperature control
- Bladder control
- Energy production
- Neurological functions

There are many different electrolytes, and each impacts the other, making it important to consider electrolyte balance as a whole system, rather than thinking about replenishing one at a time. Electrolytes also play a major role in hydration status, and both hydration and electrolyte balance can impact one another.

Without electrolytes, you wouldn't exist. You must have enough of these in your body for processes to function correctly. If one or more of these electrolytes are deficient, you're going to experience some issues. Symptoms of electrolyte deficiency include:

- Irregular heartbeat
- Feeling shaky, dizzy or weak, like you're going to pass out
- Mental and physical fatigue
- Headaches or migraines
- Brain fog
- Impaired sleep
- Mood disorders
- Leg or other muscle cramps (charley horses at night)
- Constipation and bloating
- Poor athletic performance

These are also all common symptoms of the keto flu, which can occur during induction to a keto diet when the body is adjusting to the lack of carbohydrates and switching to running on fats (ketosis). One of the primary causes of keto flu is electrolyte imbalances, which is why electrolytes are of such great importance on keto and are the first supplement we listed.

DO I HAVE TO SUPPLEMENT WITH ELECTROLYTES?

Most likely. The confusing part about electrolytes is that electrolyte demands are different for everyone and can depend on many lifestyle factors, such as the foods you eat and your activity level. Certain individuals may be able to replenish electrolytes adequately through diet alone, while others may require the support of additional supplementation. One of the best ways to determine your electrolyte needs is to listen to your body for the signs of electrolyte deficiency we mentioned earlier.

? WHY ARE ELECTROLYTES IMPORTANT ON KETO?

Remember that consuming carbohydrates leads to an increase in blood glucose, which stimulates an insulin response from our pancreas. However, when carbohydrate intake is lowered, as it is on a keto diet, our blood sugar also lowers, and our pancreas secretes less insulin. When less insulin is produced, our kidneys excrete more water and electrolytes. This makes us very prone to dehydration and electrolyte deficiencies on low-carb diets.

As mentioned, being deficient in electrolytes can cause many negative side effects such as those pesky keto flu symptoms. Replenishing electrolytes are extremely important for new keto dieters to ensure that they don't suffer from symptoms that would deter them from continuing to follow the diet. However, electrolytes are also important for any ketogenic dieter, to ensure feeling good and optimal mental and physical performance.

? HOW DO I MANAGE ELECTROLYTES?

For some individuals, optimal electrolyte replenishment can occur through diet alone. However, in some cases, such as when exercise or sweat rate is higher, there becomes an increased need for supplementation. We will discuss both.

Consider electrolytes as a system. Many of the electrolytes have the ability to impact other electrolytes. For example, potassium and sodium play an intricate role with each one affecting the absorption of the other. This means that replenishing electrolytes together is important. Luckily, many supplements contain multiple electrolytes allowing you to achieve just that.

Before we dive into the specific electrolytes to be replenished on keto, it is important to note that it is impossible to make electrolyte quantity recommendations. There are so many individual factors at play, such as your diet, exercise, sweat rate, water consumption, and more. This means that replenishing electrolytes is going to be an intuitive process. The goal will be to learn the signs of deficiency and take the necessary steps to alleviate these symptoms. This will take some practice.

? ARE THERE SPECIFIC ELECTROLYTES TO PAY ATTENTION TO ON KETO?

A particular subset of electrolytes seems to require emphasis on a keto diet:

- Sodium
- Potassium
- Magnesium
- Calcium
- Phosphorus

SODIUM

Sodium plays a big role in water retention, making it one of the main regulators of fluid balance and hydration status. Sodium also plays a critical role in many bodily functions, which is why being deficient can lead to so many side effects.

We have been misinformed about sodium. It is not harmful, and healthy people can regulate their sodium balance, meaning they do not have to worry about over-consuming sodium. Under-consumption of sodium is much more of an issue for most people than overconsumption, especially ketogenic dieters. Sodium deficiency can result in nausea, headaches, brain fog, fatigue, muscle weakness, altered mood, impaired exercise performance, and muscle cramps/spasms. Sodium is the one electrolyte that many people focus on replenishing, because keto beginners hear regularly about the importance of salting your food. When it comes to salting your foods, choose high-quality salt such as Redmond Real Salt. This is a superior source of salt because it contains additional minerals and is naturally occurring compared to table salt. However, salting your food usually is not enough! In this case, electrolyte supplements containing sodium and the use of bone broth are two additional strategies that can help you get enough sodium in.

POTASSIUM

Potassium is important for maintaining healthy blood pressure, regulating heart rate, and ensuring proper fluid balance in the body. As with sodium, we need potassium for nerve and muscle function.

Potassium consumed in very high amounts can be lethal, but this is extremely difficult to achieve via diet, and supplements are not able to contain greater than 99mg, which is much lower than the RDI or recommended daily intake. Furthermore, healthy kidneys are great regulators of potassium levels and will rapidly excrete excess potassium to help prevent toxicity.

Potassium deficiency can lead to increased blood pressure, kidney stone risk, constipation, fatigue, muscle weakness/impaired muscle function, muscle cramps, headaches, nausea, altered sodium balance, irregular heartbeat, impaired exercise performance, and impaired recovery.

Since potassium supplements tend to contain pretty low amounts, this electrolyte in particular should be a focus in your diet. There are great whole food sources out there that contain adequate amounts of potassium, including salmon, nuts, avocados, leafy green veggies, and mushrooms.

CALCIUM

Calcium is the most abundant mineral in the body and plays a big role in many functions beyond just bone health. It is required for vascular contraction and vasodilation, heart and muscle function, nerve transmission, hormonal production, blood clotting, and much more.

Serum calcium is tightly regulated and does not fluctuate as much with changes in dietary intakes. However, the body does use bone as a calcium reservoir when calcium levels are low, which is why you should consider supplementing, especially on keto.

Calcium deficiency is often asymptomatic, unless severe. However, symptoms that could occur include lack of mental clarity and muscle spasms/cramps. Severe deficiencies can result in much worse, such as mood disorders and weak bones.

You can get calcium from dairy foods, leafy greens, broccoli, fish and even non-dairy unsweetened milks like almond and coconut milk. If supplementing with calcium, make sure it includes vitamin D to ensure adequate absorption.

MAGNESIUM

Magnesium is an essential mineral, and chances are you are not getting enough of it. In fact, 57 percent of the population is not meeting the US Recommended Dietary Allowance

(USRDA) for magnesium. Why is this important? Over 300 important bodily functions depend on magnesium, one of the most important being energy production. All of our cells require energy, better known as ATP, to carry out their normal functions. ATP production is driven by mitochondria, the little powerhouses in your cells. Mitochondria plays a major role in your cells' ability to produce energy to meet demands. This means that the functioning of mitochondria is extremely important to overall health and wellness. In fact, low levels of or damaged mitochondria, also known as mitochondrial dysfunction (which subsequently means low levels of ATP), leads to chronic inflammatory cycles that are a recipe for impaired health.

There are two ways to increase our cells' ability to produce ATP: increase your total amount of mitochondria or increase the efficiency of existing mitochondria by repairing them. Both avenues depend on magnesium.

After buffering mitochondrial production, one of the important things that magnesium does is bind to gamma-aminobutyric acid (GABA) receptors in the brain and activate this important neurotransmitter. GABA is a sort of neural tranquilizer that helps the body relax for sleep. This is one reason magnesium is recommended at night.

Magnesium also plays a role in nerve and muscular function, heart rate, the immune system, and many other processes. Magnesium deficiency is commonly associated with muscle cramps and weakness, impaired sleep, weak bones, mood disorders, altered blood pressure, and even irregular heart rate.

While 57 percent of people have been estimated to be deficient in magnesium, low-carb dieters are even more prone to magnesium deficiencies. This is why it is so important to replenish this electrolyte.

Common keto food sources of magnesium include dark leafy greens and some nuts. While eating copious amounts of dark leafy greens and nuts may provide adequate magnesium for the average sedentary American, it may not be enough for the ketogenic dieter, especially an active one. Such individuals are likely to need magnesium supplementation.

High-quality magnesium supplements use only the most absorbable and bioavailable forms of magnesium—magnesium glycinate and taurinate. This may also be noted as "chelated" magnesium. Magnesium glycinate is carried with glycine, which helps the absorption and delivery throughout your body considerably. Magnesium taurinate is magnesium bound to taurine, an amino acid that calms the nervous system, to further potentiate the calming effects of magnesium.

Some magnesium supplements will pair sulfates or citrates with magnesium to make it stable, but that makes it much less available for your body to absorb. Those forms are also conveniently a lot cheaper to produce. Not a surprise that's why many companies use them.

One of the side effects of taking higher levels of lower quality magnesium is gut irritation. Magnesium will clear out your digestive system pretty easily and quickly if you take too much, so don't go too crazy. You know the laxative milk of magnesia? Magnesium is the primary driver. Supplementing with 200-300 mg per day is advised for most people who want to maximize the performance of their mitochondria, but this recommendation may vary on a ketogenic diet.

PHOSPHORUS

Phosphorus is another essential mineral, required by every cell in the body to carry out proper functions. Phosphorus plays a critical role in maintaining the structural integrity of the cell membranes. Phosphorus also plays a role in bone mineralization, energy production, cell signaling, and maintaining acid/base balance. Eighty-five percent of the body's phosphorus is found in bones and teeth.

While phosphorus is found throughout the body, it is also found in many common foods, especially meats, fish, nuts/seeds, and plants. The bioavailability of phosphorus from food sources is very high and the mineral is rarely deficient in people unless they are under conditions of severe starvation. However, phosphorus levels on a low-carb diet have not been researched frequently. Regardless, due to its high bioavailability, if you are consuming meat and nuts, chances are you are getting all of the phosphorus your need.

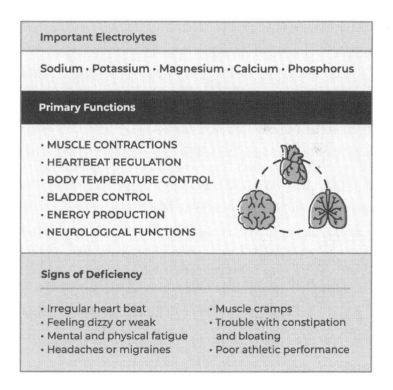

Important Electrolytes

Sodium · Potassium · Magnesium · Calcium · Phosphorus

Primary Functions

- MUSCLE CONTRACTIONS
- HEARTBEAT REGULATION
- BODY TEMPERATURE CONTROL
- BLADDER CONTROL
- ENERGY PRODUCTION
- NEUROLOGICAL FUNCTIONS

Signs of Deficiency

- Irregular heart beat
- Feeling dizzy or weak
- Mental and physical fatigue
- Headaches or migraines
- Muscle cramps
- Trouble with constipation and bloating
- Poor athletic performance

? HOW SHOULD I SUPPLEMENT WITH ELECTROLYTES?

When it comes to supplementing with electrolytes, most products contain a blend of the electrolytes you need on a ketogenic diet. The two primary types of electrolyte supplements are capsules and powders.

While both are useful for electrolyte supplementation on the go, capsules are beneficial because they make it a lot easier to adjust your serving based on your body's demands. Our recommendation for electrolyte capsules is our own product, Perfect Keto electrolytes. However, electrolyte packets are great because they have to be added to water, adding extra hydration that is already needed on keto anyway. Our recommended electrolyte powder is from Elemental Labs (LMNT).

While treating electrolyte replenishment as a whole system is beneficial, you may find that your body requires more of a specific electrolyte. For example, some people struggling with sleep on keto may require more magnesium specifically and are just fine on the other electrolytes. If this is the case, don't be afraid to add extra supplementation.

When it comes to replenishing electrolytes, you do not have to worry about consuming too much since healthy kidneys can regulate electrolyte balance and excrete any excess.

Recommendations for electrolyte maintenance:

- Salt your foods (we recommend Redmond Real Salt)
- Eat avocados, mixed nuts, and fatty fish
- Supplement with whole electrolyte products
- Know the symptoms of each electrolyte deficiency so you can add in more of a certain electrolyte if needed.

EXOGENOUS KETONES

? WHAT ARE EXOGENOUS KETONES?

Exogenous ketones are supplemental ketones that possess a very similar molecular structure to those produced by your body. When ingested, these ketones can be absorbed into the bloodstream, causing an increase in blood ketone levels similar to what we see when the liver is making ketones.

Research on these supplements is still in its infancy, but so far, we see that the body can use exogenous ketones for fuel just like it would use ketones produced naturally. This means that the increase in blood ketone levels typically seen from taking exogenous ketones demonstrates the supplement's ability to provide a readily available fuel source for the brain.

? WHY ARE EXOGENOUS KETONES BENEFICIAL ON A KETO DIET?

Since your body is already producing ketones naturally on the keto diet, why take more? One perspective that we like to offer is that your body is always producing energy; does that mean that you would never drink coffee? That is not to say that coffee is an energy source, but it does lead to an increase in energy, which you sometimes need. Exogenous ketones are similar.

HOW CAFFEINE WORKS

Caffeine actually doesn't provide the body with any energy; rather it binds to adenosine receptors, preventing adenosine from binding with these receptors through a process known as competitive inhibition. If adenosine is able to bind to its receptor, neural activity slows down, and you become tired. Caffeine's ability to bind to these receptors prevents this from happening, at least until the caffeine is fully metabolized.

Ketones are an energy source, so supplementing with them can simply provide your body with a readily available source of fuel. Ketones, when available, are actually the preferred source of fuel for the brain. In fact, research has shown that when both glucose and ketones are available, the brain will choose ketones.[55] Furthermore, ketones produce more energy per unit compared to glucose, meaning that they can provide a greater boost in cognitive function.

When you are first starting a keto diet, remember that there is a period of time while you are adapting where your energy levels are not very high. During this time, exogenous ketones can help increase the available energy to your body and especially the brain, to keep you functioning at a high level while your body is adapting.

Earlier in the book we explained the keto adaptation period and how our cells have to upregulate MCT transporters to allow for ketones to enter our cells to be effectively utilized for energy. Research has found that the presence of ketones in the blood can help stimulate this process.[56] While this has not

---

55 Joseph C. LaManna, Nicolas Salem, Michelle Puchowicz, Bernadette Erokwu, Smruta Koppaka, Chris Flask, and Zhenghong Lee, "Ketones Suppress Brain Glucose Consumption," in *Oxygen Transport to Tissue XXX* (Boston, MA: Springer, 2009): 301-306.

56 Richard L. Leino, David Z. Gerhart, Roman Duelli, Bradley E. Enerson, and Lester R. Drewes, "Diet-induced Ketosis Increases Monocarboxylate Transporter (MCT1) Levels in Rat Brain," *Neurochemistry International* 38, no. 6 (2001): 519-527.

been adequately researched, this could mean that exogenous ketones' ability to increase circulating ketone levels could aid in keto-adaptation.

? WHAT ARE THE OTHER BENEFITS OF EXOGENOUS KETONES?

To reiterate, since taking exogenous ketones can increase ketone availability, many of the perceived benefits are a result of more available energy—what we consider to be lifestyle benefits:

- More energy
- Better exercise performance
- Improved mental focus/ cognitive function
- Improved mood
- Reduced stress
- Reduced inflammation

However, exogenous ketones can provide benefits that extend far past simply increasing energy availability. Ketones, among many things, are signaling molecules, meaning that they can signal for various cascades of events that can lead to numerous changes in the body. We refer to these as physiological benefits:

- **Lower Blood Sugar:** Ketones and glucose tend to have an inverse relationship, so when ketones are high glucose is low (and vice versa).
- **Improving Mitochondrial Function:** Ketones have been found to promote mitochondrial biogenesis or increases in the size and number of mitochondria. Mitochondria are the parts of the cell responsible for burning fuel

for energy. Improving mitochondrial function can dramatically improve symptoms of many diseases as well as improve metabolism.

- **Activating Brown Adipose Tissue (BAT):** BAT is metabolically active tissue that is responsible for burning calories. Research has shown that ketones can activate this tissue,[57] which can have a profound effect on our ability to burn fat, stay lean, and stay healthy, one of the long-term benefits of having ketones available in the body.

- **Sparing the Breakdown of Muscle Proteins:** Research has long touted keto as a "muscle sparing" diet, meaning that in most cases we tend to see a retention in muscle mass on the diet despite calorie restriction. Ketones are the primary reason for the muscle sparing effect of keto. When ketones are available as fuel, the body does not need to break down muscle proteins to meet energy demands.

- **Activating Muscle Protein Synthesis:** Muscle protein synthesis, besides being Chris' favorite thing to say, is the process of making more muscle proteins to combat the breakdown of muscle proteins. A balance in the synthesis of protein and breakdown of protein is crucial for maintaining muscle mass. Exogenous ketones have been shown to stimulate muscle protein synthesis in animal models.[58] This is definitely an area of research

57 Shireesh Srivastava, Ulrich Baxa, Gang Niu, Xiaoyuan Chen, and Richard L Veech, "A Ketogenic Diet Increases Brown Adipose Tissue Mitochondrial Proteins and UCP1 Levels in Mice," *International Union of Biochemistry and Molecular Biology Life* 65, no. 1 (2013): 58-66.

58 Tijs Vandoorne, Stefan De Smet, Monique Ramaekers, Ruud Van Thienen, Katrien De Bock, Kieran Clarke, and Peter Hespel,...

that needs to be explored more but a possible added benefit to supplemental ketones.

- **Reducing Inflammation:** Ketones can reduce inflammation through several mechanisms. One is by inhibiting the NLRP3 inflammasome, which is responsible for activating the inflammatory cascade. Ketones may also be able to lower inflammation by improving antioxidant production. There is a theory that elevated ketones can allow more glucose to be shuttled to a different pathway (the pentose phosphate pathway), which is responsible for producing glutathione, one of our most potent antioxidants.
- **Appetite Reduction:** When the brain is metabolizing ketones, we tend to see a decrease in appetite signaling, leading to reduced appetite.
- **Improved Oxygen Utilization:** Ketones can improve the utilization of oxygen by the central nervous system. Exogenous ketones have been studied by famous keto researcher Dr. Dominic D'Agostino in Navy SEALs for their ability to prevent oxygen toxicity during long-duration deep-diving episodes.
- **Gene Alterations:** There is some research suggesting that ketones can also alter the expression of various genes in the body, giving these molecules an ability to offer numerous therapeutic benefits.

Outside of the physiological benefits, which are often therapeutic in one way or another, there are several additional

---

…"Intake of a Ketone Ester Drink During Recovery from Exercise Promotes Mtorci Signaling but not Glycogen Resynthesis in Human Muscle," *Frontiers in Physiology* 8 (2017): 310.

researched therapeutic implications for ketones. These we refer to as therapeutic benefits:

- **General Therapeutic Potential:** Because ketones can reduce inflammation, improve insulin sensitivity, and provide a readily available source of energy, they are able to improve overall health and improve symptoms of many diseases.
- **Preventing Neurodegeneration:** Neurodegenerative disease is due to several factors. One is insulin resistance in the brain. As we age, our brains become less efficient at using glucose for fuel and this leads to an energy crisis in the brain that can promote neurodegeneration, specifically synaptic loss and neuronal cell death. Research has found that when the brain can't use glucose, it can still use ketones.[59] This means ketones can provide fuel to prevent neurodegeneration. Additionally, reduced inflammation is neuroprotective and there is a growing body of research demonstrating that ketones may be able to slow the progression of protein deposition closely linked to Alzheimer's, amyloid and tau.[60]

---

59 Klaus W. Lange, Katharina M. Lange, Ewelina Makulska-Gertruda, Yukiko Nakamura, Andreas Reissmann, Shigehiko Kanaya, and Joachim Hauser, "Ketogenic Diets and Alzheimer's Disease," *Food Science and Human Wellness* 6, no. 1 (2017): 1-9.

60 Yoshihiro Kashiwaya, Christian Bergman, Jong-Hwan Lee, Ruiqian Wan, M. Todd King, Mohamed R. Mughal, Eitan Okun, Kieran Clarke, Mark P. Mattson, and Richard L. Veech, "A Ketone Ester Diet Exhibits Anxiolytic and Cognition-Sparing Properties, and Lessens Amyloid and Tau Pathologies in a Mouse Model of Alzheimer's Disease," *Neurobiology of Aging* 34, no. 6. (2013): 1530-1539.

- Improving Traumatic Brain Injury (TBI), or concussion, Outcomes/Treatment: We are really excited about this. A blow to the head leads to an energy crisis in the brain, so the brain starts taking in as much glucose as it can. The more glucose available, the more the brain takes in. But just like the rest of our body, the brain becomes insulin resistant and inflamed. The inflamed brain isn't able to get nutrients, making it a starving and inflamed brain. Not a good combo, and one that leads to a nasty progressive cascade. But animal research on concussion (yeah, it's not pretty research) has found that following a concussion, ketones can be taken up instead of glucose which could prevent the rapid uptake of glucose, could still solve the energy crisis in the brain, and provide antioxidant benefits in the brain.[61] Ketones should be on the sidelines at football games, not Gatorade—especially since there is evidence that ketones could be good in both the short-term and long-term treatment of TBI.[62]
- Cancer: This will take another quick lesson. One of the fundamental features of cancer cells is an increased hunger for sugar. This hunger can lead to a cascade of events that promote the growth and metastasis of cancer. If we stop providing that fuel source to cancer, we typically see therapeutic benefit; the cancer cells are being starved. There are mixed opinions on whether cancer cells can use ketones for fuel, but regardless,

61 Mayumi L. Prins and Joyce H. Matsumoto, "The Collective Therapeutic Potential of Cerebral Ketone Metabolism in Traumatic Brain Injury," *Journal of Lipid Research* 55, no. 12. (2014): 2450-2457.
62 Hayden White and Balasubramanian Venkatesh,"Clinical Review: Ketones and Brain Injury," *Critical Care* 15, no. 2. (2011): 219.

ketones can help provide fuel to our healthy cells while starving cancer cells. Other benefits include reductions in inflammation, driving down blood glucose, and improvements in mitochondrial function that could really improve cancer outcomes.

? ARE EXOGENOUS KETONES SAFE?

Despite what you may hear around the internet, there is no reason to think that taking exogenous ketones is in any way dangerous. Research to date has demonstrated that these molecules are safe and well tolerated unless consumed at very high doses, which can lead to gastrointestinal distress. Someone currently suffering from diabetic ketoacidosis likely should avoid further increasing blood ketone levels (but that doesn't mean that they shouldn't do a keto diet to get that resolved, and then start using ketones).

Supplemental ketones bound to minerals, which we will discuss in greater detail soon, provides a pretty big mineral load, if someone has damaged kidneys or any other condition that prevents them from being able to effectively balance out electrolyte levels, they should proceed with caution when taking exogenous ketones. The only side effects typically in consideration are the following:

UPSET STOMACH

It is not uncommon for people who begin taking exogenous ketones to experience upset stomach. This could be a response from the bacteria in our gut getting used to metabolizing the ketones or it could be related to the mineral load from the electrolytes found in exogenous ketone powder. Regardless, it is recommended that someone start with ¼ serving and assess tolerance before moving to a ½ and then full serving. Tolerance will improve over time.

EUPHORIA

While some may consider this to be a good thing, elevated ketone levels can result in a euphoric feeling that some may not enjoy. If this occurs, lowering the dose should do the trick.

? CAN I TAKE KETONES IF I'M EATING CARBS/NOT ON KETO?

Exogenous ketones can still be taken if you are eating carbs; however, it should be noted that the most robust benefits of using the product would occur when coupled with a ketogenic diet.

Ketones are still an energy source and taking them will still provide fuel to the brain, even when carbohydrates are consumed. Additionally, ketones can improve insulin sensitivity, which means that consuming supplemental ketones in conjunction with carbohydrates may improve the effectiveness of those carbs. However, there is much more research needed.

We would not recommend using exogenous ketones on a high-carb diet; however, using them on a low-carb but not keto diet could allow someone to experience keto like benefits at a higher total carb consumption, but this also still needs to be evaluated in research.

? WILL EXOGENOUS KETONES PREVENT MY BODY FROM PRODUCING ITS OWN KETONES?

This is one of the most common concerns you will hear about exogenous ketones. Everyone speculates that since you are consuming exogenous ketones that your body will stop producing its own, the answer is…of course they will, in the short term.

Gasp! Then why would someone take them? Easy; it's just a natural feedback mechanism that happens on a keto diet regardless of exogenous ketone use. When you have enough energy available, regulatory signals shut down the production of ketones to make sure that levels do not get too high. This is why you do not go into diabetic ketoacidosis while following a ketogenic diet. Your body shuts down ketone production when it has enough and starts it back up again when it needs more.

So, what happens when you take exogenous ketones? You see an acute increase in ketones, typically to a greater degree than achieved from a keto diet alone. After your body utilizes these ketones, your blood ketone levels return to baseline. Yes, back to baseline, not zero. Once there is another demand for ketone production, the body will turn ketogenesis back on.

? WHAT IS THE DIFFERENCE BETWEEN THE DIFFERENT TYPES OF EXOGENOUS KETONES?

There are two different types of ketone supplements on the market, ketone esters and ketone salts.

- **Ketone Salts:** Ketone molecules bound to minerals
- **Ketone Esters:** Ketone molecules bound to an alcohol group

There is a lot of science that could be discussed between the two different types of exogenous ketones, but it is pretty difficult and unnecessary for most of you to know, so we will keep it simple. The difference between the two is that the end result of one is a powder (the salts) and the other, a liquid (the esters). Research has not determined which can provide more benefit, but typically we see a more rapid and robust increase in ketones from esters and a more modest and steady increase in ketones from the salts, making both great options and potentially suggesting different uses, depending on the goal. While the price has gone down, ketone esters still tend to cost much more and have not been made as palatable as ketone salts.

In addition to the different type of ketones, some supplements within the two classifications may vary in chemical structure. The ketone molecule can come in two different forms. People who understand chemistry will get this racemic differentiation, but if not, you may hear of this as a "D" or "L" enantiomer. "D" is the version that is produced in the body while "L" is a version that is contained within some ketone supplements. The difference between the two is that one is just a mirror image of the other. Think of this as a right-hand and left-hand glove.

There has been some recent discussion whether one is better than the other, but currently there is no evidence to help us make a decision. It has also been suggested that the L version is dangerous; however, research has not actually found that either is dangerous unless you ask someone who is financially incentivized to tell you differently. In fact, for those who really want to dive into the science, there is actually evidence that shows that L enantiomer works independently of the D structure to specifically reduce inflammation.[63]

When it comes to ketone esters and ketone salts, both lead to an increase in blood ketones and as we mentioned earlier, to

---

63 Yun-Hee Youm, Kim Y. Nguyen, Ryan W. Grant, Emily L. Goldberg, Monica Bodogai, Dongin Kim, Dominic D'agostino et al., "The Ketone Metabolite B-Hydroxybutyrate Blocks NLRP3 Inflammasome–Mediated Inflammatory Disease," *Nature Medicine* 21, no. 3. (2015): 263.

varying degrees. It appears that if you are in need of a robust increase in ketone levels, like in certain therapeutic instances, a ketone ester may be the best option. However, if you are looking for a milder increase in ketones, such as to help power through your day to induce keto-adaptation, a ketone salt may be your best option. Since the minerals that ketone salts bind to typically are a blend of various electrolytes, these supplements can provide additional benefits on a ketogenic diet, where there is increased demand for electrolyte replenishment.

HOW SHOULD I SUPPLEMENT WITH EXOGENOUS KETONES?

If you are looking to induce a very high state of ketosis, the use of a ketone ester will be your supplement of choice. This could be beneficial for extreme athletes and certain therapeutic cases. For the rest of us, we recommend using exogenous ketone salts. Here are the best times to use these supplements:

- During periods of energy demand
- To improve workflow
- To provide energy for workouts
- To enhance keto adaptation
- To reduce appetite
- To minimize symptoms of being kicked out of ketosis

Referring to the last use on the list, many people think that exogenous ketones can be taken whenever you cheat on keto and the problem will be instantly fixed. However, ketones are going to increase blood ketone levels in the short-term, which means that if you are kicked out of ketosis, they are only going to acutely get you back into ketosis, which is not a long-term solution. These molecules can be relied upon to minimize symptoms of being kicked out of keto, such as brain fog and fatigue, but should not be depended on as a keto cheat aid.

Additionally, we do not know that higher ketone levels are necessarily important, so taking exogenous ketones all of the time because you believe more is better isn't necessarily right. There may be certain therapeutic instances where greater elevated ketone levels may provide benefits, but this needs more research.

Finally, it should also be noted that exogenous ketones should not be used in replacement of a ketogenic diet. They are best used in conjunction with a ketogenic diet, which will lead to more robust benefits from these supplements.

RECOMMENDATIONS FOR EXOGENOUS KETONES

- Dose of ketone ester depends on use goal (read above).
- Ketone esters are best used with extreme athletes or therapeutically.
- Single dose of ketone salts is between 11-15 g
- Use ketone salts daily during first couple of weeks of keto
- Use as needed once adapted to keto (see above for times to take ketones)

MCT OIL

? WHAT ARE MCTS?

Short answer: MCTs are unique fats that are rapidly digesting and can contribute to the production of ketones.

MCT stands for medium chain triglycerides. Triglycerides, while often considered to be bad due to a correlation between high triglyceride levels and elevated cardiovascular risk, are often misunderstood. Actually, it is just a term used for fat. Triglycerides themselves are not bad. The fats in the food we eat are called triglycerides, and the fat stored in adipose tissue also takes the form of a triglyceride. They are important to the function of the body and the production of energy, especially on a ketogenic diet.

Fat can be composed of a glycerol backbone and one-to-three fatty acids. A triglyceride is three fatty acids with a glycerol backbone made up of three hydroxyl groups, while the fatty acids are composed of a chain of 4-24 carbon atoms.

MCTs are unique fats that have a shorter chain of carbon atoms (hence the "medium chain"), which allows them to be digested differently compared to other fats, referred to as long chain fatty acids or LCTs (which have a much longer carbon chain). There are technically four fats that can be classified as MCTs:

- Caproic Acid (C6)
- Caprylic Acid (C8)
- Capric Acid (C10)
- Lauric Acid (C12)

The Cs next to each name denote the number of carbon atoms in that particular triglycerides carbon chain. Since fats are digested by removing carbon atoms two at a time; the shorter carbon chain length of MCTs makes them more rapidly digestible. In fact, the unique molecular structure of MCTs allow them to bypass typical digestion and be absorbed directly into our bloodstream.

Lauric acid (C12), by definition, should be classified as an LCT but is unique in that it possesses both characteristics of MCTs and LCTs, so it is classified as an MCT. MCTs can come from several sources, the most popular being coconut and palm oil; however, MCTs can also be found in small amounts in dairy.

? WHAT ARE THE BENEFITS OF MCTS?

MCTs provide numerous benefits to the body and in particular can provide added benefits to a ketogenic diet. Here are some of the most notable benefits:

RAPID ABSORPTION

Typically, fats are slow to digest, leading to a lag time between when they are consumed and when they are available for energy usage. MCTs, on the other hand, are able to bypass normal digestion, typically through the lymphatic system, and be absorbed directly into the portal venous system, where they can circulate to tissues to meet energy demands.

KETOGENESIS

When LCTs are digested, they are carried through the blood in lipoproteins known as chylomicrons. Since chylomicrons preferentially deliver energy to muscle and other metabolically active tissues and not the liver, the foods you eat are not able to contribute significantly to ketone production. However, MCTs can enter circulation and be delivered to the liver for ketone production. Ketone production from MCTs is minor but still significant.

IMPROVED BRAIN FUNCTION

The brain takes up ketones in proportion to their availability in the blood.[64] When the brain burns ketones for fuel, it results

---

64 Alexandre Courchesne-Loyer, Etienne Croteau, Christian-
   Alexandre Castellano, Valerie St-Pierre, Marie Hennebelle, and…

in less oxidative stress (thus lower inflammation) and greater energy production. This is one of the reasons why we say that ketones and a keto diet can improve brain function. MCTs' ability to stimulate ketone production gives them a unique ability to increase energy to the brain and improve the health and function of the brain. This has been especially noted in research in aging and neurodegenerative populations.

ANTIMICROBIAL

MCTs, specifically C12, possess potent antimicrobial, antibacterial, antifungal, and antiviral properties that give them immune-boosting potential. While the mechanism is not fully known, electron microscope studies have shown that these fats can damage the cell membrane of foreign microbes.[65] Interestingly, MCTs are found in breast milk; the described antimicrobial benefit of MCTs in this case is thought to help infants battle potential infections.

INCREASED ENERGY

The combination of rapid digestion and ketone production gives MCTs the ability to increase energy levels, particularly in the brain.

...Stephen C. Cunnane., "Inverse Relationship between Brain Glucose and Ketone Metabolism in Adults During Short-Term Moderate Dietary Ketosis: A Dual Tracer Quantitative Positron Emission Tomography Study," *Journal of Cerebral Blood Flow & Metabolism* 37, no. 7. (2017): 2485-2493.

65 Michael Shilling, Laurie Matt, Evelyn Rubin, Mark Paul Visitacion, Nairmeen A. Haller, Scott F. Grey, and Christopher J. Woolverton, "Antimicrobial Effects of Virgin Coconut Oil aAnd Its Medium-Chain Fatty Acids on Clostridium Difficile," *Journal of Medicinal Food* 16, no. 12. (2013): 1079-1085.

LOWER BLOOD SUGAR LEVELS

MCTs have been shown to improve insulin sensitivity, which would result in lower blood sugar levels. Furthermore, an increase in ketone production is typically met with a decrease in blood sugar.

IMPROVEMENTS IN NEUROLOGICAL DISORDERS

Since MCTs can improve the health and function of the brain, there has been a decent amount of research demonstrating their ability to provide benefit to neurodegenerative diseases like Alzheimer's and Parkinson's disease. This should come as no surprise, since many neuro-related disorders are a result of altered brain energy metabolism, which can be alleviated through an increase in ketone production. Furthermore, the use of an MCT-induced ketogenic diet has also been found to be beneficial for the treatment of epilepsy.[66]

There is more awareness today about the gut-brain axis, which is essentially the relationship between our gut and brain which demonstrates a potent connection between the health of these two previously considered separate organs. MCTs' anti-microbial benefit allows them to provide benefit in this case as well, which gives them the potential to benefit gut-brain related conditions such as autism.

WEIGHT LOSS

Weight loss from MCTs is not direct; however, an increase in energy, which is typically met with an increase in energy

---

66 Elizabeth G. Neal, Hannah Chaffe, Ruby H. Schwartz, Margaret S. Lawson, Nicole Edwards, Georgiana Fitzsimmons, Andrea Whitney, and J. Helen Cross, "A Randomized Trial of Classical and Medium-Chain Triglyceride Ketogenic Diets in the Treatment of Childhood Epilepsy," *Epilepsia* 50, no. 5. (2009): 1109-1117.

expenditure, coupled with fullness promoted by an increase in ketones, all together give MCTs potential to contribute to weight loss.

BLOOD LIPIDS

While optimal blood lipid levels are not fully understood (despite many cardiologists thinking they are), MCTs have been shown to increase HDL, which is no doubt a good thing.

LIVER HEALTH

Some research has suggested that MCTs may be able to reduce toxin buildup in the liver, giving them potential to improve the health of one of our most important organs.

(?) WHAT ARE THE DIFFERENT MCT-CONTAINING PRODUCTS?

> *Short answer:* MCTs can be found in both supplemental and whole food form. Each offers a slightly different composition of MCTs.

The rising popularity of MCTs has increased the number of MCT products available on the market. Here are the main products MCTs can be found in:

WHOLE FOOD

Whole food sources of MCTs, the most popular being coconut oil, are made up primarily of C12 with small amounts of C10 and even smaller amounts of C8 and C6. This makes coconut oil a great fat for antimicrobial benefits and clean energy, but not the best product for *quickly* increasing energy levels or stimulating ketone production due to the slightly longer carbon chain length of C_{12}. Whole food MCT sources also include palm oil and dairy sources like milk, cheese, cream, and yogurt.

MCT OIL

Regular MCT oil has had C_{12} removed, leaving primarily C_{10}, with minimal amounts of C8 and even less C6. This makes MCT oil much more rapidly digesting compared to coconut oil. However, this oil has been voided of much of its antimicrobial benefit.

C8 MCT OIL

As it sounds, C8 MCT oil has had C_{10} stripped away resulting in pure C8. C8 has been shown to be superior for inducing ketone production likely due to its even shorter carbon chain length.[67]

C6 MCT OIL

As it sounds, this is just C6. This product is not as common and surprisingly has not demonstrated the ability to stimulate greater ketone production compared to C8.

MCT OIL POWDER

Made by spray drying MCTs and combining with a carrier to turn into a powder form. MCT powders are typically made up of mostly C_{10} and C8, similar to standard MCT oil; however,

---

67 Camille Vandenberghe, Valérie St-Pierre, Tyler Pierotti, Mélanie Fortier, Christian-Alexandre Castellano, and Stephen C. Cunnane, "Tricaprylin Alone Increases Plasma Ketone Response More than Coconut Oil or Other Medium-Chain Triglycerides: An Acute Crossover Study in Healthy Adults," *Current Developments in Nutrition* 1, no. 4. (2017): e000257.

with a lesser amount of MCTs per serving size due to the addition of the carrier. Typically, the carriers used for MCT oil powder are fibers, or in some cases maltodextrin, which is why reading the ingredient label is incredibly important when considering an MCT oil powder. When considering MCT oil powder, look for products using beneficial fiber sources like acacia fiber. MCT oil powder tends to be a little easier on the stomach compared to MCT oil.

DIFFERENCES BETWEEN
MCT & COCONUT OIL

MEDIUM CHAIN TRIGLYCERIDES (MCTS)
- Various benefits for healthy and clinical populations
- Four main types: C6, C8, C10, an C12
- Two most common sources: **Coconut Oil** and **MCT Oil**

COCONUT OIL
- Contains **all four types** of MCTs
- Mainly C12 with small amounts of C6, C8, and C10
- Demonstrated to have greater anti-microbial effects

MCT OIL
- Contains only C8 and C10
- **Digests faster** compared to coconut oil
- Increases **energy levels** and **ketone production**

⚡ ARE MCTS SAFE?

MCTs are safe and have been researched in all age populations.[68] [69] Even high consumption of MCTs has been found to be safe; however, this is typically met with some side effects. The side effects of MCTs are well reported and commonly experienced if taken in high amounts without assessing tolerance. The rapid digestibility of MCTs can be troubling on the stomach. It is not uncommon to experience nausea, stomach pain, or diarrhea from ingesting more MCTs than your body can tolerate. Tolerance for MCTs can be acquired over time.

Someone who has never taken MCTs will have an especially low tolerance. For these individuals, starting with ¼ to ½ servings of MCTs is *crucial*. As someone gets used to taking MCTs, they will be able to better tolerate them in greater amounts without the risk of gastrointestinal distress. Additionally, the use of MCT oil powder may be a great place for beginners to start since it is less likely to contribute to gastrointestinal distress.

68 Candida J. Rebello, Jeffrey N. Keller, Ann G. Liu, William D. Johnson, and Frank L. Greenway. "Pilot Feasibility And Safety Study Examining the Effect of Medium Chain Triglyceride Supplementation in Subjects with Mild Cognitive Impairment: A Randomized Controlled Trial," *BBA Clinical* 3. (2015): 123-125.

69 Danielle AJE Lambrechts, Reina JA de Kinderen, Hans SH Vles, Anton J. de Louw, Albert P. Aldenkamp, and Marian JM Majoie, "The MCT-Ketogenic Diet as a Treatment Option in Refractory Childhood Epilepsy: A Prospective Study With 2-Year Follow-up," *Epilepsy & Behavior* 51. (2015): 261-266.

❓ HOW SHOULD I USE MCTS?

You have probably heard of people putting coconut or MCT oil in their coffee. This use is what has made MCT and coconut oil so popular. While this is a great way to add energy and satiety through your morning cup of joe, there are numerous other ways MCTs can be used.

MCTs can be used in low-carb recipes, especially shakes and smoothies. This is where MCT oil powder is commonly used and is especially beneficial due to the more recent production of flavored MCT powders. Liquid MCT oil also can make a great base for a keto salad dressing.

Coconut oil is a great cooking oil, since it can be heated to a higher temperature without oxidizing compared to other common cooking oils. Coconut oil is also used on hair and skin due to its antimicrobial benefits.

There is no right or wrong way to use MCTs. It is more important to make sure you are getting some in, even if that just means consuming pure oil—but this approach would be a lot less palatable.

RECOMMENDATIONS FOR MCTS

- Use both whole food and supplements
- Start with ¼-½ serving of MCT oil and powder and increase as tolerated
- Work your way up to 1-2 servings of MCTs per day
- Stick with powder if you are experiencing GI distress
- Use MCT powder in baking, smoothies, shakes, and coffee
- Use MCT oil as a salad dressing or in beverages (note: it's an oil so it will not mix well)

GREENS SUPPLEMENT

? WHAT IS A GREENS SUPPLEMENT?

A greens supplement is a powdered extract product that contains fruits, vegetables, and in some cases algae and grasses. These supplements allow you to acquire the micronutrients and phytonutrients found in these foods without the associated carbohydrate load.

These supplements are particularly beneficial due to their diversity; some products contain nutrients from over thirty plants, something that would be difficult to achieve on any diet, especially a keto diet.

? ARE GREENS SUPPLEMENTS NECESSARY?

The diversity that you can get from a greens supplement would be hard to achieve through food alone, making greens supplements a good option. Furthermore, since fruit contains so much sugar, greens supplements are a way to get the micronutrients from fruit without all the sugar. Finally, not everyone likes the taste of plants, especially algae and grasses. A flavored greens powder can help these people get these micronutrients a little more easily and without having to deal with the taste of these foods.

The real question is how much does your body need the micronutrients that you are getting from these products? Since meat contains many of the micronutrients that can be found in plants but in a much more bioavailable form, you may question the necessity for a greens supplement if you are consuming a diet rich in high-quality animal protein and organ meat. However, certain phytonutrients can be found in much greater form in a greens supplement than they could in any whole food version.

We like to think of greens supplements as a multivitamin that can fill in any gaps that may be left in your well-rounded, whole food, high-quality keto diet.

WHAT DO I LOOK FOR IN A GREENS SUPPLEMENT?

Seek one that has many colorful plants and not just one or two different greens. When your body gets hit with all of this nutrition at once, it is hard to absorb it all without some help, so the product should also have some fat and digestive enzymes.

Be careful with the greens you choose if you want to stay in a ketogenic state. Some supplements will add juices or other sugary ingredients to help sweeten the product. Look for a product that does not contain additives, fillers, or cornstarch. Stick to supplements made from whole raw plants. Our company has created a powder that has MCT oil powder added to it and is devoid of sugars, so you stay in ketosis while getting all the micro-nutrition you need. This is not a sales pitch for these products. We make products because we feel like there are no reasonable alternatives.

HOW SHOULD I USE GREENS POWDERS?

Specific nutrient timing for greens powders has not been established in the research so just getting them in over the course of your day is recommended. Taking greens is particularly beneficial during times when your diet lacks diversity or you are consuming lower quality foods, such as while on the road.

> ## RECOMMENDATIONS FOR GREENS
>
> - Choose a product with compounds from a variety of foods
> - Choose a product low in sugar
> - Choose a product containing fat and digestive enzymes
> - Use when your diet is lacking diversity and quality

OMEGA-3 FATS

? WHAT ARE OMEGA-3 FATS?

As you know by now, the fat you eat can play a pretty intricate role in the function of your body. There are different types of fats, and each of them can impact the body differently. Many of the healthy fats, including omega-3 fats, play a big role in cellular function.

Omega-3 fats are polyunsaturated fats found in a variety of foods, such as fish, high-quality meat, and certain nuts and seeds. The three-primary omega-3 fatty acids are alpha-linolenic acid (ALA), eicosapentaenoic acid (EPA), and docosahexaenoic acid (DHA). ALA is the primary omega-3 found in plant sources, while EPA and DHA are the primary omega-3 fats found in seafood.

ALA is an essential fatty acid, meaning your body can't produce it, that is found in certain nuts and seeds like walnuts, flax seeds, and chia seed. The majority of the benefit from ALA is in its conversion to EPA and DHA; however, it can only be converted in relatively small amounts, in fact, when you take a look at several studies you will only find a conversion of between 0-7 percent.

Omega-3 fats can be consumed in whole food version from foods like fish, high-quality meat, and certain nuts and seeds, or can be consumed in supplemental form, the most popular supplement being fish oil.

? WHY ARE OMEGA-3S IMPORTANT?

Omega-3 fats play an important role in cell membranes, which are responsible for protecting the cells in our body. They also play a big role in the heart, blood vessels, lungs, immune system, and endocrine systems. Studies have also shown that EPA and DHA play a big role in fetal development[70] and reduced risk of Alzheimer's disease.[71]

Getting enough omega-3s in the diet is important because the standard American diet is high in omega-6 fats and low in omega-3 fats, causing an imbalance in our omega-6 to omega-3 fat ratio. An improper ratio can promote inflammation, and inadequate omega-3 fat consumption has been associated with poor heart health, brain health, impaired sleep, and poor skin health.

The omega-3 index is a measure used to help determine the amount of EPA+DHA found in membranes of red blood cells and has been inversely related to risk of coronary heart disease. An omega-3 index of less than 4 percent is considered a high risk, 4-8 percent is moderate risk, and more than 8 percent

70 Sheila M. Innis, "Fatty Acids and Early Human Development," *Early Human Development* 83, no. 12. (2007): 761-766.

71 Martha Clare Morris, Denis A. Evans, Julia L. Bienias, Christine C. Tangney, David A. Bennett, Robert S. Wilson, Neelum Aggarwal, and Julie Schneider, "Consumption of Fish and n-3 Fatty Acids and Risk of Incident Alzheimer Disease," *Archives of Neurology* 60, no. 7. (2003): 940-946.

is low risk. The omega-3 index is also used to measure the absorption rate of omega-3 fats.

A high omega-6 to omega-3 fat ratio can be a big indicator of poor health. As food manufacturing has evolved, we have seen a dramatic increase in consumption of omega-6 fats, especially compared to omega-3 fats. Lower meat quality has further contributed to an increase in omega-6 and decreases in omega-3 fats in our meat. This, along with the widespread overconsumption of vegetable oils, heightens the need for food quality and omega-3 supplementation in the general population, as well as the ketogenic dieters who may consume a high amount of lower quality meat.

Since not everyone likes fish or has access to high-quality seafood sources, omega-3 supplementation is likely required for most people. That's why supplements like fish oil are among the most popular and widely used nutritional supplements.

? WHAT IS THE BEST OMEGA-3 SUPPLEMENT?

There is a bit of debate behind what is the best omega-3 supplement. To start, we can remove ALA supplementation from the conversation since on a very small portion of it is actually converted to EPA and DHA to be used by the body. Traditional fish oil contains more EPA+DHA per serving compared to other popular omega-3 sources like krill oil. However, it has been proposed that the omega-3 fats in krill oil are more bioavailable (better absorbed by the body), meaning you may be able to get the same or more benefit while consuming less. Research has demonstrated mixed results in this regard, likely due to lack of consistency in total EPA+DHA amount, source of supplementation, the possibility that bioavailability is individualized, and bioavailability may change at different doses.

Regardless, we recommend using krill oil as a source of omega-3 for a variety of reasons. First, krill is lower on the food chain, meaning that the fats are of higher quality, contain fewer contaminants, and have less chance of heavy metal toxicity. Second, krill also has natural antioxidants you get as a bonus, such as astaxanthin, which protects the structure of omega-3 and gives you some extra health benefits, which we will discuss more in a bit. Third, catching and farming krill is a much more sustainable process that is far less destructive to the ecosystem of the ocean compared to farming practices used to acquire traditional fish oil

Krill are small shrimp-like crustaceans that are the preferred meal of a lot of marine animals, especially whales. The Antarctic krill or *Euphausia superba* are most commonly used in krill supplements because of abundant supply. Krill oil is extracted through a cold vacuum process that protects the oil from degradation and helps maintain nutrient quality. This extraction process results in a concentrated phospholipid carrier of omega-3 fatty acids and the antioxidant astaxanthin. The phospholipid carrier of krill oil is what is thought to provide the increase in bioavailability, which has been demonstrated by several studies showing greater increases in the omega-3 index discussed earlier and greater decreases in omega-6:omega-3 fatty acid ratios.[72] The phospholipids found in krill oil can also provide additional health benefits independent of the omega-3 fats.

Krill oil often generates less gastrointestinal distress and "fishy" smelling burps than fish oil. Why is fish oil so popular then? Because fish oil is cheaper than krill oil.

---

72 M. Stine, Ulven and Kirsten B. Holven,"Comparison of Bioavailability of Krill Oil versus Fish Oil and Health Effect," *Vascular Health and Risk Management* 11 (2015): 511.

? WHAT ARE THE HEALTH BENEFITS OF OMEGA-3 SUPPLEMENTATION?

There are numerous health benefits associated with omega-3 fat supplementation. For this question, we will highlight both benefits of omega-3 supplementation and in some instances, krill oil specifically.

IMPROVED CARDIOVASCULAR HEALTH

It has been said that the therapeutic cardioprotective effect of omega-3 come at an effective dose of 1 gram of EPA+DHA and 2-4 grams for reductions in triglycerides. Several studies have also found the krill oil supplementation leads to an increase in HDL levels.[73]

REDUCING INFLAMMATION

Omega-3 fats possess a unique ability to combat inflammation in part due to their ability to balance the ratio of omega-3 to omega-6 fatty acids in the body.

Both omega-3 and omega-6 fats are substrates for the production of eicosanoids and share the same enzymes for the synthesis of prostaglandins and leukotrienes, which both play a role in the immune and inflammatory responses of the body. However, it is thought that omega-3 fatty acids produce compounds that are more anti-inflammatory than those produced by omega-6 fats, which tend to be more pro-inflammatory. This demonstrates a need to maintain a proper omega-6 to omega-3 fatty acid ratio.

---

73 Yoshio Suzuki, Minoru Fukushima, Keishoku Sakuraba, Keisuke Sawaki, and Kazuaki Sekigawa, "Krill Oil Improves Mild Knee Joint Pain: A Randomized Control Trial," *PloS One* 11, no. 10. (2016): e0162769.

For krill oil, it isn't just the omega-3s that give it its anti-inflammatory benefits. Krill oil provides a three-factor approach to combating inflammation. Besides the EPA/DHA being able to trigger the release of anti-inflammatory molecules and increase the release of interleukin 6 (IL-6), resulting in a decrease in c-reactive protein (CRP) and tumor necrosis factor (TNF), both markers of inflammation; the phospholipids and astaxanthin in krill oil give it additional anti-inflammatory power. The phospholipids found in krill can also play a big role in protecting cell membranes. The astaxanthin, a potent antioxidant, can further inhibit the production of TNF.

While we are at it, let's take a deeper look at Astaxanthin:

- Carotenoid commonly found in algae and some seafood (like krill)
- Powerful antioxidant functioning to reduce oxidative stress
- Has been shown to improve blood flow
- Limited evidence suggesting it may improve fatty acid oxidation and exercise performance.

One study found that four weeks of 500 mg of krill oil twice per day led to significant reductions in CRP, a common marker of inflammation.[74] Another study in patients with either cardiovascular disease (CVD), rheumatoid arthritis, osteoarthritis, or those suffering from high levels of CRP, found that after just

---

74 Arrigo FG Cicero, Martina Rosticci, Martino Morbini, Marcella Cagnati, Elisa Grandi, Angelo Parini, and Claudio Borghi, "Lipid-Lowering and Anti-Inflammatory Effects of Omega 3 Ethyl Esters and Krill Oil: A Randomized, Cross-Over, Clinical Trial," *Archives of Medical Science: AMS* 12, no. 3 (2016): 507.

seven days of 300 mg of krill oil reduced CRP by 19.3 percent compared to a 15.7 percent increase in the placebo.[74] The ability of krill oil to combat inflammation gives it the potential to contribute to improvements in symptoms of many chronic diseases, including those related to joint pain.

REDUCED JOINT PAIN

Joint pain is something we commonly see in aging populations as well as those suffering from conditions like rheumatoid arthritis. The joints of those suffering from arthritis demonstrate greater CRP production, which results in the release of pro-inflammatory cytokines (like IL-1 and IL-6), as well as tumor necrosis factor-alpha (TNF-a), which combined can contribute to the degradation of cartilage and stimulate joint pain.

There have been a few studies looking at the use of krill oil for improving joint pain, including a 30-day study that reported 2 grams of krill oil daily led to improvements in reported joint pain and stiffness.[75] There has been additional animal research further demonstrating improvements in arthritis scores in rats.

Improved heart health and reduced inflammation are the two most commonly reported benefits from omega-3 fat consumption. Since inflammation can contribute to so many chronic diseases, we can assume that there are many other conditions in which omega-3 fats could provide benefit. A few benefits that have some limited scientific evidence are improved PMS symptoms, reduced blood sugar levels, improved ADHD symptoms, cancer treatment aid, improved mental health, reduced blood pressure, and lower stroke risk.

---

75 Yoshio Suzuki, Minoru Fukushima, Keishoku Sakuraba, Keisuke Sawaki, and Kazuaki Sekigawa, "Krill Oil Improves Mild Knee Joint Pain: A Randomized Control Trial," *PloS One* 11, no. 10 (2016): e0162769.

Interestingly, cell culture research has demonstrated that krill oil can improve the intestinal barrier integrity and epithelial restitution during inflammation as a result of bacterial (specifically E-coli) invasions.[76] Another of the many potential benefits of using krill oil.

? DO I HAVE TO USE OMEGA-3 SUPPLEMENTATION?

While omega-3 supplementation is very popular, it is possible to get a lot of omega-3s from your diet. The richest sources are:

- Mackerel
- Salmon
- Sardines
- Oysters
- Herring

- Walnuts
- Anchovies
- Flax Seeds
- Chia Seed
- Grass-fed/finished beef

Note: Non-animal sources of omega-3s contain ALA, which is not converted to EPA and DHA at a high rate.

Omega-3 supplementation may not be required for those consuming enough fish and high-quality meat; however, chances are even these individuals may have challenges meeting adequate omega-3 fat intake, which is why supplementation is recommended for most people.

---

76 Manuela Costanzo, Vincenzo Cesi, Enrica Prete, Anna Negroni, Francesca Palone, Salvatore Cucchiara, Salvatore Oliva, Beatrice Leter, and Laura Stronati, "Krill Oil Reduces Intestinal Inflammation by Improving Epithelial Integrity and Impairing Adherent-Invasive Escherichia Coli Pathogenicity," *Digestive and Liver Disease* 48, no. 1 (2016): 34-42.

HOW SHOULD I SUPPLEMENT WITH OMEGA-3?

When supplementing with omega-3 fats, stick to either fish or krill oil. We recommend krill oil for all of the additional benefits previously mentioned, as well as its superior bioavailability. To reduce the potential risk of GI distress, take krill oil with a meal.
Recommendations for omega-3:

- Eat fatty fish
- 1-3 grams of krill oil daily with a meal

VITAMIN D

WHAT IS VITAMIN D?

Vitamin D is a critical micronutrient that can be made in our bodies from exposure to sunlight or it can be acquired through foods like liver, egg yolks, dairy, and fatty fish.

Most people think vitamin D does one thing—build bones. While it does play a big role in the absorption of calcium, it does much, much more. Vitamin D controls over a thousand processes in your body. When you are deficient, you end up with dysregulation of mineralization in your bones called rickets. When you're not at optimal levels, you miss out on many more benefits that could help you perform at a much higher level.

Vitamin D is hardly a vitamin. It acts like a hormone throughout the body on several important pathways. These include regulating immunity, decreasing Type II diabetes, decreasing cancer rates, decreasing dementia, increasing fertility and important sex hormones, improving gut function, and decreasing overall inflammation.

Vitamin D can also help prevent aging by reducing the shortening of telomeres.[77] Telomeres are the caps on the long strands of your DNA that essentially prevent aging. When measured, telomeres are a direct sign of cell aging. The shorter your telomeres, the older your cellular age. Safe to say, vitamin D is important!

? WHY DO I NEED TO SUPPLEMENT WITH VITAMIN D?

Over 75 percent of Americans are deficient in vitamin D.[78] This figure would be much higher if accounting for those who are not technically deficient but are still not at an optimal level. Being deficient in vitamin D can come with side effects, such as fatigue, depression, muscle pain, hair loss, and impaired hormone production.

Vitamin D deficiency is actually the primary contributor to season affective disorder, which is characterized by depression during months when exposure to sun is limited. This means that those living in states where getting outside in the winter months is difficult, the need for vitamin D supplementation is increased.

If you're a typical American who sits inside most of the day, then goes home after work and sits inside until the sun sets, you should probably supplement. Furthermore, if you're an athlete looking to make full use of recovery and reduction of inflammation, then you should supplement.

---

77 Ligi Paul, "Diet, Nutrition and Telomere Length," *The Journal of Nutritional Biochemistry* 22, no. 10 (2011): 895-901.

78 Kimberly YZ Forrest and Wendy L. Stuhldreher, "Prevalence and Correlates of Vitamin D Deficiency in US Adults," *Nutrition Research* 31, no. 1 (2011): 48-54.

If you live in an area where you can get frequent, prolonged exposure to sun *and* you take advantage of it, then supplementing with vitamin D may not be required as long as symptoms of deficiency are not occurring. The easiest way to figure out if you should be supplementing—get blood work done. Test, don't guess.

❓ HOW SHOULD I SUPPLEMENT WITH VITAMIN D?

There are many types of vitamin D you can take, and we can bore you with the chemical compounds all day, or I can just say "D3." Vitamin D3 is the form that converts the best in the body and is the one you should supplement with. Supplementation recommendations are between 400-800 IU/ day, but these recommendations are far too low. In the United States, the safer upper limit is 4,000 IU/day, but research has found that up to 10,000 IU/day is safe. If you have more fat mass, take a little more. But again, testing is important. The recommended vitamin D levels are between 40-100 ng/mL so supplementation should occur until this level is reached.

Since vitamin D is a fat-soluble vitamin, when supplementing with vitamin D, be sure to add fat. Without fat, the bioavailability is decreased, rendering the supplement useless to your body. This also means if you are overweight, you will need a higher dose than those who don't carry as much body fat.[79] The fat-soluble vitamin can concentrate in your adipose tissue and

---

79 John Paul Ekwaru, Jennifer D. Zwicker, Michael F. Holick, Edward Giovannucci, and Paul J. Veugelers, "The Importance of Body Weight for the Dose Response Relationship of Oral Vitamin D Supplementation and Serum 25-Hydroxyvitamin D in Healthy Volunteers," *PloS One* 9, no. 11 (2014): e111265.

never get to the target organs and glandular tissues to make positive changes in your body. This also means if you are losing fat and you've taken a lot of vitamin D, you probably don't need to take much more.

Pay attention when considering vitamin D supplements; many contain added vegetable oils as a fat source, these should be avoided.

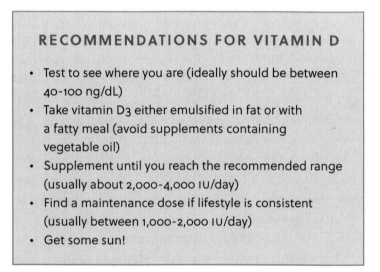

RECOMMENDATIONS FOR VITAMIN D

- Test to see where you are (ideally should be between 40-100 ng/dL)
- Take vitamin D3 either emulsified in fat or with a fatty meal (avoid supplements containing vegetable oil)
- Supplement until you reach the recommended range (usually about 2,000-4,000 IU/day)
- Find a maintenance dose if lifestyle is consistent (usually between 1,000-2,000 IU/day)
- Get some sun!

VITAMIN K

? WHAT IS VITAMIN K?

Vitamin K is under-consumed in our culture and often under-appreciated. Vitamin K was first determined to be an essential nutrient because of its ability to activate proteins important for blood clotting. There are two forms of vitamin K:

- K1 or phylloquinone, which is found in plant foods

- K2 or menaquinone, which is found in animal and fermented foods. K2 can further be classified as MK-4 and MK-7

Vitamin K also plays a critical role in promoting bone calcification and preventing the calcification of blood vessels. This means that vitamin K plays a major role in the health of your cardiovascular system.

The health benefits seem to come more from K2 than K1. Vitamin K1 is consumed in much greater amounts than vitamin K2, which may increase the need to focus on vitamin K2 supplementation. While some of K1 can be converted to K2, this process is rather inefficient. Bacteria in our gut may also be able to contribute to natural K2 production; however, it is unlikely that this is enough to get adequate K2 in the body, thus again increasing the need for vitamin K2 supplementation.

Dairy, organ meat, and egg yolks from high-quality animal sources are one way to increase your vitamin K2 supplementation. These foods will increase one of the subtypes of K2, while fermented foods like sauerkraut can help increase the other.

These foods may not supply sufficient vitamin K2. Additionally, vitamin K is a fat-soluble vitamin, so it is better absorbed when consumed with fat. If you are consuming leaner animal products, chances are you are not getting enough vitamin K in. Regardless, there appears to be a need for vitamin K2 supplementation

WHAT ARE THE BENEFITS OF VITAMIN K2 SUPPLEMENTATION?

While K1 can be converted to K2, studies using vitamin K1 typically do not demonstrate as much benefit as studies using

K2. There has been a significant amount of research around vitamin K2 and its ability to improve bone health and reduce the risk of heart disease, likely a result of the vitamin's impact on calcium deposition.[80]

There is also some research suggesting that K2 could improve kidney health by preventing calcium deposition and thus preventing kidney stones. Studies also have shown that subjects on dialysis, who supplement with K2, require less dialysis.[81]

Vitamin K is also found in the brain, primarily K2. It is thought that vitamin K2 interacts with sulfatides, a compound that has been shown to be deficient in patients with neurodegenerative diseases.

Limited research has shown that K2 may be able to strengthen the body's ability to fight cancer, but more research is needed to determine the validity in this claim.[82]

K2 may be able to improve insulin sensitivity, since vitamin K can cause bone reabsorption of calcium. This results in a release of osteocalcin, which can act on tissues to improve insulin sensitivity and lower blood glucose.[83] Again, preliminary research has only shown this in K2.

80 Katarzyna Maresz, "Proper Calcium Use: Vitamin K2 as a Promoter of Bone and Cardiovascular Health," *Integrative Medicine: A Clinician's Journal* 14, no. 1 (2015): 34.

81 Rogier Caluwé, Stefaan Vandecasteele, Bruno Van Vlem, Cees Vermeer, and An S. De Vriese, "Vitamin K2 Supplementation in Haemodialysis Patients: A Randomized Dose-Finding Study," *Nephrology Dialysis Transplantation* 29, no. 7 (2013): 1385-1390.

82 Kazuya Matsumoto, Jun-Ichi Okano, Takakazu Nagahara, and Yoshikazu Murawaki, "Apoptosis of Liver Cancer Cells by Vitamin K2 and Enhancement by MEK Inhibition," *International Journal of Oncology* 29, no. 6 (2006): 1501-1508.

83 Sarah L. Booth, Kerry E. Broe, David R. Gagnon, Katherine L. Tucker, Marian T. Hannan, Robert R. McLean, Bess Dawson-...

Vitamin K2 also plays a role in the function of other vitamins and minerals. For example, vitamins A and D both are activated by vitamin K2, allowing them to insert their function into our physiology.

Supplementation is a complex system with each ingredient impacting another. For example, vitamin K2 can play a role in the activation of vitamins A and D, which are crucial for things like gene expression. However, magnesium also plays a role in gene expression, so deficiency in this would prevent these vitamins from completing their action. This is why supplementation should be considered as a whole system and not just individual ingredients.

? HOW SHOULD I SUPPLEMENT WITH VITAMIN K2?

Much of the evidence behind the benefits of supplementing with vitamin K2 is preliminary, but since many people are deficient, it appears to be a good idea.

You can get vitamin K2 through food sources, but if those food sources are not high-quality, grass-fed animals, you will not be getting an adequate amount of vitamin K2. Furthermore, since vitamin K is fat-soluble, if you are consuming leaner cuts of meat, your need for supplementation increases.

The recommended daily intake of vitamin K is dependent on many factors, including age and gender, but 90-120 micrograms is the current recommendation. This level is

...Hughes, Peter WF Wilson, L. Adrienne Cupples, and Douglas P. Kiel, "Vitamin K Intake and Bone Mineral Density in Women and Men," *The American Journal of Clinical Nutrition* 77, no. 2 (2003): 512-516.

likely insufficient to generate improvements in heart and bone health, probably because of the inefficient conversion of K1 to K2. For this reason, K2 supplementation should be considered but the dose depends on the type of supplement used. If you do supplement with vitamin K2, be sure to consume it with fat to improve absorption.

RECOMMENDATIONS FOR VITAMIN K

- Consume high-quality meat to get vitamin K
- Supplement with vitamin K2 to increase levels
- Consume with fat to increase absorption
- Minimum effective dose for K2 MK4 is 1,500 mcg but doses up to 45,000 mcg have demonstrated being safe[84]
- Minimum effective dose for K2 MK-7 is between 90-360 mcg but more research is still needed[84]

PROTEIN POWDERS

? WHY IS PROTEIN IMPORTANT?

Proteins, or amino acids, are building blocks used by the body in many different ways, including the production and repair of muscle, tendons, skin, and organs. Amino acids also play a vital role in the production of hormones, neurotransmitters, enzymes, and other important molecules.

---

84 "Vitamin K: Proven Health Benefits, Dosage, and More," Examine. com, June 14, 2018. Accessed March 28, 2019. https://examine.com/ supplements/vitamin-k/#safety-and-toxicology_general.

There are 20 amino acids. Eleven of them are created by your body and referred to as non-essential amino acids. The other nine cannot be made by the body, meaning they must come from diet. These are referred to as essential amino acids (EAAs). If a protein source contains all 9 EAAs, it is said to be a complete protein source, which is what we should be looking for.

❓ WHY ARE PROTEIN POWDERS IMPORTANT ON KETO?

One of the primary benefits of protein powders is the convenient ability to increase total protein intake, and on a ketogenic diet low protein consumption is often a problem. Low protein consumption on keto is often a result of either fear of too much protein (leading to gluconeogenesis, which isn't a concern), or satiety leading to lower calorie intake and inherently lower protein intake.

Regardless of the reason, too low protein intake should be combatted against. Protein powders allow you to get in more protein and calories when you aren't hungry enough for a meal or if you live a life on the go.

❓ ARE PROTEIN POWDERS DANGEROUS?

Contrary to common belief, protein powders are not considered to be dangerous and are not harmful to your kidneys. Actually, we should take a step back and say that quality proteins in general are not dangerous. Certain low-quality protein powders, which many companies are putting out to cut costs, are either not beneficial or potentially harmful to your health. We discuss more about how to choose the best protein source in each individual protein type below.

The common misconception that protein powders can damage kidneys stems from the general irrational fear of high protein intake on kidney health. While high protein intake can increase pressure inside the kidneys, this does not mean that protein is dangerous. In fact, research has shown that in healthy people, high protein intake does not damage kidney health.[85] However, in individuals already suffering from kidney damage, the results are less clear. This does not mean that protein or protein powder should be avoided by these people, but it does mean that paying more attention to total protein intake may be important.

ⓘ ARE PROTEIN POWDERS OKAY ON KETO?

Also contrary to common belief, protein powders are okay on a keto diet. This fear stems from the fear of high protein consumption hindering ketosis due to gluconeogenesis. As we have discussed numerous times throughout this book, that is not a concern, besides maybe in some therapeutic uses of the ketogenic diet.

ⓘ WHAT ARE THE DIFFERENT PROTEIN POWDERS?

The most common are:

- Whey
- Casein
- Collagen
- Beef
- Egg
- Plant

---

85 Mackenzie Walser, "Effects of Protein Intake on Renal Function and on the Development of Renal Disease," *The Role of Protein and Amino Acids in Sustaining and Enhancing Performance* (1999): 137-154.

Since casein has not been shown to provide enough benefit to outweigh common sensitivities to it and we do not recommend plant protein, in this chapter we focus on whey and collagen protein.

WHEY PROTEIN

? WHAT IS WHEY PROTEIN POWDER?

Whey is one of the two primary proteins found in dairy, with the other being casein (casein: 80 percent, whey: 20 percent). Whey protein powders are made when dairy is coagulated, allowing for the separation of liquid (the whey) and solid (the casein). The liquid is spray dried to turn it into a powder and can go through various filtration techniques to get different types of whey protein, such as whey protein concentrate or whey protein isolate.

Whey protein contains all nine essential amino acids, making it a complete protein source, and is one of the most researched supplements on the market. Whey is also rich in the proteins lactoferrin, beta-lactoglobulin, alpha-lactalbumin, and immunoglobulins, all of which are antibacterial, antiviral, and antifungal, and can help reduce inflammation and improve immune function.

? IS WHEY PROTEIN DAIRY?

Yes, which is why some people with dairy intolerances may need to avoid whey proteins. However, whey protein does not contain casein, one of the two compounds found in dairy that is typically responsible for dairy intolerances. While many people have a hard time digesting lactose, a sugar contained in dairy and whey, many individuals with dairy intolerances mistake lactose as the source of their intolerance when the problem may be casein.

Regardless, many people do have difficulties digesting lactose and may need to avoid whey. However, there are several different types of whey protein containing varying amounts of lactose which may be better tolerated by some.

? WHAT ARE THE DIFFERENT TYPES OF WHEY PROTEIN?

The difference between the various types of whey protein is in the processing and filtration techniques taken after the whey is separated from casein. The three primary forms of whey protein are:

- **Concentrate:** Contains some carbs and fat. Higher in lactose
- **Isolate:** Contains more protein, less carbs and fat. Zero or close to zero lactose
- **Hydrolysate:** Pre-digested, allowing it to absorb faster, but has been shown to cause a greater spike in insulin (not preferred on keto)

If you are concerned with your ability to handle dairy, whey protein isolate may be the preferred protein powder for you, but as always you should still assess your tolerance and note that this form of protein will be stripped of much of its nutrients leaving primarily just protein behind.

❓ WHAT ARE THE BENEFITS OF WHEY PROTEIN?

While whey protein is most often touted for its muscle building capabilities, which we will still discuss, the benefits extend much further:

RAPID ABSORPTION

Whey protein is one of the fastest digesting proteins you can consume. Typically, there will be a significant rise in amino acid availability in the blood less than an hour after consumption. This rapid absorption can be good for quickly providing nutrients during times of nutrient need, such as before and/or after a workout.

MUSCLE GROWTH

Whey protein is loaded with branched-chain amino acids (BCAAs), a special group of EAAs that help regulate muscle repair and growth. One of the primary BCAAs is leucine, which is most often studied for its ability to stimulate muscle protein synthesis (MPS), or the creation of muscle proteins used for repairing and growing muscle. Whey protein is high in leucine, making it one of the preferred protein sources for muscle building. Since your body is constantly breaking down muscle proteins, especially during exercise, stimulating MPS is important to help preserve and build more muscle mass. Since whey protein is so rapidly digested, it is the preferred post-workout protein source.[86] Interestingly, human breast milk is made up of 60

---

86   Jason E. Tang, Daniel R. Moore, Gregory W. Kujbida, Mark A. Tarnopolsky, and Stuart M. Phillips, "Ingestion of Whey Hydrolysate, Casein, or Soy Protein Isolate: Effects on Mixed Muscle Protein Synthesis at Rest and Following Resistance Exercise in Young Men," *Journal of Applied Physiology* (2009).

percent whey, compared to 20 percent in cows. This is thought to help contribute to the growth and development of babies.

MUSCLE MASS RETENTION

Due to its ability to stimulate MPS, whey protein can also aid in the retention of muscle mass, which is especially important in a calorie deficit, when the body may be more likely to break down muscle proteins for energy.

INCREASED STRENGTH

Studies have found that whey protein used in conjunction with weight training is effective for increasing muscular strength.[87] This could be due to increased muscle mass and the ability of protein to be used for the contractile units of our muscles.

LOSE BODY FAT

There have been many studies suggesting that whey protein may help contribute to fat loss. There are three primary mechanisms:

- **Boost energy expenditure:** Protein is one of the most metabolically active macronutrients, meaning that the body has to burn more calories to absorb and digest protein compared to carbs and fat.[88]

---

87 Robert W. Morton, Kevin T. Murphy, Sean R. McKellar, Brad J. Schoenfeld, Menno Henselmans, Eric Helms, Alan A. Aragon et al., "A Systematic Review, Meta-Analysis and Meta-Regression of the Effect of Protein Supplementation on Resistance Training-Induced Gains in Muscle Mass and Strength in Healthy Adults," *British Journal of Sports Medicine* 52, no. 6 (2018): 376-384.

88 Thomas L. Halton and Frank B. Hu, "The Effects of High Protein Diets on Thermogenesis, Satiety and Weight Loss: a Critical Review," *Journal of the American College of Nutrition* 23, no. 5 (2004): 373-385.

- Greater muscle mass contributes to greater energy expenditure at rest: The mechanisms behind this benefit are a result of protein consumption in general, not just whey protein.
- Increased Satiety: Compared to other macronutrients, protein has been shown to promote greater satiety or fullness and for a longer period of time. This increase in fullness can contribute to greater calorie restriction and thus more fat loss. If protein intake is already adequate, added protein may not contribute to improved satiety.

In addition to the above benefits there are several other possible benefits of whey protein that are not as well studied:

REDUCE INFLAMMATION

Research has shown that whey can lower CRP, a common inflammatory marker,[89] but this benefit may only occur in individuals with already elevated CRP.

INCREASE ANTIOXIDANT PRODUCTION

Cysteine, one of the primary EAAs found in whey protein, can boost glutathione production, one of our body's most potent antioxidants.[90] Lactoferrin, another protein found in whey,

---

89 Ling-Mei Zhou, Jia-Ying Xu, Chun-Ping Rao, Shufen Han, Zhongxiao Wan, and Li-Qiang Qin, "Effect Of Whey Supplementation on Circulating C-Reactive Protein: A Meta-Analysis of Randomized Controlled Trials." *Nutrients* 7, no. 2 (2015): 1131-1143.

90 Scot R. Kimball, and Leonard S. Jefferson, "Signaling Pathways and Molecular Mechanisms through which Branched-Chain Amino Acids Mediate Translational Control of Protein Synthesis," *The Journal of Nutrition* 136, no. 1 (2006): 227S-231S.

also functions as an antioxidant. However, note that whey protein isolates have likely had most if not all lactoferrin removed in the filtration process.

IMPROVE IMMUNE SYSTEM

The presence of the proteins lactoferrin, beta-lactoglobulin, alpha-lactalbumin, and immunoglobulins found in whey may contribute to a better functioning immune system. Again, whey protein isolates may not contain these added nutrients, due to ultra-filtration techniques. However, whey protein also contains a significant amount of glutamine, which can further improve immune health and the body's ability to handle metabolic stress.

? HOW DO I SUPPLEMENT WITH WHEY PROTEIN?

The research has produced very mixed results. As it relates to muscle building and muscle retention, it has often been recommended to consume whey protein immediately after a training session due to its rapid absorption and thus ability to quickly stimulate MPS. However, additional research suggests that the timing of protein intake in this sense may be dependent on training age[91] (how long someone has exercised for), with newbies not needing to emphasize timing as much as those with more resistance training experience.

Research looking at whey protein timing for satiety has found that total protein intake for the day plays a bigger role in

---

91   Brad Jon Schoenfeld, Alan Albert Aragon, and James W. Krieger, "The Effect of Protein Timing on Muscle Strength and Hypertrophy: A Meta-Analysis," *Journal of the International Society of Sports Nutrition* 10, no. 1 (2013): 53.

perceived hunger than frequency of protein consumption.[92] In other words, consuming between your meals may not reduce hunger unless you were previously under-consuming protein, a common problem on a keto diet.

As a general rule of thumb, the best time to take whey protein is before or after a training session to allow for fuel for exercise as well as recovery through muscle repair and growth. In addition to exercise, consuming whey protein at any time to ensure adequate protein intake is logical.

On a keto diet, whey protein can be added to water, almond, or coconut milk. One of our favorite additions to a whey protein shake is a half avocado to add in some additional nutrients, calories, and provide a rich, creamy texture!

RECOMMENDATIONS FOR WHEY PROTEIN

- Consume 15-25 grams of whey protein per serving
- If lactose intolerant, experiment with whey protein isolate and assess tolerance
- Add before and/or after exercise for best results
- To add protein and calories to your diet, add an extra whey protein shake at any time of the day

---

92 Marta Lonnie, Emma Hooker, Jeffrey Brunstrom, Bernard Corfe, Mark Green, Anthony Watson, Elizabeth Williams, Emma Stevenson, Simon Penson, and Alexandra Johnstone, "Protein for Life: Review of Optimal Protein Intake, Sustainable Dietary Sources and the Effect on Appetite in Ageing Adults," *Nutrients* 10, no. 3 (2018): 360.

COLLAGEN

? WHAT IS COLLAGEN PROTEIN?

While many people recognize the importance of consuming enough protein, many of us are severely deficient in collagen, an extracellular protein that accounts for 25-30 percent of the total protein content in the body. It is the most abundant protein in the human body and the major protein involved in connective tissue, skin, tendons, and ligaments! Collagen helps your bones develop and provides your skin with structure.

One of the distinguishing characteristics of collagen is that its amino acids are wound up in triple-helices. Collagen is mainly found in fibrous tissues, including tendons, ligaments and the skin (hence why it is often referred to as the glue of the human body).

At the cellular level, fibroblasts, which are cells located in our connective tissue, create collagen. While there have been over 27 different types of collagen identified, 90 percent have been identified as Type I. Each type of collagen differs slightly in its structure and function:[93]

- **Type I:** Present in tendons, skin, bones and connective tissue
- **Type II:** Mainly present in cartilage
- **Type III:** Typically found in organs, arteries, and muscles
- **Type IV:** Found in the basal lamina, supports skin's cells
- **Type V:** Mainly found in cell surfaces and hair

---

93   Edward J. Miller, and R. Kent Rhodes, "[2] Preparation and Characterization of the Different Types of Collagen," In *Methods in Enzymology*, vol. 82 (1982): 33-64. Academic Press.

While it is apparent that collagen plays a pretty intricate role in so many different bodily processes, the problem is that our bodies slow natural collagen production as we age. This increases the need for collagen in our diets, especially as we age. Transitioning from a culture that routinely ate all parts of the animal to one that eats primarily muscle meat has skewed our collagen intake. There are foods like bone broth (which you can make at home or use a supplement like Kettle & Fire) that are rich in collagen, and if you buy high-quality animals, eating the skin, cartilage, and joint surfaces can further increase your collagen consumption. Furthermore, other foods, such as salmon and leafy green vegetables, can slow the breakdown of collagen.

Regardless, since collagen production slows as we age and getting enough via a whole food diet can be challenging, the need for supplementation increases. Collagen supplements easily dissolve in liquid and, if they are high quality, add no taste. You can effortlessly boost your collagen intake if you don't plan on eating an animal nose to tail or don't have access to the whole animal.

? WHAT ARE THE BENEFITS OF COLLAGEN SUPPLEMENTATION?

Short Answer: Collagen supplementation can improve bone, joint, gut, hair, nail, and skin health.

When taken orally, collagen appears to elicit a variety of effects. For starters, collagen has been shown to increase chondrocytes, which maintain the cartilaginous matrix and is important for maintaining connective tissue health. Supplementing with 10 grams of collagen has repeatedly been shown to decrease pain and increase range of motion in patients with osteoarthritis and osteoporosis.[94] Supplemental collagen is truly strengthening the bone at the source.

Another use of collagen supplementation is for skin health, since its peptides have been shown to accumulate in the skin and demonstrate potent antioxidant effects. Additionally, animal data has demonstrated that collagen peptides increase the migration and growth of fibroblasts located in the skin. Human trials demonstrate that collagen peptides increase skin plasticity and reduce wrinkle formation![95]

Collagen also has a fascinating ability to improve gut health. Recently, there has been an increasing interest in how gut health affects the whole body and not just digestion. Furthermore, one of the key components of a healthy gut is a strong intestinal barrier. This barrier is often referred to as the intestinal epithelium, responsible for effective nutrient absorption and protection from bile and other digestive enzymes. A compromised intestinal barrier, sometimes referred to as "leaky gut," may result in infection, inflammation, food allergy, irritable bowel syndrome, celiac disease, mental and neurological impairments, and even Type I diabetes.

The intestinal barrier is guarded by intercellular tight junctions. A variety of factors, including stress, can comprise

---

94 Alexander G. Schauss, Jerome Stenehjem, Joosang Park, John R. Endres, and Amy Clewell, "Effect of The Novel Low Molecular Weight Hydrolyzed Chicken Sternal Cartilage Extract Biocell Collagen, on Improving Osteoarthritis-Related Symptoms: A Randomized, Double-Blind, Placebo-Controlled Trial," *Journal of Agricultural and Food Chemistry* 60, no. 16 (2012): 4096-4101.

95 E. Proksch, D. Segger, J. Degwert, M. Schunck, V. Zague, and S. Oesser, "Oral Supplementation of Specific Collagen Peptides has Beneficial Effects on Human Skin Physiology: A Double-Blind, Placebo-Controlled Study," *Skin Pharmacology and Physiology* 27, no. 1 (2014): 47-55.

these junctions. Research has shown that collagen peptides can reinforce and repair a compromised intestinal barrier through modulating intestinal immune reactions![96] Other areas of interest include collagen's ability to improve nail and hair health. Brittle nail syndrome is a disorder characterized by fragile nail plates. Patients often complain that their nails are weak, soft, and dry. So far, most treatments have been deemed ineffective. Researchers began looking at collagen peptides once the literature surfaced on collagen's ability to stimulate dermal cellular metabolism. One study examined the effects of bioactive collagen peptide supplementation for four weeks on nail growth. The results demonstrated a 12 percent increase in growth rate and a 42 percent decrease in the frequency of broken nails.[97]

Studies on the effects of collagen supplementation on hair growth are preliminary.[98] However, they have discovered that a lack of collagen may result in hair thinning and hair loss, and that supplementing with additional collagen may offset these effects!

---

96 Qianru Chen, Bafang Li, Isabela Martin, Jeffrey B. Blumberg, and CY Oliver Chen, "Collagen Peptides Derived from Alaska Pollock Skin Protect against Tnfα-Induced Dysfunction of Tight Junctions in Caco-2 Cells." *The FASEB Journal* 30, no. 1_supplement (2016): 125.5.

97 Doris Hexsel, Vivian Zague, Michael Schunck, Carolina Siega, Fernanda O. Camozzato, and Steffen Oesser, "Oral Supplementation With Specific Bioactive Collagen Peptides Improves Nail Growth And Reduces Symptoms Of Brittle Nails," *Journal of Cosmetic Dermatology* 16, no. 4 (2017): 520-526.

98 Hiroyuki Matsumura, Yasuaki Mohri, Nguyen Thanh Binh, Hironobu Morinaga, Makoto Fukuda, Mayumi Ito, Sotaro Kurata, Jan Hoeijmakers, and Emi K. Nishimura, "Hair Follicle Aging is Driven by Transepidermal Elimination of Stem Cells via COL17A1 Proteolysis," *Science* 351, no. 6273 (2016): aad4395.

ⓘ DO I NEED TO TAKE COLLAGEN IF I AM TAKING OTHER FORMS OF PROTEIN?

Collagen's amino acid profile is unique compared to other popular proteins such as whey, casein, and soy. Collagen is composed of glycine, proline, hydroxyproline, and hydroxylysine, and lacks the common branched chain amino acids (BCAAs) such as leucine, isoleucine, and valine. Although BCAAs are typically regarded as the most effective for stimulating muscle protein synthesis, collagen's amino acid profile still packs some unique benefits.

In addition to all of the benefits previously listed, collagen's amino acid profile has demonstrated the ability to maintain a positive nitrogen balance in subjects following a low protein diet. Nitrogen balance is a good way to determine whether the individual is in a state of anabolism (building up) or catabolism (breaking down). If a positive nitrogen balance is identified then there is greater nitrogen intake than what is being excreted, indicating that there is a state of anabolism; the environment is optimal for muscle growth. On the contrary, if nitrogen loss is greater than intake, this is considered a catabolic state or a state of muscle loss. Research has not supported that collagen is superior for actual muscle gain, but these results do indicate that it can play a factor in muscle growth or the maintenance of muscle mass.

Additionally, collagen contains high amounts of arginine and glycine, which are important substrates for the synthesis of creatine in the human body. Creatine is regarded as one of the most popular and researched backed supplements and has been shown to increase power production, strength, and lean body mass. Recent research has shown creatine may have some neurological benefits as well and that collagen's amino acid profile may provide the building blocks to increase creatine production naturally.[99]

Regardless of the stance on muscle building, collagen's unique amino acid profile allows it to produce different effects in the body compared to other proteins, increasing the need for supplementation even if you are already supplementing with or consuming plenty of protein.

? HOW DO I SUPPLEMENT WITH COLLAGEN?

Collagen supplements can be either flavored or unflavored. If you are using an unflavored collagen supplement, you can add it to most drinks since it does not impact flavor. Flavored collagen powders can make for great shakes, can be added to coffee, and can even be used to cook with! Collagen can also be consumed alongside other protein sources due to its different amino acid profile.

There are no recommendations on the timing of collagen protein intake so simply getting collagen in your day is enough to experience the benefits.

RECOMMENDATIONS FOR COLLAGEN PROTEIN

- Consume 10-15 grams of collagen per day from food or supplements
- Look for collagen coming from grass-fed bovine
- Add to other protein sources for additional benefits

---

99 M. Flint Beal, "Neuroprotective Effects of Creatine," *Amino Acids* 40, no. 5 (2011): 1305-1313.

? HOW DO I CHOOSE THE BEST PROTEIN SOURCE?

The best protein source for you depends on your goal. If your primary goal is muscle building, then considering a supplement like whey protein may be a better approach. However, if you are looking at other aspects of your health like bone, skin, hair, nail, and gut health, supplementing with collagen is recommended. The point here is that you do not necessarily have to choose; each protein has its own purpose and place in your diet.

If you are looking to build muscle but are concerned with the lactose found in whey, you could also consider proteins like egg or beef protein each of which may provide a bit of their own added benefits. While some think protein sources like egg or beef may be better for preventing increases in blood sugar compared to whey, we have not found that in our personal research and self-experimentation.

Collagen	Whey
IMPROVES **GUT FUNCTION**	STIMULATES **MUSCLE GROWTH** AND RECOVERY
PROMOTES HEALTHY **SKIN, NAILS, AND HAIR**	FASTER **DIGESTING**
REDUCES JOINT PAIN/ IMPROVES **JOINT HEALTH**	INCREASES **STRENGTH**

INSULIN SENSITIZING AGENTS

? WHAT ARE INSULIN SENSITIZING AGENTS?

At this point you should understand the importance of keeping insulin and blood glucose low. While keto is great for keeping insulin and blood glucose low, several supplements can improve insulin sensitivity and also help you keep your blood glucose levels lower.

While prescription drugs such as metformin have displayed an incredible ability to lower blood sugar,[100] there are also natural, over-the-counter ingredients and formulated products that have shown pretty good evidence of producing similar effects on the body.

? WHAT ARE THE BENEFITS OF INSULIN SENSITIZING AGENTS?

The benefits of insulin sensitizing agents lie in their blood glucose lowering and subsequent insulin lowering effect. While we are still learning about these agents, some of them may be able to produce an effect in both the short term and the long term.

As we have discussed, the benefits of lowering blood sugar are widespread, from lowering HbA1c, a common marker of diabetes, to reducing inflammation and improving blood lipid profiles. Additionally, as it relates to keto, lower blood sugar is important for stimulating ketone production.

---

100 Michael Stumvoll, Nurjahan Nurjhan, Gabriele Perriello, George Dailey, and John E. Gerich, "Metabolic Effects of Metformin in Non-Insulin-Dependent Diabetes Mellitus," *New England Journal of Medicine* 333, no. 9 (1995): 550-554

? WHAT ARE THE BEST INSULIN SENSITIZING AGENTS?

Since we are fond of insulin sensitizing agents, Anthony formulated one for his company, Perfect Keto. While there are many ingredients out there that may be able to improve insulin sensitivity and lower blood glucose, our formulation, Keto Blood Sugar Support Capsules, contains the ingredients that we feel have the most potent ability to do so. Let's dive into each:

BIOTIN

Biotin is also commonly referred to as vitamin B-7. Like other B vitamins, Biotin plays a role in metabolism, especially helping metabolize carbohydrates.[101] Biotin can be found naturally in the body and is also present in common food sources such as eggs, almonds, cauliflower, and spinach. Biotin is water soluble and generally nontoxic, but it has been found to interact with some medications, specifically seizure medications.

CHROMIUM PICOLINATE

Chromium is a mineral found in the body that plays a role in helping insulin perform its actions. Chromium picolinate is absorbed better than traditional chromium and is thus used in most supplements. As you know, insulin plays an important role in shuttling blood sugar into the cells of the body. This function is compromised in people with diabetes. Several studies have demonstrated that chromium supplements can

---

101 J. P. Bonjour, "Biotin in Man's Nutrition andT--A Review," *International Journal for Vitamin and Nutrition Research. Internationale Zeitschrift fur Vitamin-und Ernahrungsforschung. Journal International de Vitaminologie et de Nutrition* 47, no. 2, (1977): 107-118.

improve blood sugar regulation for those with diabetes.[102] Most research uses 200 ug of chromium daily. Currently, there is no upper tolerable limit available for chromium. Chromium picolinate may negatively interact with beta blockers and NSAIDs.

GYMNEMA SYLVESTRE LEAF POWDER

Gymnema sylvestre is a forest shrub found in India, Africa, and Australia. The leaves have been used in ancient medical practice, as they have been suggested to inhibit sugar absorption and improve symptoms associated with diabetes. One of the main components in gymnema sylvestre leaf powder, gymnemic acid has been shown to block sugar receptors and suppress sweetness. Research has also shown that gymnema sylvestre leaf powder can block receptors in your intestines, lowering sugar absorption and post-prandial (following a meal) blood glucose levels.[103] While it is regarded as safe it probably should not be combined with other blood sugar lowering medications like metformin.

BITTER MELON EXTRACT (MOMORDICA CHARANTIA)

Bitter melon is a common supplement recommended for diabetics, as it has been shown to act in synergy with insulin bringing glucose into the cells. The magnitude of the effect of bitter melon extract is still up for debate, but several studies have found that bitter melon extract reduced glucose levels in

---

102 William T. Cefalu, and Frank B. Hu, "Role of Chromium in Human Health and in Diabetes," *Diabetes Care* 27, no. 11 (2004): 2741-2751.

103 Pragya Tiwari, Khurshid Ahmad, and Mohammad Hassan Baig, "Gymnema sylvestre for Diabetes: from Traditional Herb to Future's Therapeutic," *Current Pharmaceutical Design* 23, no. 11 (2017): 1667-1676.

Type II diabetics.[104] Consuming bitter melon extract in excess can result in several side effects.

CINNAMON EXTRACT

Cinnamon is a common spice made from the inner bark of a certain tree species. Cinnamon contains a large number of antioxidants such as polyphenols, which protect the body from free radicals. Cinnamon has been shown to reduce insulin resistance and lower blood sugar levels.[105] Cinnamon appears to interfere with digestive enzymes which break down carbohydrates in your digestive tract, thus preventing sharp increases in blood sugar following carbohydrate consumption. Typically, these effects are demonstrated when consumed at 1-6 grams per day. Ceylon cinnamon is often regarded as the best source of cinnamon. Cassia cinnamon contains a greater concentration of coumarin compared to Ceylon. Consuming too much coumarin may cause liver toxicity and increase risk of cancer.

BERBERINE BARK EXTRACT

Berberine is a bioactive compound extracted from a group of shrubs known as berberis and has been used in ancient Chinese medicine. Berberine acts as an alkaloid and is one of

---

104 Anjana Fuangchan, Paveena Sonthisombat, Tippawadee Seubnukarn, Rapeepan Chanouan, Pontap Chotchaisuwat, Viruch Sirigulsatien, Kornkanok Ingkaninan, Pinyupa Plianbangchang, and Stuart T. Haines, "Hypoglycemic Effect of Bitter Melon Compared with Metformin in Newly Diagnosed Type 2 Diabetes Patients," *Journal of Ethnopharmacology* 134, 2 (2011): 422-428.

105 Bolin Qin, Kiran S. Panickar, and Richard A. Anderson, "Cinnamon: Potential Role in the Prevention of Insulin Resistance, Metabolic Syndrome, and Type 2 Diabetes," *Journal of Diabetes Science and Technology* 4, no. 3 (2010): 685-693.

the only natural compounds demonstrated to be as effective as pharmaceutical drugs at lowering blood glucose. In fact, berberine has been shown to be equally as effective as metformin, which is the most commonly prescribed drug to reduce blood sugar levels.[106] Part of the reason why berberine is so effective is because it travels directly into cells and activates enzymes causing a downstream effect. One of the enzymes berberine activates is AMPK, which regulates metabolism. Berberine decreases insulin resistance by increasing the effectiveness of insulin. Additionally, berberine increases the breakdown of glucose as well as decreases sugar production in the liver.[107] Berberine appears to be tolerated very well with minimal side effects; however, if you're taking any current medications to lower blood sugar, consult with a physician.

BANABA LEAF EXTRACT (LAGERSTROEMIA SPECIOSA)

Banaba leaf extract is a tropical tree native to the Philippines that has been demonstrated to have some anti-diabetic effects. The extract contains three main components credited with these effects: corosolic acid, lagerstroemia, and gallotannins. Supplementing with banaba leaf extract has been demonstrated to decrease blood sugar levels by 13-30 percent when

106 Hui Dong, Nan Wang, Li Zhao, and Fuer Lu, "Berberine in The Treatment of Type 2 Diabetes Mellitus: A Systemic Review and Meta-Analysis," *Evidence-Based Complementary and Alternative Medicine* 2012 (2012).

107 Yun S. Lee, Woo S. Kim, Kang H. Kim, Myung J. Yoon, Hye J. Cho, Yun Shen, Ji-Ming Ye et al., "Berberine, a Natural Plant Product, Activates AMP-Activated Protein Kinase with Beneficial Metabolic Effects in Diabetic and Insulin-Resistant States," *Diabetes* 55, no. 8 (2006): 2256-2264.

supplementing at 100 mg for six months.[108] There have been several clinical trials investigating the effects of banaba leaf extract and no adverse effects have been noted. Additionally, some suggest that supplements like fenugreek and garlic may enhance the effects of banaba leaf extract. Most studies have used 30-50 mg of banaba extract daily.

There is still a lot more research that needs to be done on this class of supplements, but early evidence demonstrates that they could be something to be excited about and definitely something we should be continuing to study.

In addition to the ingredients listed above, there are other insulin sensitizing agents out there, such as moringa, which have demonstrated early evidence of efficacy but still require additional research and a greater understanding.

❓ HOW SHOULD I SUPPLEMENT WITH INSULIN SENSITIZING AGENTS?

It appears that some agents may be able to lower your blood glucose response to carbohydrate containing meals; however, it has not been established if the best time to take these products is before or after eating so we suggest consuming them with a meal.

Taking these supplements daily over time has been shown to improve blood sugar and insulin levels, meaning that simply getting these supplements in, regardless of timing, likely produces an effect.

---

108 Guy Klein, Jaekyung Kim, Klaus Himmeldirk, Yanyan Cao, and Xiaozhuo Chen, "Antidiabetes and Anti-Obesity Activity of Lagerstroemia speciosa," *Evidence-Based Complementary and Alternative Medicine* 4, no. 4 (2007): 401-407.

While it has not been tested, we believe that taking these supplements during initiation to a ketogenic diet may lead to an enhanced ability to keto-adapt. This is something we are definitely looking more into.

While these supplements can be used to manage the impact carbohydrates have on your body, we do not recommend using them as a crutch to do so, unless you have a strategic reason. If your fasted blood glucose is high while on a ketogenic diet, we recommend using insulin sensitizing agents to help improve this reading. If your blood glucose levels are already in a normal range, you may not require this supplement.

RECOMMENDATIONS FOR INSULIN SENSITIZING AGENTS

- Consume with a carb containing meal
- If not eating carbs, simply consume daily
- Look for supplements that contain a blend of ingredients that can work together
- Measure your blood sugar to ensure that these supplements are not causing your blood sugar to go too low

---

DIGESTIVE ENZYMES

WHAT ARE DIGESTIVE ENZYMES?

During digestion, our body secretes enzymes that are important for breaking down food and extracting nutrients. Normally, these enzymes are produced in response to food intake; however, as we age our body may lose its ability to produce a sufficient amount of digestive enzymes. This can lead to gastrointestinal distress, poor nutrient absorption, and potentially intolerances to those foods.

While impaired digestive enzyme function can be a result of age, it may actually be a result of prolonged poor diet. Thus, improving your diet is a great way to improve gut health, likely limit reductions in digestive enzyme production, and maybe even improve digestive enzyme production.

The most common types of digestive enzymes are:

- **Proteases:** breaks down protein
- **Amylases:** breaks down carbs
- **Lipases:** breaks down fat

These enzymes, among others, are produced in your intestines, but can also be acquired through certain foods. Keto-friendly foods containing digestive enzymes include avocados, ginger and fermented foods like kefir, sauerkraut, kimchi, and miso.

While getting these digestive enzymes in through your diet can help, some people may require the aid of digestive enzyme supplementation.

WHAT ARE THE BENEFITS OF SUPPLEMENTAL DIGESTIVE ENZYMES?

Better absorption of micronutrients is at the top of our list. Other benefits include lifestyle factors such as limiting gas, abdominal cramping, nausea, and loss of appetite. Additionally, your body does not make certain digestive enzymes like cellulase, the enzyme responsible for digesting fiber. This is why high fiber consumption can be associated with gastrointestinal pain; however, supplementing with digestive enzymes that contain cellulase may limit or avoid these symptoms. If you frequently feel bloated or have other digestive discomfort after a meal, chances are you are either intolerant to that food or you could use the support of a digestive enzyme.

? HOW DO I SUPPLEMENT WITH DIGESTIVE ENZYMES?

Supplementing with digestive enzymes appropriately depends on what your diet consists of. Since this is a ketogenic diet book, we are going to cover the digestive enzymes that are relevant to the foods you will be eating on keto. Look for supplements containing lipase (for fat), proteases and pepsin (for protein). If your keto diet is rich in fiber, look for digestive enzymes containing cellulase. In the case that you are consuming limited amounts of fruit on keto, look for pectinase in your digestive enzyme supplement. Additionally, if you have a deficiency in stomach acid production, supplementing with betaine hydrochloride (betaine HCL) can also be beneficial.

RECOMMENDATIONS FOR DIGESTIVE ENZYMES

- Look for supplements containing enzymes needed for the foods you are eating
- Consume 20 to 30 minutes before a meal for optimal benefits

PROBIOTICS AND PREBIOTICS

? WHAT ARE PROBIOTICS?

Probiotics are living organisms that support a healthy digestive system. Our gut is comprised of trillions of bacteria. Some bacteria are good, and some are bad. If you couldn't guess it, the foods you eat play a big role in which type of bacteria dominate your gut. Probiotics are supplements meant to promote the growth of healthy bacteria, which could improve the health of your gut.

? WHAT ARE PREBIOTICS?

Prebiotics feed the beneficial bacteria in our guts. This is still a fairly new concept that is being researched. Prebiotics may be important to help beneficial bacteria thrive and grow in your digestive tract. An example of a prebiotic is soluble fiber, which is fermented by the bacteria in your gut.

? WHAT ARE THE BENEFITS OF PREBIOTICS AND PROBIOTICS?

Probiotics can impact gut health, a key regulator to so many aspects of health, including blood lipids, mood, brain health, inflammation levels, and more. Theoretically, supplementing with probiotics can be a great way to improve gut health, but there are two things to consider here.

If you have a ton of gut bacteria, especially bad bacteria, probiotics may not provide much benefit. Instead, it may be better to follow an elimination diet to help kill off the bad bacteria in your gut so you can re-populate it with healthy bacteria through the use of probiotics.

If you are not feeding the beneficial bacteria, then they cannot grow and populate your gut. This is why prebiotics are so important; they need to be incorporated into your diet to ensure that you are feeding these microbes you are trying to grow in your digestive tract.

? WHEN ARE PREBIOTICS AND PROBIOTICS BENEFICIAL?

Following the completion of an elimination diet is a great time to incorporate pre- and probiotics to help populate your gut with good bacteria again. Once you have populated your gut with good bacteria, the continued use of prebiotics ensures that those bacteria stay well fed. Note that returning to a poor diet can damage these bacteria and remove any benefit you may have gained.

Additionally, after taking antibiotics, which completely destroy your gut, consider resetting your gut with a pre- and probiotic combination.

HOW DO I CHOOSE THE BEST PROBIOTIC?

It is important to get a quality probiotic, which can be a challenge, since there is a lot of garbage out there. There are three types of probiotics to look for: Lactobacillus, Bifidobacterium, and saccharomyces boulardii. We recommend finding a probiotic that contains 15-30 billion CFU of bacteria from sources such as the following:

- Lactobacillus helveticus
- Bifidobacterium longum
- Bifidobacterium lactis
- Lactobacillus breve

- Bifidobacterium infantis
- Lactobacillus ramnosus
- Lactobacillus acidophilus
- It is also beneficial to have a fungi source, such as S. boulardii.

The problem with most probiotics is that they are destroyed before they make it to the small intestine, so having a delivery mechanism, such as a phospholipid bilayer, to ensure proper delivery is important.

? HOW DO I CONSUME PREBIOTICS?

Prebiotics can come from a variety of food sources like chicory root, asparagus, onions, garlic, leeks, Jerusalem artichoke, and various fermented foods. Consuming these foods is a great way to feed the healthy bacteria you are trying to grow in your gut.

If you do not have access to all of these foods or do not like them, supplementing with a prebiotic supplement may be advisable.

RECOMMENDATIONS FOR PREBIOTICS AND PROBIOTICS

- Take a probiotic after an elimination diet or following antibiotic use
- Choose a probiotic containing the above list, with S. boulardii and a phospholipid bilayer
- Continue to consume prebiotic foods to help feed the beneficial bacteria
- Avoid processed carbohydrates to maintain improvements

ADAPTOGENS

? WHAT ARE ADAPTOGENS?

Adaptogens are a unique class of plants and herbs that impact your adrenal system and improve your body's ability to respond to stress. Their effects include altering hormone production, increasing energy, improving brain function, reducing stress and anxiety, and improving overall health and wellness. Adaptogens are a form of ancient medicine that has been used by many different cultures for many different therapeutic effects. If you look up what adaptogens can do for you, it may seem as if they are a panacea because of their ability to impact so many different aspects of health. This isn't necessarily the case but their ability to impact our adrenals and hormones make them broadly beneficial.

? WHICH ADAPTOGEN SHOULD I BE TAKING?

That depends on why you are taking them. Different adaptogens can produce similar benefits, but you may react to each individual adaptogen differently. Here are our favorite adaptogens and experiences with each of them.

ASHWAGANDHA

This is probably the most common adaptogen, most notably used to reduce stress and anxiety. Ashwagandha has also been shown to lower inflammation, reduce cortisol, improve brain health, and improve muscle mass and exercise performance.[109]

---

109 Ruchi, Tiwari Sandip Chakraborty, Mani Saminathan, Kuldeep Dhama, and Shoor Vir Singh,"Ashwagandha (Withania Somnifera):

Ashwagandha will not likely produce effects that you will notice the way a cup of coffee would, but that does not mean it is not working. This supplement is something Chris has been taking for a long time. We highly recommend to most people using ashwagandha as a multivitamin of sorts, especially those suffering from mood disorders.

When supplementing with ashwagandha be sure to use the KSM-66 version, which is the most widely researched extract. We recommend supplementing with 300-600 mg of ashwagandha per day, but this dose could increase depending on the person.

RHODIOLA ROSEA

Rhodiola produces similar effects to ashwagandha but with better reported results in fighting fatigue. In Chris' experience, this herb provides a greater cognitive boost compared to ashwagandha, which is why he takes it.

The recommended type of rhodiola is the SHR-5 extract. Dosing will vary, with the lowest effective dose being 50 mg, up to 300-680 mg for managing stress. Research has found that exceeding 680 mg is ineffective.

ADAPTOGENIC MUSHROOMS

Several mushrooms have adaptogenic properties, including lions mane, chaga, cordyceps, and reishi.

Lion's mane is now being researched as an ingredient for improving brain health and function and limiting cognitive decline, likely due to its impact on BDNF or brain-derived

---

Role in Safeguarding Health, Immunomodulatory Effects, Combating Infections and Therapeutic Applications: A Review," *Journal of Biological Sciences* 14, no. 2 (2014): 77-94.

neurotrophic factor, a protein that has many brain health related benefits. Chaga may play a role in cancer prevention. Preliminary research suggests it could suppress tumor growth and limit DNA damage due to its potent antioxidant potential. Cordyceps are commonly used for improving exercise endurance but have also been shown to combat fatigue, reduce inflammation, and improve brain function. Reishi is a unique mushroom that can provide your immune system with a boost and may be able to help detox your body and fight cancerous cells along the way.

There are numerous adaptogens out there, like holy basil, panax ginseng, bacopa monnieri, astragalus, and others. While these each show promising preliminary research as well, we do not have as much experience in supplementing with these particular adaptogens.

? SHOULD I BE TAKING ADAPTOGENS?

We have not found any reason to think that adaptogens are dangerous or should be avoided, and due to existing research highlighting their benefits, we think they make a great addition to a supplement routine.

Since there is still limited research and each adaptogen may impact you differently, we suggest doing your homework and self-experimenting to see which adaptogens provide you with the benefit you are seeking.

? HOW SHOULD I TAKE ADAPTOGENS

Optimal intake timing has not been established for adaptogens. While some adaptogens, like lions mane or rhodiola, may provide a big cognitive boost thus providing an optimal time to take them, others do not display as noticeable effects. For this reason, most adaptogens can be taken anytime throughout the day.

RECOMMENDATIONS FOR ADAPTOGENS

- Experiment with adaptogens to determine which one you react best to
- Use the recommended dose for each when consuming

NOOTROPICS

? WHAT IS A NOOTROPIC?

Nootropics are supplements designed to enhance cognitive function. Nootropics can come from a variety of sources, including herbs, amino acids, and lipids. Nootropics can support mental alertness, clarity, concentration, creativity, and most importantly brain health.

There are both natural and over-the-counter supplements (which we will be discussing here), and prescription nootropics like Adderall and Modafinil (which we will not be discussing).

There are so many different nootropic products out there. Many either using poorly researched ingredients or good ingredients but at too low a dose to get all of the benefits. For this reason, Anthony made his own nootropic formula to include the ingredients that he likes at the doses he finds to be optimal for supporting a healthy and well-functioning brain.

Another big difference between the product Anthony made versus others on the market is that his focuses on more than just stimulating the brain to improve cognitive function. Anthony's formulation also focuses on brain health by targeting contributors to cognitive decline like oxidative stress. Here is a list of our favorite brain enhancing ingredients:

- Exogenous Ketones
- MCTS
- Phosphatidylserine
- Alpha-GPC
- Ginkgo biloba

- ALA
- L-theanine
- DHA
- Cat's claw
- Adaptogenic mushrooms

? ARE NOOTROPICS SAFE?

The ingredients that we have just laid out are safe; that's why we picked them! However, not all nootropic supplements are. Some products contain a ton of caffeine or other, less studied and potentially harmful ingredients that should be avoided.

If you are looking at nootropic supplements, review each ingredient to determine if it is safe for you to consume.

? ARE NOOTROPICS ADDICTIVE?

Some nootropics can definitely be addictive, by either binding to opioid receptors or causing dopamine release. If you are reviewing a particular nootropic ingredient, be sure to check for the potential for addiction.

Even though some nootropics may not physiologically cause addiction, since they can improve the way you feel and perform, some people may become dependent. For this reason, we recommend using nootropics strategically and not having them a part of your everyday life.

? **HOW SHOULD I TAKE NOOTROPICS?**

Nootropics can be taken whenever you are in need of improved focus and mental clarity. Our favorite time to take nootropics is before a deep work session, where we are attempting to work with very intense focus, like we did while writing this book.

Each nootropic will have time to onset of action. Note that this could also vary from person to person so again, self-experimentation is key.

RECOMMENDATIONS FOR NOOTROPICS

- Find which safe nootropic or combination of safe nootropics works best for you
- Check out the Perfect Keto Nootropic (we are pretty proud of its formulation)
- Avoid using everyday

ORGAN MEAT CAPSULES

? **WHAT ARE ORGAN MEAT CAPSULES?**

Just what they sound like: capsules containing nutrients from organ meat. Organ meat capsules are becoming more popular as the benefits of consuming organ meat are becoming more widely known and most people do not particularly enjoy eating organ meat.

Organ meat capsules can contain vitamins, minerals, healthy fat, and essential amino acids from individual organs like liver, heart, brain, lung, tongue, bone, kidney, pancreas, and spleen or a combination of any of the organ meats.

⑦ WHAT ARE THE BENEFITS OF ORGAN MEAT CAPSULES?

If you recall from earlier in the book, organ meat is extremely high in bioavailable micronutrients and something we should include in our diet. However, not everyone enjoys the taste or even the thought of consuming organ meat. This is where organ meat capsules can come into play.

While organ meat capsules can provide you with many of the nutrients from organ meat, these are a fairly new class of supplements, so how effective these supplements are at increasing micronutrient consumption still needs to be evaluated.

⑦ HOW SHOULD I TAKE ORGAN MEAT CAPSULES?

There is no specific intake timing recommended for organ meat capsules. We suggest using organ meat capsules as a daily multivitamin since they are so dense in micronutrients. Consume them daily with a meal.

If you do supplement with organ meat capsules, look for capsules containing nutrients from grass-fed bovine. Just like the food you eat, the quality of the source of your supplement matters as well!

RECOMMENDATIONS FOR ORGAN MEAT CAPSULES:

- Use like a daily multivitamin
- Check out the Equip Grass-Fed Liver Capsules

? ARE THERE ANY SUPPLEMENTS I SHOULD AVOID?

There are a lot of supplements out there and companies are very good at making them appear to be beneficial and in some cases a necessity. However, most of this is just marketing and we hate this. (That's why Perfect Keto was created, to get past the garbage and put out quality products.)

Several nonsensical supplements that you should avoid:

- Meal replacements
- Raspberry Ketones
- Fat Burners
- High caffeine products

MEAL REPLACEMENTS

Meal replacements are shakes containing a high quantity of calories. While these may be an effective strategy for increasing overall calorie consumption, most times these products contain a lot of fillers, carbohydrates, and are typically devoid of the beneficial nutrients found in whole foods.

RASPBERRY KETONES

Ever since Dr. Oz promoted raspberry ketones on his show back in 2012, they've been all the rage and hailed as the biggest fat-burning miracle supplement. You've likely seen the Google ads, the advertisements on TV, and the online "testimonials" talking about this supplement's amazing weight loss benefits. But how true is all of this, really? And do these raspberry ketones actually have anything to do with real ketosis?

The truth: raspberry ketones are pointless when it comes to ketosis. Even though they sound fancy and contain the word "ketones," raspberry ketones really have nothing to do with entering or keeping the body in ketosis. It's easy to get pulled into the appeal of the product due to the name's association with the fat-burning and health benefits of a low-carb diet. However, these ketones are completely different than those made by our bodies, so they have no relation to or function within ketosis or the ketogenic diet.

In its true form, a raspberry ketone is found naturally in trace amounts in red raspberries and other fruits like blackberries, cranberries, and kiwis. It's what gives berries their nice, appealing scent and flavor. Before they were sold as supplements, raspberry ketones were mostly used in processed foods like ice creams and soft drinks, and in perfumes and cosmetics. The claim from proponents is that raspberry ketones help the body burn fat faster and more effectively because they supposedly increase levels of adiponectin, which is a hormone that regulates metabolism and blood sugar levels.

This is appealing because adiponectin typically increases when you lose weight, and those with low levels of the hormone tend to have a higher risk of suffering from Type 2 diabetes, obesity, heart disease, and fatty liver disease. Also, the molecular structure of raspberry ketones is close to molecules that have been shown in studies to boost metabolism: synephrine (a stimulant), and capsaicin (a component in chili pepper). The claim here is that raspberry ketones can also boost metabolism because of the similarities.

However, there are several problems with these claims. There is no human evidence. Those selling the supplements will cite a few studies with rats and mice to establish credibility, but those aren't as impressive as they'd have you believe. In one study, fat cells were isolated from rats and grown by researchers in a test tube with raspberry ketones added.[110] This

---

110 Kyoung Sik Park, "Raspberry Ketone Increases both Lipolysis and Fatty Acid Oxidation in 3T3-L1 Adipocytes," *Planta Medica* 76, no. 15 (2010): 1654-1658.

made the cells release more adiponectin and increased the breakdown of fat, but this doesn't demonstrate that the same could happen in a living human, or even a living rat.

Another study involved feeding mice an unhealthy version of a high-fat diet for six weeks. Some were given raspberry ketones while others weren't. At the end of the six weeks, the mice given the raspberry ketones weighed 50 grams while those not given the ketones weighed 55 grams. Neither group lost any weight; the first one just gained 10 percent less than the second group.[111]

In a third study, 40 rats were given a fattening diet along with raspberry ketones.[112] Their adiponectin levels were increased, but they were given the raspberry ketones in *huge* amounts— much higher (over 100 times) than would be feasible (or likely safe) for a human to take at all, much less on a regular basis.

We also need to recognize that there are better, more natural ways to increase adiponectin in the body and reduce fat, like eating a very low-carb diet, getting regular exercise, and even drinking coffee!

We can't be completely sure raspberry ketones are safe to consume. They were recognized by the us Food and Drug Administration (FDA) as a "Generally Recognized as Safe" food additive, but that was back in the 1960s before people were taking them in much larger amounts as a supplement.

Before the Dr. Oz show, only a few people made a supplement with real, natural raspberry ketones powder because the

111 Chie Morimoto, Yurie Satoh, Mariko Hara, Shintaro Inoue, Takahiro Tsujita, and Hiromichi Okuda, "Anti-obese Action of Raspberry Ketone," *Life Sciences* 77, no. 2 (2005): 194-204.

112 Lili Wang, Xianjun Meng, and Fengqing Zhang, "Raspberry Ketone Protects Rats Fed High-Fat Diets against Nonalcoholic Steatohepatitis," *Journal of Medicinal Food* 15, no. 5 (2012): 495-503.

cost of the raw ingredients was so high. Now, most have to use fillers and fake ingredients to keep the supplements affordable. In fact, many of these products use mostly ground up anise seeds with just a touch of real raspberry ketone and add flavor artificially.

FAT BURNERS

Fat burners are some of the most popular supplements because people want a short-term answer to losing weight. Fat burning should be regulated by shoring up nutrition, movement, stress, and sleep, not by taking a magic pill. While some products on the market may be able to stimulate some type of fat burning most of them can be dangerous and only provide short-term minimal improvements and potentially long-term complications.

HIGH CAFFEINE PRODUCTS

There are many supplements out there that will simply use a ton of caffeine to make you feel something, thus thinking the product works. There is a particular group of energy drinks out there right now that not only contains harmful ingredients but uses 300 mg of caffeine, which is like three or more strong cups of coffee. This is much more than is needed and can promote anxiety, increase heart rate, and decrease caffeine sensitivity over time, increasing your need for more! Avoid these products.

Remember, supplements are meant to support and fill the gaps in a well-formulated diet. They are not meant to replace what you should be getting from consuming high-quality whole foods. We mentioned a lot of supplements in this chapter. Not everyone will require using all of these supplements. However, it is important to know which of the many supplements out there actually work and how and when they can be implemented into your diet to provide the most benefit.

When it comes to supplementation, do your homework. Always look for the best quality products with the right ingredients at the right doses. If you are looking for more information on the specifics of a certain supplement, we recommend checking out the websites examine.com and selfhacked.com. Both of these websites present information in a pretty easy to digest manner and provide citations for the benefits listed.

CHAPTER 9

FASTING AND KETO

Fasting is another dietary practice that has grown in popularity over the last few years due to its weight loss potential, especially intermittent fasting. However, there is nothing new about fasting. In fact, fasting is mentioned numerous times in the bible and has been used as a form of medicine for thousands of years.

Hippocrates, considered the father of modern medicine, frequently prescribed fasting back during BC times and even wrote, "To eat when you are sick, is to feed your illness." The ancient Greek historian Plutarch in early AD also wrote, "Instead of using medicine, better fast today." Fasting was also one of the first dietary methods for treating epilepsy as far back as the early 1900s. Furthermore, our ancestors frequently had to fast due to limited food availability. The point here is that fasting is not a new practice and can provide a lot more than just weight loss.

Fasting and keto are often in the same conversation because of the similarities between these two dietary principles. If you recall from earlier in the book, the ketogenic diet was actually created as an alternative to fasting due to its ability to impact epilepsy symptoms through very similar mechanisms.

However, a ketogenic diet does not have to be followed as an alternative to fasting. In fact, as we will get into more in this chapter, fasting and keto can actually pair very well and lead to even more robust benefits. Let's dive into one of the most ancient dietary practices.

? WHAT IS FASTING?

Short Answer: Fasting is the abstinence of food and in some cases drink for a certain period of time. Fasting has been shown to be therapeutic for numerous health conditions.

Fasting is a pretty simple concept—you don't eat. When your body goes without food for an extended period of time, it has to adapt to find another fuel source. Sound familiar? It's very similar to a ketogenic diet. In fact, the ketogenic diet was created for its ability to mimic fasting. Fasting provides numerous benefits, but as it relates to keto, fasting can lower blood glucose and increase ketone production.

Without the body's ability to switch into a ketogenic state to burn body fat for fuel, we would have died out as a species long ago. I know it is probably hard for anyone in a developed country to think about going without food for more than three hours, but stints of three days or more between meals were routine throughout most human history. If we couldn't switch to using fat for fuel, we would have gone extinct. Good work, body.

While fasting evolved as a survival mechanism, it is becoming a commonly used dietary practice for managing weight, promoting weight loss, and numerous other health improvements.

Fasting for these purposes rarely includes extended fasting, typically focusing on intermittent fasting, or intermittently avoiding food within your day. We will get more into the various fasting methods later in this chapter.

? HOW DOES FASTING WORK?

Fasting, similar to keto, induces a transition in fuel utilization. Your body is continually running; it doesn't shut off. It has to have energy available to some degree at all times. When you eat food, you provide the body with many of the things it needs to function, including energy and that energy can be used or stored away for later. Once it is stored, it can be accessed during periods of fasting. Since carb stores are limited, they can only contribute a small amount of energy during fasting. The rest comes from the body's ability to burn fat and produce ketones. This sounds just like ketosis because it is. While there are many other benefits that happen during fasting, the way it operates is essentially through ketosis.

You can experience some fasting benefits without having to refrain from eating for too long. This can be done through intermittent fasting, which we will get more into later in this chapter but is a shorter method of fasting used strategically and typically frequently.

? WHAT IS THE DIFFERENCE BETWEEN FASTING AND KETO?

Fasting and keto both induce several of the same physiological states in the body, particularly lower insulin and blood glucose and greater fat burning and ketone production. The difference is that you get to eat during one of them and you don't on the other. Keto was invented to allow for food consumption but still experience a similar physiological state to fasting.

While the human body can sustain fasting for a surprisingly long period of time with minimal side effects, it is not a sustainable way to live. Insert the ketogenic diet. You can consume calories and nutrients on keto. Choosing the right keto foods will lead to you flooding your body with beneficial nutrients while still maintaining a similar physiological state as fasting—the best of both worlds.

It is important to point out that despite keto being a more practical method for receiving some of the benefits of fasting, there are still added benefits to fasting that make it an incredibly useful dietary tool, especially in conjunction with a keto diet.

? WHAT ARE THE BENEFITS OF FASTING?

Fasting is somewhat like working out. When you're working out, you're not actually doing good things to your body. You are breaking down your tissues and sending a signal to your body that they should be stronger next time you face that stress. This is what is called a hermetic stressor. Your body is responding positively to a stress. When you are fasting, you are telling your body that you need to adapt and make sure you are more resilient. Your body is forced to recycle old cells and ones that aren't working that well in order to make new cells and improve function.

Fasting benefits include lower blood sugar, increase in blood ketones, improved energy, decrease in inflammation, improved immune function, enhanced weight loss, and improved overall health. Fasting, depending on the length, also offers a particularly useful benefit known as autophagy. Autophagy is a process that results in the recycling of damaged cells and replacing them with new healthy cells. This is a process that is crucial to make sure that damaged or mutated cells are not replicated and is a great way to rid the body of potentially precancerous cells.

Fasting can also be used therapeutically to weaken cancer cells. As we will get into more later in the book, cancer cells thrive on glucose. Lowering glucose through fasting is a great way to weaken cancer cells, thus making them more susceptible to standard care cancer treatments like radiation and chemotherapy.[113]

Fasting may also be able to promote longevity. If your body is constantly metabolizing nutrients it is much more prone to accelerated aging. Fasting for brief periods of time can help slow this cycle. Furthermore, research looking at calorie restriction, a feature that typically accompanies fasting, has also been shown to slow aging.[114]

? DO YOU HAVE TO FAST WITH KETO?

While it is true that keto was born from fasting, that does not necessarily mean that they have to go together. Starting a keto diet can be tough enough for some people; the addition of fasting may only make it harder. That being said, fasting and keto together can lead to more robust benefits and should be

---

113 Brittany A. Simone, Colin E. Champ, Anne L. Rosenberg, Adam C. Berger, Daniel A. Monti, Adam P. Dicker, and Nicole L. Simone, "Selectively Starving Cancer Cells Through Dietary Manipulation: Methods And Clinical Implications," *Future Oncology* 9, no. 7 (2013): 959-976.

114 Edda Cava and Luigi Fontana, "Will Calorie Restriction Work in Humans?" *Aging* (Albany, NY) 5, no. 7 (2013): 507-514.

considered once you are adapted to keto. Fasting can further stimulate ketone production, so using them together typically leads to higher ketone production.

Fasting is often part of the natural progression of keto, with many people introducing fasting down the road as they adapt to the diet and start to experience satiety and more stable blood sugar levels making fasting much easier.

That said, fasting can provide a lot of benefit when starting keto as a way to help stimulate greater ketone production, thus aiding in keto adaptation. But again, if you are new to keto, the diet may be a big enough change and adding fasting may only increase your likelihood of poor adherence. In this case, it is not worth adding it at the beginning and may be better to hold off until it can be more easily stuck to. Moral of the story: no, you do not have to fast on keto.

HOW DO YOU FAST?

Don't eat.

All right, fine, fasting is a little more complex than that. Like keto, there are strategies to either maximize the benefits or manage any potential side effects. Most notably, water and electrolyte replenishment are important, especially for longer duration fasts.

There are several different protocols for fasting, with each providing slightly different benefits. Selecting the right one will be critical for ensuring that you are not only going to reach whatever goal you have, but also that you are going to be able to sustain the practice. How you fast depends on what type of fasting you're doing, and why you are doing it.

Due to the blood sugar crashes and subsequent energy dips and hunger pangs, fasting when not on a keto diet is typically much harder than fasting while on keto. Since you are already in a state of ketosis on a keto diet, stable blood sugar, sustained energy, and reduced hunger makes adding in fasting easier. It can take some adjusting, but if you give it a little time you might just find that (for example) breakfast has been a habit that society has (literally) shoved down your throat since you were a little kid.

? WHAT ARE THE DIFFERENT TYPES OF FASTING?

While fasting is a pretty simple concept, there are several different variations that can be followed. Most are time dependent and have different benefits for different lengths. Here is a breakdown of the different fasting variations:

OVERNIGHT FAST

An overnight fast is just the time from your last meal at night to your first meal the next day. Typically, an overnight fast is only 8-12 hours for most people. While this may be able to induce a very minor state of ketosis in more insulin sensitive people, it will not provide many of the benefits of fasting.

A proper overnight fast is important for self-experimentation, but we will get more into that in Chapter 13.

INTERMITTENT FASTING

Intermittent fasting is like it sounds, intermittent bouts of food restriction implemented strategically. These bouts are referred to as the "fasting window," which is followed by a period of eating, called the "eating window." Typically, people eat right when they wake up and right before they go to bed, leading to an eating window of anywhere from 12-16 hours. Intermittent fasting employs much shorter eating windows, 8, 6, 4 or even 2 hours within the day. This means you'll be fasting for 16, 18,

20 or 22 hours. Fasting for 16+ hours is a significant enough time for your body to tap into stored energy sources, meaning that intermittent bouts of these fasting windows can…well, intermittently provide benefits.

It doesn't really matter when your eating windows are. Some science has shown that it may be better to time eating windows for when the sun is shining, which means no late-night meals. However, the research is not definitive. We recommend fasting through the morning, the easiest way to implement an intermittent fasting protocol. The morning provides a few different benefits. One of the main benefits we like is not having to think about food, cooking, or cleaning when we first wake up. We both like to do deep work in the morning and fasting can contribute to greater ketone production during that time, thus improving mental focus. We also find that a nice dinner at night with family or friends is much more enjoyable and not something we want to skip.

Intermittent fasting is easier to do and thus easier to incorporate into life than longer fasts, especially on keto. All you do is skip breakfast and you are basically intermittent fasting. Our favorite intermittent fasting protocol is:

- Dinner 7 p.m.
- Fast 16-20 hours
- Lunch between 11 a.m. and 3 p.m.
- Dinner 7 p.m.

While intermittent fasting is extremely easy to implement and can lead to robust benefits, especially in conjunction with keto, there may be additional benefits to longer fasts. Rigorous randomized controlled trials investigating the effects of intermittent fasting are rare. However, a recent systematic review demonstrated that intermittent fasting can improve several clinical outcomes, including decreases in fat mass, triglycerides, and inflammatory markers.[115] Preliminary data also suggest intermittent fasting may also improve cognition.

WHOLE DAY FASTING

Whole day fasting is as it sounds, a whole day of not eating. Twenty-four hours. Many things happen in the body during a fast and some of the benefits that occur may be more robust the longer you fast, such as cell recycling, autophagy, and immune system regeneration.

Since whole day fasting is a little more intense than intermittent fasting, it is not done as frequently. Some individuals may report doing this once a month or a little more aggressively at once a week. The data is not out on how frequently to do these fasts for maximum benefit, but incorporating them occasionally will provide health benefits.

If you are adapted to keto, a whole day fast, like intermittent fasting, is likely not very challenging. Whole day fasts may be a good induction to a keto diet to enhance keto-adaptation; however, due to the challenging nature of this approach, it may not be advisable to new keto dieters.

ALTERNATE DAY FASTS

Alternate day fasting means alternating whole days of fasting with eating days. Alternate day fasting is pretty simple and looks like:

- Wake up
- Fast all day

---

115 Benjamin D. Horne, Joseph B. Muhlestein, and Jeffrey L. Anderson,

- Wake up
- Don't fast

While this is a simple approach, research has shown positive health outcomes. One research group had thirty-two normal weight and overweight individuals perform either alternate day fasting or maintain their normal dietary patterns. On fasting days, subjects in the alternate day fasting group were provided with one meal by the researchers which met 25 percent of their daily caloric needs. After twelve weeks, subjects in the alternate day fast group decreased their body weight by an average of 5.2 kg (6.5 percent) compared to control! Fat mass was reduced by 3.6 kg and muscle mass values did not change versus control. These researchers concluded that alternate day fasting is effective for weight loss and cardio protection.[116]

This approach is a bit more extreme than the previously mentioned fasting methods and is not recommended for those who are new to fasting. This approach should be worked up to.

EXTENDED FASTS

Extended fasts last longer than three days. Like whole day fasting, the benefit here is in the longer duration. Also, like whole day fasting, the greater intensity of this approach implies infrequent use, unless for therapeutic intervention.

"Health Effects of Intermittent Fasting: Hormesis or Harm? A Systematic Review," *The American Journal of Clinical Nutrition* 102, no. 2 (2015): 464-470.

116 Krista A. Varady, Surabhi Bhutani, Monica C. Klempel, Cynthia M. Kroeger, John F. Trepanowski, Jacob M. Haus, Kristin K. Hoddy, and Yolian Calvo, "Alternate Day Fasting for Weight Loss in Normal Weight and Overweight Subjects: A Randomized Controlled Trial," *Nutrition Journal* 12, no. 11 (2013): 146.

Extended fasting is where you would start to really see improved immune function and autophagy occurring which is why one recommendation, made by the great cancer researcher Dr. Thomas Seyfried from Boston College, is to do an extended fast quarterly to rid your body of precancerous cells. The glucose ketone index (GKI), which as we will get into in Chapter 13, is a calculated relationship between your blood glucose and ketone levels. Fasting for 2-3 days can induce a GKI that is conducive of autophagy.

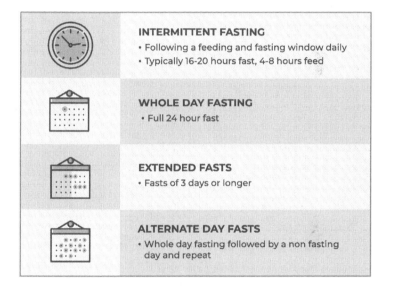

INTERMITTENT FASTING
• Following a feeding and fasting window daily
• Typically 16-20 hours fast, 4-8 hours feed

WHOLE DAY FASTING
• Full 24 hour fast

EXTENDED FASTS
• Fasts of 3 days or longer

ALTERNATE DAY FASTS
• Whole day fasting followed by a non fasting day and repeat

? WHAT BREAKS A FAST?

Short Answer: This answer is depending on the goal but for most people, breaking a fast is consuming anything of caloric value.

By definition, fasting is the absence of food and drink. While you may be able to fast without water (known as dry fasting), and there may even be some potential benefits to doing it this way, we believe that water is good, and dehydration is bad. We don't think this approach is advisable, at the very least not frequently. The longer you fast, the more important drinking water becomes. Some call this a water fast, which is a fair way to classify it.

To optimize performance and limit potential side effects of fasting, we believe that supplementing with electrolytes is also advantageous and is more important in longer fasts. This may be referred to as a supplemental water fast. This line of thinking leads to the definition of fasting as "not consuming anything of caloric value." This is the most widely accepted and also typically allows for black coffee.

However, there is another view on the definition of fasting based on the principle that the major benefits of fasting are a result of lower blood glucose and insulin, and greater ketone production. This line of thinking leads to the definition of fasting as "not consuming anything that spikes blood glucose or insulin levels." This is most often referred to as fat fasting. We will get more into this shortly.

Each of these definitions of what breaks a fast is valuable. This means that the strategy you use for fasting is based on which benefits you are looking for. If your main goal is autophagy, immune system reboot, digestive cleanse, therapeutic intervention, or other benefits from longer term fasts and you want to absolutely maximize these benefits, then consider doing a water only or supplemental water fast. If you are just looking to increase ketone production, promote some weight loss, and increase mental focus, fat fasting may be a better approach for you.

? WHAT IS A FAT FAST?

A fat fast means consuming fat or exogenous ketones during the fasting window. Yes, fat has calories and yes, fat can trigger an insulin response. However, fat consumed in small amounts only triggers insulin to a minimal amount and has minimal to no effect on blood glucose, making this approach a possible alternative method of fasting.

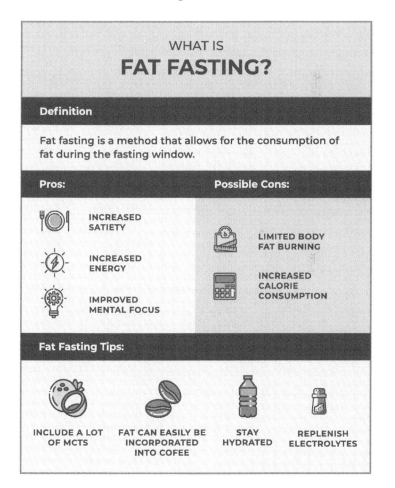

WHAT IS
FAT FASTING?

Definition

Fat fasting is a method that allows for the consumption of fat during the fasting window.

Pros: **Possible Cons:**

INCREASED SATIETY

                                                 LIMITED BODY FAT BURNING

INCREASED ENERGY

                                                 INCREASED CALORIE CONSUMPTION

IMPROVED MENTAL FOCUS

Fat Fasting Tips:

INCLUDE A LOT OF MCTS | FAT CAN EASILY BE INCORPORATED INTO COFEE | STAY HYDRATED | REPLENISH ELECTROLYTES

When choosing the best fasting technique, it is important to consider what is most optimal vs. what is most sustainable. For example, if your main goal is fat loss, maybe consuming no calories is most optimal, but you can only fast for 12 hours this way. If fat fasting allows you to extend that to 16+ hours, maybe that is more sustainable and may even produce similar benefits.

Also consider whether consuming strategic foods that do not spike insulin or glucose, such as MCTs and exogenous ketones, may allow you to experience the benefits of no-calorie fasting to a lower degree but with additional benefits, such as increased energy and cognitive focus.

? IS THERE A WRONG WAY TO DO FASTING?

We're wary of those who approach fasting with a fad mentality. Fasting is not a quick fix "detox" to erase all of the bad decisions you've made. Your body has detoxification pathways that are always running, whether or not you are fasting. For them to work properly, modify the food and lifestyle you lead on a day-to-day basis so that your body can work the way it is supposed to. No amount of juice cleansing or fasting will help if you just go back to making terrible decisions you know you shouldn't be making in the first place. The best cleanse or detox plan is eating real food, moving a lot, getting high-quality sleep, and decreasing stress. All of the time.

Fasting is not a last-minute fat loss plan. While fasting will put you in ketosis, which can lead to using body fat for energy, this isn't a diet only meant to shed pounds before beach season. If you want to lose fat, using a ketogenic diet and making good choices over a long period of time is the best approach you can take. Maybe this book would sell more if we sold a magic pill, but there are simply no shortcuts to fat loss. Put in the work if that's what you want.

? IS FASTING SAFE?

Chronic under eating can lead to health problems like malnutrition and hormonal issues. For this reason, if fasting leads to calorie restriction, be sure to track this over time to ensure that you are not restricting calories too much for too long. The longest documented fast was over a year, with minimal supplementation.[117] The individual thrived without food for over 382 days. This is an extreme example and was heavily monitored, so don't go out and try to mess around with fasting for a year without medical supervision. It is, though, good evidence that the human body can survive some pretty incredible stress.

This goes without saying, Anthony is a doctor, but he is not your doctor. Talk with your physician about the risks of fasting and how they apply to your current situation. If they completely dismiss fasting without thinking about how it can be used as a tool, you should probably find another doctor.

Fasting does have some inherent risks and certainly isn't for everyone. The majority of this is common sense, but just in case you aren't sure, fasting is *not* for the following:

CHILDREN

Kids are growing and need an excessive amount of various nutrients to thrive, produce hormones and grow. Going

---

117 W. K. Stewart and Laura W. Fleming, "Features of a Successful Therapeutic Fast of 382 Days' Duration," *Postgraduate Medical Journal* 49, no. 569 (1973): 203-209.

without food for extended periods of time will stunt growth and mess up metabolism. Feed your kids.

ELDERLY

Conversely, those late in age should probably not worry about fasting either. Maintaining lean body mass is especially important in elderly populations and becomes harder as you age. Fasting could lead to severe calorie restriction, which may not be advised for this population.

PREGNANT, TRYING TO GET PREGNANT, OR NURSING

Just as with the whole children thing, babies and fetuses are growing rapidly. You need to feed them.

WHAT IF I FEEL AWFUL DURING FASTING?

If you just feel sluggish and foggy, that can be normal as you switch from burning carbs to burning fat. If you feel you are truly sick and that you are going to pass out or die (but know that you're not going to), then eat something. This is the great thing about fasting—you control everything. If you're not digging it, then eat. Don't be a fool and push yourself into unsafe territory.

It may take some time to get used to fasting. You may have to experience some negative side effects for a while as you get accustomed to this. If you start feeling a little low energy on an intermittent fasting protocol, the first step is to check your food tracking app and make sure that you are getting enough to eat. Your hormones will be pretty pissed at you if you're not routinely getting enough food. Humans are animals that have thrived on variance in the past. It also probably is a good idea to pepper in this protocol instead of religiously executing it on a day-to-day basis for years on end. Mix it up!

Also note that not feeling well during a fast may be a result of dehydration or electrolyte depletion, and treating these two factors can make a big difference. This can be managed through consuming salt during the fasting window, using electrolyte supplements, or adding exogenous ketones, which will not only provide additional electrolytes but also a fuel source to help energize you.

? CAN I EXERCISE WHILE FASTING?

Exercise while fasting can be a great way to improve insulin sensitivity, induce greater ketone production, and promote more fat burning. However, someone who is new to fasting may have a hard time with this approach, so this is likely better for someone who is a little more accustomed to fasting.

When deciding if fasting and exercise is right for you, consider what will allow you to train at a higher intensity and enjoy your training. This is likely a greater determinant of your success.

Below is an example of what an intermittent fasting and exercise protocol with a four-hour eating window would look something like:

- Wake up at 7 a.m.
- Workout at 1 p.m.
- Eat at 2 p.m.
- Stop eating at 6 p.m.
- Repeat

In summary, the ketogenic diet was created to stimulate similar changes in the body as fasting. While the two do not have to be used together, fasting does tend to be a natural progression of keto dieting since reduced hunger and cravings on keto make it easier to skip a meal in the morning. Fasting and keto together can lead to more robust benefits. Fasting also provides some additional benefits like autophagy, which is why incorporating several of the different types of fasts mentioned in this chapter can be beneficial. We do not recommend practicing fasting when starting keto since the transition into keto can be challenging enough for some.

CHAPTER 10

DIFFERENT TYPES OF KETO

By now you have probably realized that there is no one size fits all approach to nutrition. To think that everyone is going to thrive on the same foods or even the same macronutrient ratios misses the understanding that no two people are the exact same.

The same holds true for the ketogenic diet. Lowering your carbohydrates, increasing your protein and fat consumption, and focusing on a variety of quality foods will provide benefit for everyone. However, there are tweaks that can be made to a ketogenic diet to better suit an individual or to help achieve a particular goal. This is why we are seeing a variety of other diets being born out of the ketogenic diet.

Before we dive into the different variations of the ketogenic diet, we recommend that anyone new to the diet start with a traditional ketogenic diet. Starting with the principles we have been preaching throughout this book is a great way to lay a strong nutritional foundation that you can further build on with the different variations of keto we are going to discuss in this chapter. These variations include:

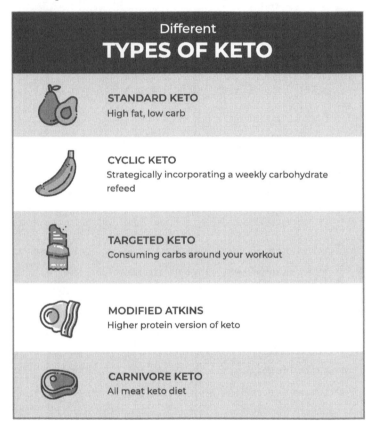

Different
TYPES OF KETO

STANDARD KETO
High fat, low carb

CYCLIC KETO
Strategically incorporating a weekly carbohydrate refeed

TARGETED KETO
Consuming carbs around your workout

MODIFIED ATKINS
Higher protein version of keto

CARNIVORE KETO
All meat keto diet

CYCLIC KETO

? WHAT IS CYCLIC KETO?

The cyclic keto diet consists of consuming carbohydrates one or two days a week and following a ketogenic diet for the other days.

There are several reasons why someone may take this approach, including wanting a break from keto, to replenish glycogen, having a goal of building muscle, improving exercise performance, or attempting to limit the side effects of keto.

? IS CYCLIC KETO AN EFFECTIVE STRATEGY?

Short Answer: Cyclic keto may be an effective strategy for those who are looking to maximize performance or muscle building, but the diet has not been studied extensively.

While cyclic keto is practiced by many, it has not been studied or reported on very frequently in the literature. Instead we have to rely on interpreting related research and anecdotal evidence, both of which provide conflicting results. We would love to see more research looking directly at cyclic keto because while we love to speculate, speculation is only so effective.

Cyclic keto means cyclic ketosis. You will be in and out of ketosis using this strategy. Being in ketosis is not the end all be all of health, but ketosis provides a lot of benefits. If you take this approach, you are going to be frequently kicked out of ketosis which could lead to some unwanted side effects, such as fatigue, brain fog, and difficulty becoming keto-adapted.

For this reason, we do not recommend cyclic keto for beginners. If your first day of keto is Monday, you will start to have significantly elevated ketones by, let's say, Wednesday or Thursday. But then you have carbs on Saturday and are kicked out of ketosis. If you start back up Sunday, it takes at least another two or three days to get those ketones elevated again—but then you consume carbs again and are again kicked out of ketosis. This cycle will prevent you from fully keto-adapting.

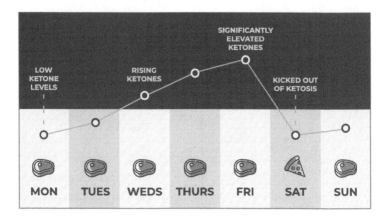

Furthermore, while hunger and cravings are reduced on a ketogenic diet, research has demonstrated that when carbs are reintroduced, hunger tends to come back. A cyclic keto approach may prevent you from feeling the satiety effects of keto and make you more prone to falling completely off the wagon following a carb refeed.

In addition, if you are frequently being kicked out of ketosis and it takes you a couple of days to get back in, you may be at a greater risk of losing muscle, as you will not have as much benefit from the protein-sparing effect of keto.

For someone who is keto-adapted, the story may be different. A keto-adapted individual can typically transition back into ketosis quicker, so if they have a carb refeed on Saturday, they may be back into ketosis by mid-day Sunday. This means that any side effects of being kicked out of ketosis will not last as long compared to someone who is new to keto.

While a keto-adapted individual may be able to better follow a cyclic keto diet, we have yet to determine if using the diet is beneficial. As we mentioned in Chapter 5, carbs are not needed for exercise performance or muscle building; however, they can help. For this reason, one of the only potential uses of the cyclic keto diet that we would consider is if the *primary* goal is exercise performance or muscle growth.

There is also some anecdotal evidence that a cyclic keto diet may be useful around a woman's menstrual cycle; however, more research is still needed to determine the effectiveness of this strategy. To reiterate, there may be some uses of a cyclic keto diet but for most people, following a standard ketogenic diet is going to be better for long-term adherence and success. This is especially true for someone who is insulin resistant, prediabetic, or diabetic. These individuals do not effectively utilize carbs so even strategically implementing them is unlikely to be beneficial.

❓ HOW DO I FOLLOW A CYCLIC KETO DIET?

If cyclic keto is effective, there is definitely a right and wrong way to do it. Cyclic keto does not mean eating keto for five days, followed by a weekend of pizza, beer, ice cream, and pancakes. That is just a poor attempt at keto and an inability to control cravings.

Cyclic keto should be the strategic consumption of carbohydrates from quality, nutrient dense sources such as sweet potatoes or plantains, and it should be limited. If we were going to recommend an approach to cyclic keto, this is what it would look like:

- Keto Monday-Friday
- Fasted Saturday morning, intense training session
- Higher carb + protein, lower fat meal (Ex. Chicken, sweet potatoes.)
- Higher protein, lower carb, moderate fat dinner
- Sunday back on track, maybe another workout

We recommend that the carbs be consumed around exercise. Exercise can increase insulin sensitivity, improving your ability to utilize those carbs for recovery and reduce the likelihood of them causing damage within the body.

We also recommend using this approach less frequently. We don't think that a consistent weekly cyclic keto approach is a great idea. The best approach would be doing weekly cyclic keto for a set period of time (i.e., during a 4-6-week intense exercise program), or only using the approach a couple of times a month.

TARGETED KETO

? WHAT IS TARGETED KETO?

Targeted keto is the strategic consumption of carbohydrates around a training session or competition and keto all other times. Targeted keto is used by those who exercise frequently or at high intensities, particularly athletes.

The purpose of this approach is to either stimulate greater exercise performance, promote greater recovery from exercise or competition, and/or stimulate muscle growth.

? IS TARGETED KETO AN EFFECTIVE APPROACH?

Short Answer: Targeted keto, if done right, may be an effective approach for someone who is keto-adapted and has the primary goal of improving exercise performance.

Before we dive in, we must again point out that targeted keto has not been adequately studied, so most of what we will be discussing is anecdotal and theoretical.

Once keto-adapted, your body is in a physiological state that allows for the transition between carbohydrates and fat and ketones for fuel based on availability and the demand of the body. This is what some people refer to as the "dual-fuel" benefit of keto. To explain a different way, someone who has properly followed a keto diet for an extended period of time is typically more insulin sensitive, meaning they can better utilize ingested carbohydrates and easily transition back to burning fat and producing ketones once these carbohydrates have been used.

Again, we have to decide if being able to better utilize carbohydrates actually warrants their use. While the exact mechanism is not fully understood, carbohydrates can act as an ergogenic aid and have been shown to improve exercise performance.[118] However, many of these studies are in carb-adapted athletes whose primary fuel source is carbohydrates. Carbs provided to a keto-adapted individual may not produce the same improvements or to the same degree. As it relates to muscle building, consuming carbohydrates after a workout will stimulate insulin, which can aid in but is not essential for muscle growth.

Together this means, like the cyclic keto diet, targeted keto is for someone who is looking to maximize performance, recovery, or muscle growth. If you are an average Joe (and don't lie to yourself, many of us are and we both are), then this principle likely doesn't apply to you. Again, this strategy should be for someone who has one of the three above goals as their *primary* goal.

If your goal is to stay in ketosis, either for therapeutic purposes, the desire to maintain enhanced cognitive function, or the

118 Asker E. Jeukendrup, "Carbohydrate Intake During Exercise and Performance," *Nutrition* 20, no. 7-8 (2004): 669-677.

goal of maximizing fat loss, then anything that may hinder this, such as the consumption of carbohydrates, is not advised. Like cyclic keto, we do not recommend targeted keto for beginners. Furthermore, there is plenty of research in the general population that demonstrates the ability to maintain or improve exercise performance while on a keto diet, even while completing training higher in intensity, such as CrossFit.[119] Additionally, as we pointed out in Chapter 4, there have also been studies and anecdotal evidence demonstrating muscle can be gained on keto. Targeted keto may help but it is not essential.

? HOW WOULD TARGETED KETO AFFECT FAT LOSS?

Since this approach has not been extensively studied, we have to speculate again. Since insulin impairs fat burning and consuming carbs after exercise can prevent improvements in insulin sensitivity, the consumption of carbs before or after exercise is probably not advantageous for fat loss.

Thus, if your primary goal is weight loss, we suggest forgetting about targeted keto until a good study in keto-adapted athletes demonstrates otherwise.

? HOW DO I DO TARGETED KETO?

As with cyclic keto, there is a difference between strategically consuming carbohydrates and eating poorly while using exercise as an excuse. If used, targeted keto should be consuming a

---

119 Rachel M. Gregory, H. Hamdan, D. M. Torisky, and J. D. Akers, "A Low-Carbohydrate Ketogenic Diet Combined with 6-Weeks of Crossfit Training Improves Body Composition and Performance," *International Journal of Sports Exerercise Medicine* 3 (2017): 1-10.

moderate amount of the appropriate carbohydrates, not crushing Pop-Tarts before or after your workout. Since there is no research on targeted keto, it is hard to make an exact prescription. If you are following targeted keto for the sake of competition, it may be best to take the approach of "train low-compete high." That means avoid the carbs during training and use them strategically for competition. The reason for this is that you are training your body to become an effective fat burner, which will come in handy during the competition, especially if the competition is long enough or intense enough to require an additional fuel source outside of the ingested carbohydrates.

If you do take this approach, do not go into competition blind, unfamiliar with how your body will respond to the ingested carbohydrates. Run a mock trial of your competition with various carbohydrate types and amounts to find out what your body responds to best.

If you are using targeted keto as a method of improving your training sessions, consuming around 20-30 grams of carbs 30 minutes prior to exercise from nutrient dense carb sources like sweet potatoes, rice, or fruit may provide some benefit.

If you are following targeted keto with the goal of stimulating muscle mass, consuming carbs during the post-exercise window would be the best approach. Again, the carb type, amount, and timing of ingestion are dependent on the person and should be experimented with. When I had the chance to ask keto trainer Jane Downes, who uses this approach to gain muscle, she recommended 30-50 grams of carbs from sweet potatoes post-workout and has found that using fruit during this time is not advantageous.

We recommend self-experimenting with this approach to see how it affects not only your performance but also your recovery after performance. Save this self-experiment for when you are keto-adapted to get a better idea if it will actually provide you with benefit.

MODIFIED ATKINS

? WHAT IS MODIFIED ATKINS?

> *Short Answer:* Modified Atkins is a higher fat version of the traditional Atkins Diet, making it a higher protein ketogenic diet.

You may have heard this term while searching for keto. The Modified Atkins Diet (MAD) is, like it sounds, a modified version of the formally popular Atkins Diet. Dr. Robert Atkins was close to nailing it with his diet; he just failed to focus on food quality and increasing fat intake to better provide energy to the body.

MAD was first introduced to Chris at a conference a few years ago by the great Dr. Eric Kossoff, professor of neurology and pediatrics at Johns Hopkins Children's Center. MAD can be an effective alternative to a ketogenic diet, especially for those with more muscle mass, training at a high intensity, or looking to bust through a weight loss plateau.

? IS MAD AN EFFECTIVE APPROACH?

Anecdotally, we often find that once someone is keto adapted, lowering fat a bit and increasing protein tends to promote fat loss, especially in those who are stuck at a weight loss plateau. Again, there is not a whole lot of research to support this, but the thought here is that once adapted to keto, lowering dietary fat may promote an increased reliance on body fat burning, especially if there is a lot of stored fat available.

Additionally, if you recall from earlier in this book, low protein on keto can lead to muscle loss, which can be prevented using a MAD approach. Furthermore, for those who have an increased demand for protein, such as those exercising at a high intensity or those who have more muscle mass, this approach can be effective for maintaining or gaining muscle mass.

Several studies have also found this approach to be effective for seizure control, demonstrating its ability to provide similar therapeutic benefits to the traditional "high-fat-moderate protein" keto diet.[120]

Some people may find MAD a little easier, since consuming enough fat is a common complaint of new keto dieters. However, we tend to recommend this approach for someone who is a little more experienced with keto. When you first start keto, your body may require the additional fat for energy, since it is not yet adapted to efficiently burning fat and producing and utilizing ketones.

? HOW DO I DO MAD?

This approach does not mean that you should pay no attention to protein intake. Rather, strategically increase it to achieve your goal. The traditional MAD is based on a 1:1 fat to protein ratio, making it higher protein and lower fat compared to a

---

120 Eric H. Kossoff, Jane R. McGrogan, Renee M. Bluml, Diana J. Pillas, James E. Rubenstein, and Eileen P. Vining, "A Modified Atkins Diet is Effective for the Treatment of Intractable Pediatric Epilepsy," *Epilepsia* 47, no. 2 (2006): 421-424.

traditional keto diet. However, we use MAD as an umbrella term to describe all higher protein variations of keto.

A MAD approach can be achieved through macronutrient counting or just the incorporation of higher protein, lower fat meats which can be found in Chapter 7. Removing oils and adding more protein is another effective way to accomplish the MAD shift in macronutrients. If you feel like your energy is low, you may be going too low with your fat. In this case, tracking your macros can be beneficial.

Additionally, if you are following this approach, you should pay attention to your total calorie intake. Fat provides 9 calories per gram while protein only provides 4. That means that decreasing your fat intake and increasing your protein consumption can lead to a drop in total caloric intake. Remember, drastically under consuming calories for too long is not beneficial.

CARNIVORE DIET

WHAT IS THE CARNIVORE DIET?

The boom we saw in keto several years ago is now hitting the carnivore diet. We're sure you could guess this: the carnivore diet is either a strictly meat-based diet or animal-based diet. Just as when keto was starting to get popular, it is often met with much controversy.

This carnivore diet has been popularized by folks like Dr. Shawn Baker and Jordan Peterson and has been a topic of discussion on several popular Joe Rogan podcast episodes. While both of us have tried it and like it, just like keto, there is a right and wrong way to follow this approach.

Like most of the variations of keto mentioned in this chapter, there is limited scientific evidence on carnivore, but that doesn't mean that it isn't effective. There are many benefits associated with carnivore, such as decreased inflammation, improved insulin sensitivity, improved blood lipid profiles, increased energy, improved gut health, improved cognitive function, better hormone production, and the most popular, weight loss. There are also many potential therapeutic uses of the carnivore diet.

? IS CARNIVORE AN EFFECTIVE APPROACH?

As stated, this diet has not been evaluated much in research, so exact mechanisms behind its benefits have not been fully established. However, we can speculate on several mechanisms behind why a carnivore diet tends to work.

Like keto, carbs are cut out, but in the case of carnivore they are reduced to a greater degree. Since carnivore is strictly animal based, it is functionally a no-carb diet, with the exception of organ meat. We know that cutting out carbs leads to improved insulin sensitivity and reduced inflammation.

Second, carnivore is essentially an intense elimination diet, even more than keto. On carnivore, you are limiting your food choices to meat alone, and like most elimination diets, there are short-term benefits to this, primarily the improvements in gut health. Removing all other foods out of your diet leads to the death of many gut bacteria and a sort of "gut reset." This can be extremely beneficial since the overgrowth of "bad bacteria" can lead to a wide variety of health problems. Resetting the gut allows you to re-populate it with "good bacteria," which can have a profound effect on numerous aspects of overall health and wellness.

Third, since the carnivore diet is limited to meat, it allows for more protein in the diet, which can be beneficial for a lot of people and for particular goals.

The weight loss potential of carnivore is one of the main reasons this diet is popular. While there are several mechanisms in play, the reduction in hunger and cravings are a huge contributor. It is hard to overeat on the carnivore diet, even more so than a traditional keto diet. Of course, we do not think that calories are the end all be all for weight loss, but they do play a role, and overeating calories can be counterproductive for weight loss.

Why does carnivore have a stronger ability to reduce hunger and cravings? Primarily because it lacks "hyper-palatability." The diet does not have a ton of flavor compared to a standard keto diet; lack of flavor can limit hunger and cravings. Furthermore, meat has a texture that is a little chewier compared to many other foods, which can promote fullness thus preventing overeating.

On a carnivore diet you consume a lot of red meat, which also means an increased intake of saturated fat. Contrary to conventional wisdom, saturated fat will not kill you and can be a good way to improve hormone production, which is why this diet is promoted for its libido boosting capabilities.

IS CARNIVORE SAFE?

Short Answer: There is limited research on carnivore, but so far, we have not seen a reason to fear using it strategically.

The carnivore diet has not been evaluated by researchers. We cannot definitively say that this diet is either safe or unsafe. However, on a properly formulated carnivore diet, you are eating real food, and there is nothing to suggest that this would be particularly dangerous.

However, there are several things wrong with the way some people approach carnivore. As with keto, food quality matters, and this is especially true when following a diet based on the consumption of one food group. If the only food you are eating is low quality, then you are only putting low-quality foods in your body. As mentioned earlier, low-quality meat can mean increased consumption of pro-inflammatory fats, preventing many of the benefits that should come from carnivore. A carnivore diet centered around bacon and grain-fed meat is probably not the best approach. A carnivore diet centered around grass-fed and finished beef and maybe incorporating high-quality fish is a different story.

At the time when we were writing this book, if you typed "carnivore diet" into Google, you would primarily find people saying how unhealthy and unsafe it is. However, none of it is useful evidence, even if it does come from registered dieticians. Don't get caught up in titles; not reading or understanding research is still not reading or understanding research, whether you are an RD, MD, or PhD. The point here is that the majority of the reasons people are saying that carnivore is bad is because of the stigma that meat is bad, fat is bad, red meat is bad, or saturated fat is bad. All of which we know is not true.

Another reason why some speculate that carnivore is unhealthy is because of the dogma that vegetables are incredibly healthy. While it is true that vegetables can provide some benefits, they are not as necessary as many people think. As mentioned previously in the book, yes, vegetables are high in micronutrients; however, the micronutrients found in vegetables are not very bioavailable—they are not absorbed very well. While consuming vegetables may mean that you are taking in a high amount of micros, you may not actually be efficiently utilizing many of these micros.

Micronutrients are also found in meat, particularly high-quality meat. If an animal is eating greens, its muscles are saturated with the micros you are trying to get from consuming vegetables—except the micros in this muscle tissue is much more bioavailable for humans. Long story short, you don't need vegetables to survive so removing them, at least in the short term, does not appear to be harmful.

The only relevant argument we have heard against long-term carnivore is gut health. Since carnivore is essentially an elimination diet, the complete removal of all other bacteria may not be the best approach for an extended period of time. Dr. Rhonda Patrick has expressed concern that having only amino acid (protein) fermenting bacteria in the gut could promote the production of harmful compounds. However, it has yet to be determined what the threshold for this is and when this problem would outweigh the benefits of carnivore.

Although we cannot say whether or not a carnivore diet is safe for everyone nor recommend it for everyone, we can say that we have both tried it, and when done right have seen numerous benefits from it.

? HOW DO I FOLLOW A CARNIVORE DIET?

If you have read this, conducted your own research and decided that carnivore is something you want to try, check out our recommendations. Again, if you are new to keto, we do not recommend this approach. Although carnivore could be the best approach for a beginner (because it would allow for a gut reset followed by a reintroduction of foods that would promote the production of healthy gut bacteria), it is extremely restrictive and likely will be much harder for a beginner to stick to. The best approach is to start with a traditional keto diet and become adapted prior to giving carnivore a try.

Here are a few laws to stick with if you try the carnivore diet:

RULE #1: HIGH-QUALITY MEAT

100 percent grass-fed/grass-finished is the gold standard, but at the very least your meat should be primarily grass fed.

RULE #2: INCLUDE ORGAN MEAT

Yes, organ meat is not the most appetizing thing to eat but it is one of the most nutrient dense foods. Organ meat contains many bioavailable micronutrients. We view organ meats as a must on carnivore. That does not mean you have to eat them everyday, but a couple of times a week is recommended.

RULE #3: LIMIT PORK

Yes, pork is meat, but it is very difficult to get high-quality pork, so it should not be your primary source of meat on any diet, including a carnivore diet. Yes, that means not going crazy with bacon.

RULE #4: INCLUDE SOME HIGH-QUALITY FISH

Fish offers its own benefits, particularly the omega-3 fatty acid content. Add fish occasionally into your carnivore diet to increase the consumption of these anti-inflammatory fats.

RULE #5: DON'T FRY YOUR MEAT

If you fry the heck out of your meat you can burn off a lot of the beneficial nutrients and oxidize the fats, causing them to be harmful to your health. To maintain the nutrient profile of your meat, cook on lower heat.

RULE #6: STICK TO THE PRINCIPLES OF GENERAL KETO

Carnivore is very similar to keto, so stick to the same basics: supplementing with electrolytes, staying hydrated, managing stress, getting some movement in, and focusing on sleep quality.

Outside of these rules, there are some other aspects to consider. When it comes to oils, a true carnivore diet would mean using butter or lard for cooking; however, we think that the use of other keto-friendly oils, like coconut oil, isn't going to hurt and will likely provide some additional benefits.

Dairy, while it does come from animals, should probably be limited on carnivore, especially if you are doing this diet with the goal of resetting your gut. We like to cycle the use of pasture-raised locally sourced eggs into carnivore, but some may benefit from completely cutting these out, especially if they were previously consuming a lot of eggs.

We do not know the most effective duration to follow a carnivore diet, but we speculate that benefits from the diet can be experienced between 2-6 weeks, after which we recommend getting some blood work done and paying attention to how your body reacts to determine if you should continue following the diet or transition back to a traditional keto diet.

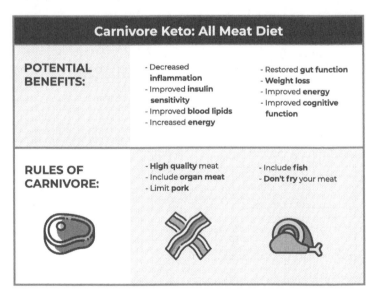

Carnivore Keto: All Meat Diet

POTENTIAL BENEFITS:	- Decreased inflammation - Improved insulin sensitivity - Improved blood lipids - Increased energy	- Restored gut function - Weight loss - Improved energy - Improved cognitive function
RULES OF CARNIVORE:	- High quality meat - Include organ meat - Limit pork	- Include fish - Don't fry your meat

We have both experimented with each of the variations of keto discussed in this chapter. Currently, we both follow closer to a MAD diet and often like to incorporate the carnivore approach. Once we became adapted to the keto diet, we found these approaches to be the best for meeting our goals and the demands of our bodies.

Do not let yourself become overwhelmed with the different types of keto diets discussed in this chapter. Again, if you are new to keto then you need to start with the basics by following keto the way we mapped it out in Chapter 7. Once you have become adapted to keto that way, you can begin experimenting with different variations of the diet based on the goal you are looking to achieve.

CHAPTER 11

KETO FOR WOMEN

There are a lot of questions specific to women that come up frequently when starting a ketogenic diet. As we will get into in this chapter, the way the body responds to keto is similar between men and women, but there are some differences and certain use cases of the diet that are specific to women. For this reason, the ladies are getting their own chapter.

Before we dive in it is important to point out that women are not used as research subjects as often as men because of variables like shifting hormones over the course of a month, which make inferring conclusions from a study more difficult. However, we are starting to see more research demonstrating the efficacy of keto for women. We need to continue to improve our understanding of how exactly the diet impacts women and how it can be best used for various conditions.

? IS KETO SAFE FOR WOMEN?

Ketosis is a safe state of metabolism for adults of all shapes and sizes and has many health benefits. Many people argue that keto is not safe for women. We think those people are sad and need some help. While women are extremely different from men, there is no reason to speculate that keto is unsafe for women. In fact, when it comes to nutrition, for many women, a ketogenic diet is the best option.

In addition to some of the use cases we will be highlighting throughout this chapter, we do have plenty of research demonstrating improvements for women following a keto diet, including improvements in blood pressure, lipids, fasting glucose, and insulin[121] and improvements in body composition when used in conjunction with resistance training.[122]

? IS KETO DIFFERENT FOR WOMEN?

> *Short Answer:* Women and men may see different degrees of response to the diet but the general response to the diet is the same.

The physiological changes that occur on a ketogenic diet, such as increased ketone production and lower blood glucose, insulin, and inflammation, occur in women just as they do in men. However, it is common to see men respond a little better to any dietary change compared to women. Many times, we have

---

121 Bonnie J. Brehm, Randy J. Seeley, Stephen R. Daniels, and David A. D'alessio, "A Randomized Trial Comparing a Very Low Carbohydrate Diet and a Calorie-Restricted Low Fat Diet on Body Weight and Cardiovascular Risk Factors in Healthy Women," *The Journal of Clinical Endocrinology & Metabolism* 88, no. 4 (2003): 1617-1623.

122 Pal T. Jabekk, Ingvild A. Moe, Helge D. Meen, Sissel E. Tomten, and Arne T. Høstmark, "Resistance Training in Overweight Women on a Ketogenic Diet Conserved Lean Body Mass While Reducing Body Fat," *Nutrition & Metabolism* 7, no. 1 (2010): 17.

spoken to a woman who has started keto with her male counterpart and is frustrated that he is feeling amazing and losing weight while she is not seeing as much progress and not feeling so well.

One thing to point out here is that the difference in weight loss between men and women at the start of keto is a result of greater water and glycogen loss in men. Typically, men are bigger and more muscular, which means their bodies can hold more water and glycogen. They have more, so they have more to lose.

Regardless, we still tend to see that women respond a little different to keto compared to men and while we do not have a great explanation of why this happens, it is likely that hormone fluctuation is a key factor.

Women's hormones fluctuate more frequently and to a greater degree than men's, and hormone levels can impact responses to the food you eat. Furthermore, any drastic dietary change can result in hormone alterations, which appear to impact women a little more than men. For this reason, some people speculate that a slower transition into keto for women may be the best approach; however, currently we do not have any evidence that this approach is better.

A bigger factor than the dramatic change in carbohydrate consumption when switching to keto is the subsequent reduction in calories that tends to accompany this dietary change—and it is not uncommon to see this happen to a greater degree in women. We suggest that women not severely calorie-restrict when starting keto, since this, in combination with a big dietary change, may cause adverse side effects when starting keto.

We recommend starting a whole food, high-quality version of a keto diet that optimizes your micronutrient intake while keeping your calorie intake high enough to meet the demands of your body.

If calories and food quality are dialed in, transitioning to keto should be a lot easier for women. However, another factor that makes keto different and a little more difficult for women is menstrual cycles due to some of the common PMS symptoms. During menstrual cycles, it is common to experience increased cravings and trouble digesting foods, among other common symptoms like cramps, headaches, bloating, and impaired mood. These can make sticking to a big dietary change that much harder. For this reason, it may not be advisable for a woman to start keto around their menstrual cycle.

? WHAT ARE THE BEST SITUATIONS FOR WOMEN TO DO KETO?

Keto is beneficial for most women under most conditions. However, there may be some specific situations when keto is especially beneficial for women, such as:

- Looking to experience weight loss
- Weight loss plateaus
- Impaired sex hormone profiles
- During or prior to menopause
- Frequent irregular periods
- Individuals who are planning on becoming pregnant

Keto can be helpful in these situations primarily because of the way the diet impacts hormones. Women can also follow a keto diet simply for the benefits in overall health and wellness.

? WHAT IMPACT DOES KETO HAVE ON HORMONES IN WOMEN?

Keto has a unique ability to impact hormones. Typically, as women become adapted to a keto diet, they begin to experience more balance in their hormones, which can be beneficial for women of all ages. Women who are menstruating may experience reduced PMS symptoms as well as more regular cycles. Women who are perimenopausal or menopausal may also see reduced side effects during this time.

This is likely a result of lowering insulin and improving sex hormone production, which also provides potential therapeutic benefit for women suffering from polycystic ovary syndrome (PCOS), which we will discuss more soon.

Furthermore, when it comes to hormones, the HPA axis is also important to consider. The HPA axis is a complex relationship between your hypothalamus, pituitary, adrenal glands. The hypothalamus sends signals to your pituitary and adrenal glands to stimulate hormone production. Contrary to common belief, keto does not mess this up. In fact, there is some evidence that keto could improve hypothalamus signaling, thus improving this mechanism.

? DOES KETO DESTROY YOUR THYROID?

Thyroid function is another common concern people have regarding keto dieting for women. Two important hormones secreted by the thyroid are T3 and T4. These hormones play a big role in regulating metabolism, amongst many other bodily functions. While keto has been reported to reduce thyroid hormone production (typically thought of as a bad thing), there have not been any well-controlled studies in humans to confirm this. Most of the reports are anecdotal, meaning that there could be plenty of other factors at play.

The truth is, interpreting changes in hormones is different on a keto diet. It is speculated that your body improves signaling and response to hormone production, decreasing the need to stimulate more production of a particular hormone. In this case that would mean increased thyroid hormone sensitivity. Seem impossible? It's widely accepted that keto improves insulin sensitivity, meaning you don't need to produce as much insulin to manage carbs, due to improved insulin and cell communication. A similar mechanism could apply to other hormones like those produced by the thyroid, but more research is still needed.

❓ WHAT ABOUT WOMEN WHO ARE COLD, LOSE THEIR HAIR, AND MISS THEIR PERIODS ON KETO?

Women certainly can experience adverse side effects on a ketogenic diet. However, with every woman we've worked with we've found that this is not a problem from being in ketosis, but rather doing keto incorrectly.

It is not uncommon for many women to start a ketogenic diet and fall victim to one or all three of the following problems:

- Extreme caloric restriction
- Undereating protein
- Overtraining in an attempt to lose more fat

Any of these issues alone can cause problems with your hormones, especially your thyroid. All three together is a recipe for disaster. Again, it's important to eat enough protein on keto (remember, don't fear gluconeogenesis) and that you eat enough overall food to make sure your body can thrive.

If you're just switching to a ketogenic diet, you don't need to be extreme and do thirteen CrossFit classes a week. Changing your entire metabolism is a stressful event and adding an unnecessary amount of physical stress to that isn't going to speed up your results—it will hamper them. If you're a woman and experiencing any of the above problems, take a step back and make sure that you are eating enough food, especially enough protein, and that you're not running yourself into the ground with exercise.

? CAN I GET PREGNANT ON A KETO DIET?

Yes! In fact, ketosis might be the best nutrition strategy to help get pregnant. The opportunity to improve fertility through a low-carb, high-fat diet is widely ignored but has solid applications. Sex hormones, the uterus, and everything else needed for reproduction requires fat—especially saturated fat.

If you are looking to improve fertility, make sure you are getting enough fat. The body will not want to reproduce if it can't even take care of itself. Calorie restriction is common on a ketogenic diet—not on purpose, but because fat is so filling and satiety signaling is commonly a result of ketosis. For this reason, tracking your food in an app to make sure you're eating enough is a good idea. You may find it appropriate to overeat slightly, since the body will be much more likely to reproduce in times of plenty. This doesn't mean go overboard and guzzle down a gallon of coconut oil per day. We're talking maybe about 200-250 kcal above what you might normally need.

Don't be hungry, be satisfied. We also recommend avoiding fasting during this time. Again, you're trying to signal to your body that it has everything it needs to make an entirely new human.

You should also be mindful of eating real foods. The foods you eat should be additive to your body's health, not subtractive. Prioritize the absolute highest quality of fats. This means grass-fed animal products, high-quality oils, etc.

In addition to fat consumption, keto's ability to lower insulin levels and reduce insulin resistance further contribute to improved fertility via increases in sex hormone production. Reducing inflammation and improving body composition can also have a positive impact on fertility.

? IS KETO A GOOD OPTION FOR PCOS?

If you've had irregular periods, infertility, somewhat "masculine" features, anxiety, fatigue, or low sex drive, you could be suffering from a condition known as polycystic ovarian syndrome, or PCOS. It is a common condition that affects women, usually in their teen years. The biggest problem with PCOS is that while research has reported that between 12-21 percent of women in their reproductive years have the condition, it is estimated that 70 percent of women with PCOS go undiagnosed.[123]

Another problem with PCOS is that it is named a "syndrome." Syndromes are just collections of symptoms that we call such because there is no other easy way to describe them. It can be difficult to know of the root cause of syndromes, which means they can be hard to treat. PCOS is thought to be caused by hormonal imbalances between luteinizing hormone (LH) and follicle stimulating hormone (FSH). When LH production is too high, the body will start producing testosterone which can lead to the slew of symptoms typically experienced

---

123 Jacqueline Boyle and Helena J. Teede, "Polycystic Ovary Syndrome: An Update," *Australian Family Physician* 41, no. 10 (2012): 752-756.

on PCOS, such as ovarian cysts, excessive body hair, irregular menses, acne, weight gain, infertility, and low sex drive.

In addition to the altered sex hormones, PCOS is also characterized by insulin resistance and inflammation, which offers up the hypothesis that a ketogenic diet could be beneficial for this condition. This is especially important since most treatment modalities for PCOS have proved to be ineffective. While the research is limited, a 2005 study put keto to the test by investigating the effects of the diet on patients with PCOS.[124] In this study, 11 obese women with PCOS were instructed to follow a ketogenic diet for 24 weeks. Participants returned to the clinic every two weeks for measurements and help sticking to the diet.

At the end of the study, those who completed the program lowered their body weight by an average of 12 percent, their testosterone by 22 percent, luteinizing hormone/follicle stimulating hormone ratio by 36 percent and fasting insulin by 54 percent. Researchers also reported non-significant decreases in glucose, HbA1c, triglycerides, and perceived body hair. In addition, two women became pregnant during the study despite previous infertility problems (a little support to the previous question on fertility)! If that doesn't tell you there is something to look at, then we don't know what will.

The primary reason why the keto diet can offer therapeutic value to PCOS is the improved insulin levels, lower inflammation, weight loss, and improved metabolism, all of which provide a positive impact on PCOS symptoms.

124 John C. Mavropoulos, William S. Yancy, Juanita Hepburn, and Eric C. Westman, "The Effects of a Low-Carbohydrate, Ketogenic Diet on The Polycystic Ovary Syndrome: A Pilot Study," *Nutrition & Metabolism* 2, no. 1 (2005): 2:35.

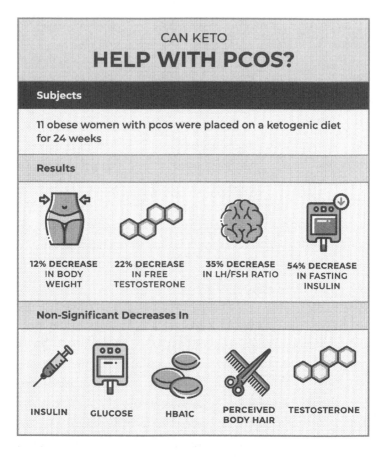

CAN KETO
HELP WITH PCOS?

Subjects

11 obese women with pcos were placed on a ketogenic diet for 24 weeks

Results

| 12% DECREASE IN BODY WEIGHT | 22% DECREASE IN FREE TESTOSTERONE | 35% DECREASE IN LH/FSH RATIO | 54% DECREASE IN FASTING INSULIN |

Non-Significant Decreases In

| INSULIN | GLUCOSE | HBA1C | PERCEIVED BODY HAIR | TESTOSTERONE |

Additionally, because fat is the precursor to our sex hormones, it makes sense that many of the hormone imbalances associated with PCOS are remedied by a (healthy) high-fat diet. Other things to prioritize if you're addressing PCOS are exercise, stress reduction, and restful sleep.

? IS KETO SAFE FOR WOMEN DURING PREGNANCY?

There is no valid reason to think that ketosis and low-carb dieting during pregnancy is unsafe. Before you troll us by saying we don't have research to back this up, we know. We do not have research studies on pregnant women on a keto diet because that is not an ethical study; pregnant women should not be used as test subjects.

When anyone talks about ketosis being unsafe in pregnancy, they're likely referencing studies on diabetic ketoacidosis (DKA) which have demonstrated DKA being harmful to fetal brain development.[125] Remember, DKA is dangerous but much different from nutritional ketosis, which is safe and beneficial. DKA is extremely rare in pregnancy and is a result of either a Type I diabetic pregnancy or gestational diabetes. DKA will not occur on a ketogenic diet. Regardless, misunderstandings like this has led to a widely accepted belief that ketosis during pregnancy is harmful to the baby.

Let's look at some actual facts. Women accumulate stored fat in the first half of gestation that can be utilized for energy and ketone production in the latter half of gestation.[126] Most pregnant women suffer from morning sickness, at least in the beginning of their pregnancy. Between that, nausea, low appetite and food aversions, it's not uncommon for women to eat sporadically and lightly, at least during the first trimester. This will naturally take pregnant women temporarily in and out of ketosis, and is one of the reasons why research has demonstrated that healthy pregnant women have ketone levels that are three times higher than women who are not pregnant.[127]

---

125 D. Kamalakannan, V. Baskar, D. M. Barton, and T. A. M. Abdu, "Diabetic Ketoacidosis in Pregnancy," *Postgraduate Medical Journal* 79, no. 934 (2003): 454-457.

126 G. E. Shambaugh 3rd, "Ketone Body Metabolism in the Mother and Fetus," *Federal Proceedings*, vol. 44, no. 7 (1985): 2347-51.

127 Mary CJ Rudolf, and Robert S. Sherwin, "Maternal Ketosis and its Effects on the Fetus," *Clinics in Endocrinology and Metabolism* 12, no. 2 (1983): 413-428.

These ketones are not just used by the mother but also by the baby to contribute to development, especially in the brain.[128]

The point here isn't that expecting mothers need to go keto; the point is that ketosis naturally occurs during pregnancy and appears to be beneficial for the baby so we should not fear it. As registered dietitian Lily Nichols has said, it seems safe for women to eat lower carb during pregnancy as long as they are still eating certain foods for proper nutrition. Fetuses require both glucose and ketones to grow, so a balance is key. What's important is to ensure the mother has normal blood sugar levels and is getting enough calories.

Here are some things to keep in mind for those who are pregnant, whether following keto or not:

DON'T AIM FOR WEIGHT LOSS
The ketogenic diet is effective for weight loss, but pregnancy is not the time to pursue it. Getting enough calories and proper nutrition is most important.

EAT WHOLE FOODS
Good nutrition is especially vital when you're growing a baby. Get high-quality whole foods dense in micronutrients

AVOID REFINED GRAINS, ADDED SUGARS, AND PROCESSED FOODS
If you are consuming carbohydrates, the quality of carbohydrates is important to ensure the diet is nutrient-dense and both mom and baby are getting the good stuff they need to thrive.

---

128 Emilio Herrera and Encarnación Amusquivar, "Lipid Metabolism in the Fetus and the Newborn," *Diabetes/Metabolism Research and Reviews* 16, no. 3 (2000): 202-210.

DON'T DO INTERMITTENT FASTING

While intermittent fasting has a variety of benefits for the average person, it's not appropriate during pregnancy when it's most important to listen to your own hunger cues and ensure mother and baby are getting enough nutrients for growth.

An important point we want to make is that if you are fearing that a low-carb diet is unsafe for your baby but are following a standard American diet, your line of thinking is flawed. It is extremely important to take precautions with the foods you are eating during pregnancy and many pregnant mothers fail to do this. There have been numerous times where we have heard expecting mothers say that they were following a low-carb or ketogenic diet prior to pregnancy but stopped once they became pregnant because they heard it was unsafe. Yet they consume massive amounts of processed carbohydrates and other low-quality foods without even a second thought. We feel pretty confident in saying that a low-carb diet is going to be more beneficial for your baby than a diet chock full of Oreos and gummy bears.

To reiterate, we are not necessarily recommending that you try keto while pregnant. In fact, you likely shouldn't change anything major while you're pregnant since drastically altering nutrition is stressful to the body no matter what the diet is. If you have never done low-carb or keto dieting, starting during pregnancy may not be advised. Sticking to a low-carb approach is probably a better approach. If you are keto leading up to pregnancy, then it appears that continuing your diet or making some small adjustments can be beneficial. As always, consult with a keto-understanding physician to ensure that you are on the path toward the most optimal pregnancy.

❓ IS KETO SAFE DURING BREASTFEEDING?

Another common fear is that keto will impair breastfeeding, but again there is not much validity to these concerns either. As with pregnancy, the current scientific literature surrounding the ketogenic diet and breastfeeding is extremely limited. A literature review looking at the evidence of the impact of maternal nutrition on breast milk composition concluded that "the available information on this topic is scarce and diversified. Most of the evidence currently used in clinical practice to make recommendations is limited to studies that only reported indirect associations."[129] This tells us that there is reason to question current recommendations.

One study comparing a high-fat/low-carb diet, to a high-carb/low-fat diet in breastfeeding women found that regardless of the diet, daily breast milk production and daily infant breast milk intake remained the same.[130] Neither diet had an effect on milk lactose or protein concentration; however, milk fat concentration and the energy content of milk were higher during the low-carb diet than the high-carb diet. Infants' energy intake was also higher for babies whose mothers were on the low-carb diet.

----

129 Francesca Bravi, Frank Wiens, Adriano Decarli, Alessia Dal Pont, Carlo Agostoni, and Monica Ferraroni,"Impact of Maternal Nutrition on Breast-milk Composition: A Systematic Review," *The American Journal of Clinical Nutrition* 104, no. 3 (2016): 646-662.

130 Mahmoud A. Mohammad, Agneta L. Sunehag, and Morey W. Haymond, "Effect of Dietary Macronutrient Composition under Moderate Hypocaloric Intake on Maternal Adaptation During Lactation," *The American Journal of Clinical Nutrition* 89, no. 6 (2009): 1821-1827.

Besides the fact that the low-carb diet did not impair milk production, it increased fat concentration in milk. Interestingly, breast milk contains a high percentage of MCTs, which is one of the reasons why babies are born and remain in a state of ketosis until they are introduced to carbohydrates. Both the fat and ketones present in an infant's body are important for growth and development, especially for the brain.

Although there are anecdotal reports that some mothers have had reductions in milk production after going keto, this is most likely due to factors, such as dehydration, lack of adequate calories or nutrients, and possible lack of adjustment in cases of rapid carbohydrate restriction, which is why certain strategies should be used to ensure success when breastfeeding on a keto diet.

TIPS FOR SUCCESSFUL BREASTFEEDING WHILE FOLLOWING A KETOGENIC DIET

Breastfeeding your baby is important, and most mothers don't want to do anything that might risk their supply. We've already demonstrated that you can follow a ketogenic lifestyle while breastfeeding (and it could even help you shed some of the baby weight), but you need to do it properly. Here's how:

#1: Start Keto Early

When you first start keto, your body needs to go through an adjustment period, and you may feel flu-like symptoms. This is called the "keto flu," and if you've never experienced it before, you may feel as if there's something wrong. You don't want to have to go through this adjustment period while you're trying to learn the particular art of breastfeeding, so being adapted to keto going into pregnancy may be best to ensure that you limit keto-flu side effects if you are doing keto while breastfeeding.

#2: *Avoid Dehydration*
One of the biggest culprits of scarce milk supply is not drinking enough water throughout the day. Your body uses extra water to produce breast milk and heal from labor and delivery. Hydration is especially important for mothers on keto, due to the higher excretion of water from lower carbohydrate intake.

#3: *Don't Forget Your Nutrients and Electrolytes*
Consuming enough vitamins and minerals is extremely important to avoid any negative side effects, such as headaches, loss of energy, or light-headedness.

#4: *Consume Enough Calories, Especially High-Quality Fats*
The most important nutritional factor when breastfeeding is the quality of food being eaten. You should, without question, prioritize making the right choices around food. Make sure you have a steady supply of energy throughout the day for both yourself and your baby. Consuming adequate calories and enough good quality fats will be other keys to producing healthy quantities of milk and fueling both you and the baby.

#5: *Try a Moderate Low-Carb Diet Rather Than Strict Keto*
If you're having trouble producing adequate milk, try starting with 50-75 grams of carbs per day and slowly lowering the carbs each day (say 5-10 grams), tracking how it affects your milk supply. Make sure you are getting your carbs from healthy sources such as vegetables, nuts, seeds, and berries. Avoid bread, pasta, and other refined carbage (carbs + garbage = carbage).

#6: *Track Your Food/Drink Consumption and Daily Milk Production*
Use an app, such as MyFitnessPal or My Macros+, to keep track of the foods and drinks you are consuming—this will

make it easier to track your calorie and fat consumption as it relates to how much milk you are producing each day, so you can adjust accordingly. Also try to track your daily milk production. This might mean pumping and feeding your baby expressed breast milk for a couple of days. You can use an app like Baby Connect to track your production. Do remember that babies extract more milk than a pump, and the quality of your breast pump also impacts your output.

While weight loss should not be a primary goal during breast-feeding, many women do like to begin making strides at losing weight during this time. Interestingly, in the above study, women on the low-carb diet actually burned more calories compared to women on the high-carb diet. This offers the possibility that keto may be the best diet for ensuring optimal breastmilk production but also tackling that baby weight.

Despite what the internet tells you, women should not fear keto dieting. While some situations may require a little more care and attention to detail, there are actually a lot of reasons why women should follow a keto diet.

A big call out to science is to start conducting more research in women. While these studies can be a little more challenging, we simply cannot apply what we see happen in men over to women. Especially as it relates to conditions that only occur in women, such as PCOS and menopause. We look forward to more research shedding light on how a ketogenic diet can best help the ladies out there.

CHAPTER 12

HOW TO STAY KETO

Keto can provide its most robust benefits when it is adopted as a lifestyle and not a short-term diet. The problem is that around 90 percent of diets fail so if you are going to succeed at adopting the ketogenic diet long term, then it is crucial that you find the best ways to incorporate keto into your lifestyle. Diets suck—if you make keto a diet, it will also suck.

This means finding a balance between what is most optimal and what is most sustainable. Thus far we have discussed the most optimal approaches to implementing keto; however, what is most optimal is not always most sustainable. In order to make this a sustainable lifestyle, you must figure out how to best make the diet fit your life. This means learning to eat in different situations, learning when it is okay to cheat, how to manage dietary slip ups, and how to replace your favorite non-keto foods.

Note that if you are following this diet for therapeutic reasons, depending on the condition, some of this chapter may not apply to you. Optimizing your treatment may require constant

100 percent attention to detail. This would be something you would discuss with a keto-approved physician.

TRAVELING ON KETO

? CAN I TRAVEL WHILE ON KETO?

Traveling can make following a diet a little harder. However, staying in ketosis while you travel is very possible, as long as you plan ahead and make a commitment to yourself to make the best choices available. While you may not be able to control some things like food quality (try your best though), you can still make keto food choices and that is part of making this diet a lifestyle.

Follow these tips to set yourself up for success on keto while traveling.

PLAN AHEAD
Book a hotel or vacation rental with a kitchen, kitchenette, or at least a mini fridge. This will allow you to cook some of your own meals. When you arrive at your destination, head to a local farmers market or grocery store and stock up on all the keto essentials. This is especially important for longer trips to avoid eating every meal out for an extended period of time.

Research keto-friendly restaurants in your destination. No matter where you are traveling, you can search for keto-friendly restaurants in your area. Keep reading to see our keto restaurant advice!

PACK ACCORDINGLY
Whether you are on the road or in the air, strategically packing can be a great way to help you stay the course. If you are traveling by plane, pack items that don't need to be refrigerated.

If you are going on a road trip, pack a small cooler full of pre-made meals and snacks.

Packable Keto Options
- Perfect Keto Bars
- Keto Base single packs
- MCT single packs
- Collagen single pack
- Perfect Keto Coffee
- Biltong or beef jerky
- Beef or meat sticks
- Raw nuts
- Hard-boiled eggs
- Fresh celery and nut butter (think ants on a log... without the ants)
- Fat bombs
- Nut butter individual packs
- Sardines
- Seaweed snack
- Kale chips
- Pork rinds
- Boxed bone broth
- Olives
- Small bottled olive oil or other healthy oils (great alternatives for dressing)

ROAD TRAVEL

If you are on the road traveling, the package options above will be especially useful since on the road you are more susceptible to being stuck with hunger and lack of keto options.

If you forget to pack snacks or run out, don't fear, even gas stations contain some keto-friendly snacks. While the quality is typically not ideal, you can still find keto snacks in almost every gas station. Here is a list of the most common keto-friendly gas station snacks:

- Hard-boiled eggs
- Nuts (best choices don't contain vegetable oils)
- Pork rinds (best choices don't contain vegetable oils)
- Beef jerky (most contain too much sugar so check labels)

AIR TRAVEL

Air travel can present its own challenges to anyone, especially those on a ketogenic diet. Here are some of our best hacks for air travel.

Fasting

Fasting is a fantastic tool to use when traveling via airplane. Besides preventing you from eating those plane peanuts coated in hydrogenated oils, fasting can also help alleviate jet lag symptoms and give your immune system a must needed boost while flying.

Hydration

Being on a plane increases the need for hydration. Plane cabin humidity levels are very, very low which promotes dehydration. Pack a water bottle, increase your water intake, and supplement with electrolytes while you travel. Dehydration also exaggerates jet lag, so drink up!

Airport Navigation

Similar to gas stations, airports have some keto-friendly options, but again, the quality may not be ideal so choose wisely. Here are some of the best options you can find at airport convenience stores:

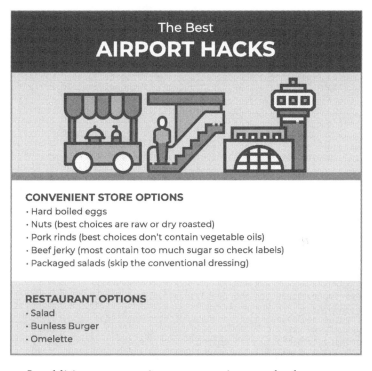

The Best
AIRPORT HACKS

CONVENIENT STORE OPTIONS
· Hard boiled eggs
· Nuts (best choices are raw or dry roasted)
· Pork rinds (best choices don't contain vegetable oils)
· Beef jerky (most contain too much sugar so check labels)
· Packaged salads (skip the conventional dressing)

RESTAURANT OPTIONS
· Salad
· Bunless Burger
· Omelette

In addition to convenience stores, airports also have restaurants where keto options can be found. Continue reading to the next section to get tips on dining out while on keto.

DINING OUT ON KETO

? IS IT HARD TO DINE OUT ON KETO?

Dining out can feel stressful for some ketogenic dieters, especially when first starting. There are a lot of bad food choices, usually less keto-friendly options, more temptations, and a greater risk for hidden carbs.

Did that scare you? Don't let it. Eating out at restaurants does not have to be feared. While the majority of restaurants' menus are not filled with keto-friendly options, there are plenty of ways for you to hack the menu to stay in ketosis and still enjoy eating out with friends and family. Taking certain steps prior to dining out is a great way to limit, or in some cases completely avoid, damage done from dining out.

The problem with many restaurants is the quality of food or cooking methods. Many restaurants may make sacrifices in quality of meat or cooking oils to increase profit. It's hard to know this ahead of time, and if you aren't choosing the restaurant, then you may not have any control in this situation. Don't panic, just make the right food choices.

If you are in charge of picking the restaurant, search for farm-to-table restaurants in your area. Simply Google "Farm to Table + Your Location." Other search terms that can lead you in the right direction:

- "grass-fed burger near me"
- "serves fresh local eggs near me"
- "serves sustainable local cuisine"

If you do have the luxury of checking out a restaurant ahead of time, browse the menu online to find entrees and sides that are on your approved list of food (see the following for suggestions on what to order). Avoid restaurants that state "No Substitutions."

Quality of dressings is also often sacrificed at restaurants, typically leaving you with vegetable oil-containing options. You can, of course, sub these dressings out for more keto-friendly options like olive oil and vinegar, but if you want a creamy salad dressing, plan ahead and bring your own dressing!

? WHAT CAN I EAT AT A RESTAURANT?

Staying keto while dining out starts as soon as you sit down at a restaurant. If you are dining alone or everyone at your table is keto, ask the server to hold the bread or tortilla chips. This will help you avoid temptation and not waste food. If you are with people who do enjoy these pre-dinner foods, don't be afraid to avoid them!

- When it comes time to order, don't be embarrassed to ask your server questions like:
- What oils are used to cook? Ask for your meal to be cooked in ghee, coconut oil, avocado oil, or olive oil.
- Are there sugars added to the sauce, dressing, or condiments?
- Are thickeners (flour, corn starch, etc.) added to the sauce, soup, dressing, or condiments?
- What oil is used to make the sauce, dressing, or condiment?

Be specific and polite with the server about your restrictions. Most every restaurant is willing to accommodate your needs. When it comes to choosing the best foods, consider the following:

- Order grass fed, pasture raised, wild caught, organic, and locally sourced when possible. Don't be stressed if you can't control this.
- Don't be scared to make several substitutions. Swap out the starch or bread for a side of vegetables, avocado, or a side salad.
- Ask for a side of healthy fat (olive oil, avocado oil, grass fed butter, grass fed ghee, coconut oil).
- Avoid "crispy" or breaded items.

If you didn't bring your own salad dressing, ask to substitute conventional dressings and sauces for healthier alternatives such as olive oil, vinegar, fresh lemon slices, or organic mustard, or only use salad dressings in moderation.

Remember, if you are unable to control some of the food quality factors, do not allow this to prevent you from dining out. Stick to keto foods and enjoy yourself; you will be just fine. Just don't make a frequent habit out of it!

Of course, there is going to be a lot of variety in your options from restaurant to restaurant. Here are some of our favorite keto options that are commonly seen at most restaurants:

BREAKFAST

Tip: Always ask for your meal to be cooked in a healthy fat (coconut or olive oil are common options).

Our Favorite Options:
- Omelet with vegetables and meat
- Eggs Benedict; substitute avocado for the English muffin
- Steak and Eggs
- Poached Eggs and Avocado (*Poached eggs are cooked without oil and can be a good option if the restaurant cannot substitute the cooking oil)

AMERICAN

Tip: Make sure to ask for no fruit, croutons, crispy wontons, cheese, or fried tortillas. Substitute for conventional dressings with a side of olive oil and balsamic vinegar.

Our Favorite Options:
- Cobb Salad

- Caesar Salad
- Burger, no bun and a side salad
- Baked buffalo wings (not breaded)

MEXICAN

Tip: Ask for no rice, beans, or tortillas. Always ask for your meal to be cooked in a healthy fat.

Our Favorite Options:
- Salad with grilled steak, chicken, or shrimp
- Add any of the following: tomatillo-red, guacamole, and a side of olive oil and vinegar
- Carnitas with a side of guacamole

SUSHI

Tip: Avoid imitation crab meat and soy sauce. Bring your own coconut aminos, which make a much healthier alternative to soy sauce for dipping.

Our Favorite Options:
- Rolls made with cucumber wraps
- Sashimi

ITALIAN

Tip: Avoid meatballs and meatloaf because they are usually made with breadcrumbs. Always ask for your meal to be cooked in a healthy fat.

Some Italian places may have zucchini pasta or the option to have the paste entree served over spinach or other greens. Be careful when ordering anything with red pasta sauce because it is typically made with added sugars.

Our Favorite Options:
- Steak and a double side of vegetables
- Fish and a side salad
- Zucchini pasta

INDIAN

Tip: Always ask for your meal to be cooked in a healthy fat. Ask for a side of ghee, which is a staple in Indian cuisine. Skip the rice and naan.

Our Favorite Options:
- Kabobs
- Curries made without added sugars

BARBECUE

Tip: Avoid barbecue sauce and ask if the rubs used are sugar-free. Always ask for your meal to be cooked in a healthy fat.

Our Favorite Options:
- Brisket
- Sausage
- Ribs
- Pulled pork
- Pulled chicken
- Collard greens
- Side salads

CHINESE

Tip: Ask about added sugars and thickeners (particularly cornstarch) in curries, stir-fries, and other sauces. Always ask for your meal to be cooked in a healthy fat.

Our Favorite Options:
- Beef and broccoli
- Curry
- Lettuce wraps

At the end of the meal always be sure to show your appreciation and thank the server and the cook and consider tipping a little extra.

? IS IT OKAY TO CHEAT ON KETO?

Short Answer: Yes, but you should be aware of potential side effects that come with cheating and how to limit the damage.

What?! Cheat on keto, how dare you? Just kidding—it happens, right? As we wrote this chapter, Chris daydreamed about his honeymoon in Italy, where he spent a week enjoying some of the most delicious carb-heavy meals Italy has to offer. Safe to say that he cheated on keto. Was this okay? Of course, it was okay! Because he doesn't cheat often, and he has strategies to limit the damage.

Remember, we want you to follow keto long term. We would much rather have someone follow a high-quality keto diet for two months, decide they need a pizza, crush a pizza, and get back to a high-quality keto diet—versus following keto for two months, having an intense desire for pizza, and deciding that since they fell off the keto wagon, they should give up altogether. Or maybe even worse, spend a lot of time debating if they can have that pizza or what the consequences will be, decide to eat it anyway, feel guilty after, and decide that keto isn't for them. Think "keto lifestyle." If that means you need to have a cheat every once in a while, that's fine, but don't let a cheat spiral out of control or be used frequently.

You probably think that we are going to tell you that when it comes to a cheat meal on keto, planning is important, right? Actually, quite the opposite. What if it comes time to "cheat" and you aren't even craving the junk you're about to eat? Planning on the meal likely will mean you will have the meal regardless of whether or not you're experiencing the craving. Don't plan your cheat meals; take them as they come and try to limit them as much as possible.

A common goal in adhering to a healthy lifestyle is breaking previous negative habits. Science has proven how addictive sugar can be; recent studies suggest refined sugar could be even more addictive than cocaine. If you were dependent on drugs or alcohol, a once a week planned relapse wouldn't be considered. This means that if you are someone who is suffering from severe food addictions and are attempting to break a habit, then a cheat may be counterproductive. Feeding current addictions will sabotage your ability to completely dismiss them.

With that being said, of course there are going to be times in your life where you are going to want to enjoy non-keto-friendly foods, and that is okay (unless being therapeutically used). However, it is important to not let this be a frequent occurrence and to know whether or not you are in a position where a cheat meal may be okay. For beginners, we recommend sticking to keto for at least 4-6 weeks before considering a cheat meal.

? WHAT HAPPENS IF I CHEAT?

Short Answer: You will be temporarily kicked out of ketosis and may not feel well afterwards.

In most cases, you get kicked out of ketosis. When you are first starting a ketogenic diet, this is not a good thing. Think of ketosis like a fire. When you first start a fire, any little rain or wind may put the fire out and make it hard to start again. This is true for beginners on keto. A cheat meal means that ketosis fire is going to be put out, making it harder for you to adapt. If you are new, don't cheat, stay diligent.

However, as a fire gets bigger, it can take a little more rain and wind without going out. If the rain and wind does impact the fire, it recovers quickly. This is what we see for people who have been following keto for a long time. They become a little more *metabolically flexible* meaning that they may be able to transition back and forth between using carbs and fat, and this allows them to get back into ketosis more quickly following a cheat.

Health isn't just about being in ketosis though. Being kicked out of ketosis every once in a while, unless you are doing it for certain therapeutic cases, is not that big of a deal. However, there are other consequences that accompany a cheat.

Typically, when people cheat, they aren't cheating with healthier non-keto options; typically they are cheating with processed carbs or the feel-good foods that can do quite a number on our gut health. These foods can rip little holes in the gut like chainsaws, letting undigested food particles into your bloodstream, giving them an opportunity to drive up inflammation and impair our overall health.

These holes in your gut take, on average, seven days to heal. If you are planning a once-per-week cheat meal, your gut is continually damaged, and you are constantly overloading your system with inflammation and possible autoimmune symptoms.

The point is that depending on the severity of your cheat, you can experience some adverse side effects and damage.

There will be a big difference in a cheat meal of a hot fudge sundae versus a sweet potato. The former is going to cause many negative side effects than the latter. However, most people will be able to recover quickly regardless.

? HOW CAN I LIMIT THE DAMAGE OF A CHEAT MEAL?

Again, cheat meals can be okay, but limiting the damage of a cheat meal will play a big role in your body's journey back to ketosis. Since carbs can be addictive and stimulate hunger, a carb cheat meal can lead to spiraling out of control and completely falling off of the keto wagon. This will make the consequences of a cheat meal much more dire.

Instead, a cheat meal should be just that—a single meal, not a whole day, and not frequent. Every time you eat a cheat meal you are making an informed decision to put lower quality and potentially harmful foods in your body. While this may not have a huge impact when done rarely and responsibly, it can be harmful if blown out of control and done frequently.

There are also a couple of supplements that can be strategically used to limit the damage of a cheat meal. Supplementing with insulin sensitizing agents, like we mentioned in Chapter 8, can ensure you are limiting the glucose and insulin response from a cheat meal. Exogenous ketones can further reduce symptoms from a carb cheat. While they will not "get you back into ketosis," they can boost ketones to prevent fatigue and brain fog, which may accompany your cheat meal.

Many people think that fasting is a great way to prepare for a cheat meal. While fasting can improve your insulin sensitivity, which improves your ability to manage the carbs, it still may not be the best approach. Gary Taubes, famous nutrition journalist, framed the question this way: If I were to tell you that tonight we are going to be going to enjoy cuisine from the best chef in your city so bring your appetite, what would you do? You would likely fast to make sure you show up with an appetite! And typically, it works! The same thing can happen with fasting before a cheat; fasting may give you a bigger appetite and thus a greater capacity to damage your body with your cheat meal. Instead, follow your day as normally planned and just have your cheat meal. Your calories may be higher but for a day, this is not a huge deal.

Fasting plus exercise after a cheat meal is also a commonly used strategy. While this may be a good approach for stimulating your body to start producing ketones a little quicker, it is also a rather unhealthy way of looking at your diet. You should not punish yourself for a cheat meal by fasting and pounding your body in the gym. This can induce a dangerous cycle of binge eating and fasting, which is not the relationship we want you to have with your diet.

It is also worth mentioning that you do not have to cheat on Keto. That is completely okay, too! Or you may be able to swap out a full-blown cheat for a keto snack or even a dirty keto cheat, such as some keto pancakes or a little bit of low-carb ice cream.

? SHOULD I DO A CARB REFEED?

A carb refeed is a word that many people will use to justify a cheat, but that is not what the intention of a carb refeed is. A carb refeed is essentially a planned meal or day of consuming carbohydrates. The purpose of this approach is typically to "ramp up metabolism" or help replenish glycogen. While in theory this sounds nice, this is not necessary on a keto diet and, in fact, is counterproductive for most.

We already mentioned in Chapter 5 how replenishing glycogen is not a high priority on a ketogenic diet. The idea of using a carb refeed to ramp up metabolism was born from individuals practicing carb cycling and eating low calorie diets. Since we know that chronic, severe calorie restriction is not the best for your metabolism, many assume this can be alleviated through a carbohydrate refeed that would also lead to a higher calorie intake. On a ketogenic diet, you are already improving your metabolism through many other mechanisms so the need to implement such a strategy is not needed.

In addition, just like a cheat meal would kick you out of ketosis, so would a carb refeed so this should again be especially avoided by keto beginners. However, there may be times when doing a *calorie* refeed could be beneficial for the same reason as not keeping your calories too low for too long. This can be done by sticking to keto-friendly foods but eating more of them. We suggest choosing the most nutrient-dense foods you can if taking this approach so you can get a double whammy of more calories and more nutrients!

It is worth mentioning here that a carb refeed strategy may be used by those on a cyclic keto diet. While this approach could serve a purpose for these people, for the average person, especially someone just starting a keto diet, a carb refeed will not provide benefits. Refer to Chapter 10 to learn more about cyclic keto diets.

❓ HOW LONG SHOULD I STAY KETO?

Very little research has been done on the long-term effect of a ketogenic diet, but currently there is no reason to think that there is harm in following the diet long term. Your goal for the keto diet should determine the length of the time you maintain the diet. If you are following keto for therapeutic applications, it could be something you maintain for the rest of your life. If your goal is fat loss, mental clarity, or any other non-therapeutic application, keto might be a tool that you use off and on throughout your life.

In general, a keto dietary approach can provide many health benefits and help keep certain diseases at bay, so following it long term is a great approach!

? DO I HAVE TO STAY KETO FOREVER?

This is a question we get all of the time and the answer is... *of course!!!*

Actually, that's not the answer, we are just firm believers in the benefits of ketosis. The truth is, you do not have to do keto forever, nor can you expect to. There are going to be times in your life when you are going to want to take a break from keto. Maybe it's a vacation or a holiday or you just flat-out want to eat pizza. While we should always focus on at least maintaining a low-carb lifestyle, it is inevitable that people will take a break from keto at some point, and that is fine unless stopping the diet will drastically alter your disease management.

The reason why many people think you must follow a ketogenic diet forever is because of what typically happens after someone stops the diet. Many people who stop keto tend to make up for that period of time of not having carbs by drastically over-consuming carbs. This leads to weight regain, fatigue, mood swings, and much more. This leads many to think that the keto diet must be followed forever to maintain your results. However, this is not the case. It must be realized that regardless of the progress you have seen on keto, if you go back to a poor diet and lifestyle, you are going to go back to feeling how you did before. This should be common sense. The keto diet is powerful but it's not magic!

Again, unless you are following the diet for disease management, you do not have to be keto forever. However, how you come off of keto is very important.

? WHAT IS THE BEST WAY TO COME OFF OF KETO?

The way you come off keto is important for not only maintaining any results you experienced on the diet, but also continuing to improve. In our opinion, the best way to do this is through a slow carbohydrate reintroduction. If you are flooding your system with excess carbs after your body has not seen carbs for a period of time, you are going to have some complications. Go easy on the carbs and give your body some time to adjust.

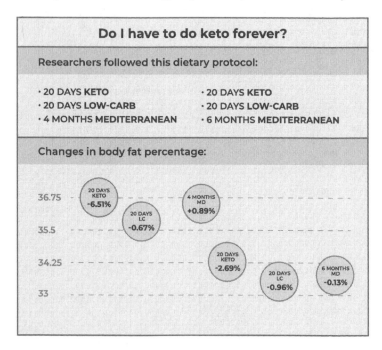

Do I have to do keto forever?

Researchers followed this dietary protocol:

· 20 DAYS KETO
· 20 DAYS LOW-CARB
· 4 MONTHS MEDITERRANEAN

· 20 DAYS KETO
· 20 DAYS LOW-CARB
· 6 MONTHS MEDITERRANEAN

Changes in body fat percentage:

36.75	20 DAYS KETO -6.51%
	4 MONTHS MD +0.89%
	20 DAYS LC -0.67%
35.5	
34.25	20 DAYS KETO -2.69%
	6 MONTHS MD -0.13%
	20 DAYS LC -0.96%
33	

One study put this theory to the test by having subjects transition off of keto by going to a low-carb diet and then to a Mediterranean diet. This approach allowed the subjects to maintain most of their improvements in body composition and even jump-start further improvement once they started keto again![131]

We follow keto the majority of the time because we love the way it makes us feel, but we have experience with coming off of the diet. Here is the approach we recommend:

1. Track your food for a couple of days, eating as you have been to determine your typical macronutrient range. From there, convert some of your fat consumption over to protein consumption and follow this strategy for one to two weeks. You can either keep your calories the same or allow yourself to fall into a caloric deficit to ensure you keep the weight off. This would look something like:
   - *Keto:* 70 percent Fat, 25 percent Protein, 5 percent Carb (based on percent of total calories)
   - *Transition 1:* 40 percent Fat, 55 percent Protein, 5 percent Carb

2. After protein has been increased, swap out more fat for some carbs and follow for an additional one to two weeks. We recommend starting with lower glycemic

---

131 Antonio Paoli, Antonino Bianco, Keith Grimaldi, Alessandra Lodi, and Gerardo Bosco, "Long Term Successful Weight Loss with a Combination Biphasic Ketogenic Mediterranean Diet and Mediterranean Diet Maintenance Protocol," *Nutrients* 5, no. 12 (2013): 5205-5217.

carbohydrates during this time like oatmeal, sweet potatoes, and carrots. This could look something like:
- *Transition 2:* 30 percent Fat, 55 percent Protein, 15 percent Carb

3. At this point, we recommend not going much lower on fat, since it is so crucial to many functions in the body. If you are looking to go higher with your carbs, instead convert more protein over to carbs. This could look something like:
   - *Transition 3:* 30 percent Fat, 40 percent Protein, 30 percent Carb

4. From here, decide how high you want your carb intake to be. If you are trying to go much higher, you may need to lower fat further, but this is not something we recommend. Regardless of being keto or not, at least being low-carb is going to be important for your health so going higher than 20-30 percent is not advised. Self-experiment with different macronutrient ratios so you can see what works best for you.

② IF I GO OFF OF KETO, WILL I HAVE TO GO THROUGH KETO ADAPTATION AGAIN WHEN I START BACK UP?

Anyone who has followed keto remembers the not-so-great feelings that occur while adapting to the diet. The fear is that if you have a carb cheat meal or decide to take a break from keto, you will have to go through adaptation again. Whether that's true depends on how long you have been keto for and the degree of departure from the diet. If you have been adequately keto-adapted previously, your body will more easily adjust back to using fat for fuel. The amount of carbohydrates you eat, the duration you spend not eating keto, and your individual metabolism will determine the amount of time it will take for you to readapt to keto. Here are some tips you can use to help transition back into ketosis:

- Reduce carbohydrate intake to less than 20 total grams
- Implement fasting
- Increase your physical activity
- Supplement with ketones and MCTs

It is important to be responsible with the above strategies. Do not let them become a crutch. If you are cheating all the time, it doesn't matter what techniques you use; you are not going to see results. Additionally, we do not recommend the "binging and purging" approach to handling dietary slipups. Too many people think it is okay to cheat on the weekend and combat that with a long fast and punishing exercise. To us, that seems like a trend toward an unhealthy relationship with food and is not something we recommend.

COOKING REPLACEMENTS

When it comes to cooking on keto, things are a little different. Many of the typical ingredients you are accustomed to using to prepare your food are not going to cut it under this new dietary lifestyle. This can be a big adjustment for some, especially those who have a little more passion for the cooking. If you do like cooking (even a little), you might enjoy the challenge.

When Chris's sister, who has a degree in culinary arts, first started keto she was frustrated because all she had learned about achieving certain textures, flavors, and preparing common dishes was challenged. However, as she followed the diet, she learned how to make adjustments to achieve her desired result. Now she is so good at cooking keto that she prepares foods for other people who are trying to stick to the diet as well.

Just because you can't use flour, sugar, and milk doesn't mean you can't create some pretty awesome dishes on keto— some of which can replace your favorite carbohydrate containing foods. Bear in mind, though, that just because you can make keto pancakes does not mean that you should have them all the time. One of the purposes of a ketogenic diet is to kill off sugar and carb cravings; if you are making things like fat bombs and keto cupcakes the staple of your diet, not only will you not achieve this, you also will miss out on the nutrients found within whole foods.

Cook the foods in this section when you are having a house party or guests over, at holidays, or to reward yourself for reaching a health goal. Do not let these ingredients and recipes become something that you are consuming every day. This would be what we consider a "dirty keto" diet, which we will discuss before diving into cooking replacements on keto.

? WHAT IS DIRTY KETO?

> *Short Answer:* Dirty keto is a version of the diet that fails to emphasize the importance of food quality.

Unfortunately, dirty keto is how many people are introduced to the diet. Lately, keto has put such an emphasis on macronutrients that it has failed to stress the importance of food quality and micronutrient density. This emphasis has led many to believe that anything low in carbs is keto-friendly, thus safe to consume on the diet.

What exact foods are we referencing here? Foods like pork rinds, bacon, loads of butter, cheese sticks, lunch meats, and "low-carb" treats laced with a ton of sugar replacements, of which many are not that keto-friendly. Because these foods have low-carbs or low-net-carbs, they are considered to be healthy. While consuming these foods *will* allow you to get into ketosis, that does not mean they are the healthiest foods to be consuming, especially in excess.

Just because a food is low-carb does not mean that it isn't pro-inflammatory. Pork rinds fried in vegetable oil? Pretty inflammatory. Grain-fed processed beef with its higher omega-6 fat content? Pretty inflammatory. Cheese sticks...well hell, they are hardly even real food.

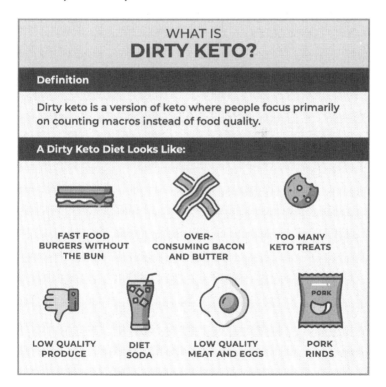

WHAT IS
DIRTY KETO?

Definition

Dirty keto is a version of keto where people focus primarily on counting macros instead of food quality.

A Dirty Keto Diet Looks Like:

| FAST FOOD BURGERS WITHOUT THE BUN | OVER-CONSUMING BACON AND BUTTER | TOO MANY KETO TREATS |
| LOW QUALITY PRODUCE | DIET SODA | LOW QUALITY MEAT AND EGGS | PORK RINDS |

Can you see results by following keto this way? Absolutely—especially at first. This approach is likely better than your previous diet, especially if it was a diet chock-full of processed and refined carbohydrates. You may see some results because your metabolism gets a bit of a break without having to process so many carbs and sugars. Yes, you will also lose weight and improve many health markers, but you are definitely not optimizing your health or receiving as many of the benefits as you could be. There is more to your body than your metabolism.

Many people will think we are snooty keto advocates trying to fearmonger people into eating higher quality food. That's just not the case. We will admit that dirty keto may be okay to use strategically. In fact, dirty keto is what we do instead of having a carbohydrate filled cheat meal. Super Bowl party? Let's have a few low-carb beers and some of those pork rind nachos. Home with family for a birthday party? We may make a keto cake. The point here is that dirty keto can be okay in moderation but isn't something you should do frequently.

❓ WHAT ARE THE BEST REPLACEMENTS FOR FLOUR?

The commonly used flours, such as all-purpose, bleached, unbleached, white, and wheat flour, all contain a lot of carbohydrates and are all out on keto. A few flours are better suited for a ketogenic diet:

COCONUT FLOUR
Coconut flour is made from the pulp of coconut, which is formed as a by-product during the creation of coconut milk. A quarter cup of coconut flour contains 16 grams of carbs, with 10 of these grams coming from fiber, and is gluten-free. While this

is a little higher in carbs compared to other low-carb flour alternatives, because it can be absorbed in recipes, it is a fan favorite.

When using coconut flour, use 2 tablespoons of water for every 2 tablespoons of coconut flour to prevent your dish from becoming too dry. Eggs can also be used to help combat this.

ALMOND FLOUR

Almond flour is also gluten free but contains much less carbohydrate compared to coconut flour. A quarter cup of almond flour contains 14 grams of fat, 6 grams of protein, and only 6 grams of carbs, with 3 of these grams coming from fiber. Almond flour is a great source of vitamin E, iron, manganese, magnesium, potassium, and calcium.

You can also use almond meal. The only difference is that almond flour is made from blanched, ground almonds with their skins removed, while meal is made from almonds with the skin still on. This gives almond meal a slightly grainy texture but doesn't change much else. You can make your own almond meal or flour in the food processor.

When using almond flour, consider the amount you are consuming. A full cup of almond flour is the equivalent of 90 whole almonds. While this amount in a recipe that feeds several people would be okay, if a single person consumes that much, they would be overdoing it.

FLAX MEAL

Flax meal is ground flaxseed. It contains 6 grams of carbs, all of which come from fiber, as well as 4 grams of protein and 8-9 grams of fat. Flax meal is rich in omega-3 fats (from ALA) and possesses antioxidant potential.

Flax meal has a bit of a gritty texture, so bear this in mind when incorporating it into a recipe. Some people have intolerances or allergies to flax, so if you have never had it, be sure to not overdo it the first time.

Other flours that can be used on your keto diet include nut flours like walnut flour and seed flours like sunflower seed flour, but these flours are a little less commonly used in keto recipes you may find on the internet.

? WHAT ARE THE BEST REPLACEMENTS FOR SUGAR?

Yes, there are replacements for sugar, but no, you shouldn't make them a staple of your diet. While many sugar replacements do not contain significant caloric value, that does not make them a good choice for your health. They should be used infrequently.

It is worth mentioning that most studies that demonstrate sweetener alternatives damaging the gut or other health markers are animal studies in which the human equivalent of the amount of sweetener the animals consume is much higher than what a human would actually consume. This tells us that in moderation, most sweeteners can be okay.

The problem is that sweeteners are still sweet, in some cases even sweeter than sugar itself. This can stimulate hunger and cravings which make the ketogenic diet a much less enjoyable experience. Furthermore, many keto sweeteners can cause stomach pain due to differences in digestion. So, don't overdo it.

There are many sweeteners out there; we feel the best are monk fruit and stevia. These sweeteners are typically better tolerated, especially as they relate to gastrointestinal distress, and they can actually provide a few health benefits. If you are going to be using sweeteners, try using them individually and in combination to find out which you prefer. Note that both stevia and monk fruit are significantly sweeter than sugar, so determining the amount to achieve a desired level of sweetness may take a little experimenting.

? HOW DO I THICKEN OR ADD TEXTURE TO MY FOOD WHEN COOKING?

When altering recipes to make them keto, texture is a common struggle. Carbohydrates help hold things together and often produce a more desirable texture in certain recipes. However, there are a few substitutes that can help. The two most popular are:

- **Psyllium Husk:** Comes from the seeds of the *Plantago ovata* plant and is commonly used to help give bread-like textures to certain foods. Psyllium husk is a prebiotic and good source of fiber.
- **Xanthan Gum:** A thickening agent that can be used in very small amounts to induce texture changes.

? WHAT ARE THE BEST REPLACEMENTS FOR MILK?

Milk is typically a no-go on keto, due not only to its sugar content but also the processing that most available milk has gone through. There are a few alternatives, such as various nut and seed milks. Our favorites are:

- Almond Milk
- Coconut Milk/Cream
- Hemp Milk
- Flax Milk

Get the unflavored versions, since most contain added sugar for taste. These milks typically have a much different texture and taste compared to dairy milk, so unless a recipe specifically calls for one of these milks, you may have to experiment to achieve a desired taste or texture.

? ARE THERE WAYS TO REPLACE BREAD?

Ah yes, bread, a fan favorite. While traditional bread must be avoided on keto (and really should be on any diet), there are plenty of keto bread recipes out there. While these recipes can be great, they can also be a little challenging and expensive. For this reason, it may be better to look for bread replacements. If you are trying to replace a bun or bread for a sandwich, mushroom caps and lettuce wraps are a great alternative. If you wish to add breadcrumbs to something, ground pork rinds are a better alternative.

You can also just skip the idea of bread, because in most cases you don't need it. Even in the case of a big burger, there is nothing wrong with going bunless and eating it with a fork.

? ARE THERE WAYS TO REPLACE RICE?

Rice is another no go on keto. Yep, even brown rice, which everyone likes to say is so much better, is not on the plan. However, there is the magical cauliflower you can use in its place. Cauliflower rice can substitute for traditional rice and even tastes very similar! You can make your own cauliflower rice, or you can buy pre-riced cauliflower.

? ARE THERE WAYS TO REPLACE CHIPS?

Chips are obviously not keto, but that does not mean that you won't want to enjoy some chips and guacamole every once in a while. Pork rinds, again not a very nutritious choice, are a better alternative to chips, if you are looking for a little crunch or something to dip into a keto-friendly sauce. Look for pork rinds not cooked in vegetable oils.

? ARE THERE WAYS TO REPLACE TORTILLAS?

There are a few low-carb tortilla options out there, and while they may be "keto macro-friendly," they contain ingredients that we would want to avoid on keto. Instead, try replacing your tortilla with lettuce wraps or, if you are okay with some dairy, there are some recipes out there to make cheese taco shells! Not the most health-conscious, but a safe alternative to be used in moderation.

? ARE THERE WAYS TO REPLACE PASTA?

For those with Italian roots, like Chris, you likely grew up on a diet of pasta and bread. And really, who doesn't love pasta? Obviously, neither of these are keto friendly, but lucky for you, there are several alternatives out there. Here are the main three:

GLUCOMANNAN NOODLES

Also known as shirataki noodles or miracle noodles, these noodles are made from glucomannan, a fiber found in the root of the konjac plant. These noodles are made up of mostly water and fiber and are pretty low carb. This makes them a decent option for replacing spaghetti noodles on keto; however, not everyone likes the texture, so give it a try and see what you think.

SPAGHETTI SQUASH

Spaghetti squash is a hard winter squash. After roasting or steaming, you can scoop the flesh out into delicious, noodle-like strings that can be seasoned and eaten alone or incorporated into another dish. Spaghetti squash is a little higher in total carbs, about 10 grams, with about 2 of those coming from fiber.

ZUCCHINI NOODLES

Zucchini noodles are our personal favorite. Zucchini can be spiralized, turning this summer squash into a noodle that can be used in various recipes. This is a super simple process and tastes pretty good. A full zucchini has about 10 grams of carbs but makes a pretty big portion size.

The Best
KETO SWAPS

BUNS	→	MUSHROOM CAP OR LETTUCE WRAP
RICE	→	CAULIFLOWER RICE
CHIPS	→	PORK RINDS
PASTA	→	ZUCCHINI NOODLES "ZOODLES"
POTATOES	→	CAULIFLOWER RICE

If you are trying to replace pasta, consider the sauce. Most pasta sauces contain a surprisingly high amount of added sugar. Check the labels for the lowest sugar options or consider making your own.

? ARE THERE ANY WAYS TO REPLACE POTATOES?

Neither white nor sweet potatoes are keto friendly, but who doesn't want a little mashed potato every once in a while? You can make a cauliflower mash that, if done right, is a pretty good substitute to mashed potatoes. This is one of our favorite things to do around holidays like Thanksgiving. If you are looking for a replacement for a full potato, though, you won't find it.

? ARE THERE KETO-FRIENDLY DESSERTS?

Lucky for you ketogenic lifestylers, there are lots of wonderful recipes for keto-friendly desserts. Ingredients like almond flour, coconut flour, stevia, monk fruit, heavy cream, and coconut cream can create mouth-watering treats without all the sugar and carbohydrates.

However, remember that these foods should especially not become a staple. A diet full of keto cupcakes may allow for ketosis but it will not optimize your health. Perfectketo.com has a long list of great keto recipes that use approved ingredients and cut out the garbage.

? CAN I HAVE "SUGAR-FREE" SNACKS?

With the rise in the popularity of low-carb dieting, we are also seeing many more sugar-free food options. Just as not all low-carb foods are the best for a keto diet, the same is true for sugar-free foods.

Remember, continuing to eat sweets will impair your ability to prevent hunger and cravings. Furthermore, it is possible that your body could respond to sweet tasting foods with an insulin response, regardless of actual sugar content.

Sugar-free foods are also typically very low quality, contain too many strange ingredients, and replace sugar with other sweeteners that, while they may be "calorie-free," could still come with negative side effects, such as disruptions in the gut microbiome and digestive distress when consumed in high amounts.

Even worse, we have tested a lot of "sugar-free" snacks and have seen huge increases in blood sugar. A notable brand here is SmartSweets, which provides gummy versions of our favorite candies and markets them as only having 3 grams of sugar per serving. The catch? They use 30 grams of low-quality fiber syrups that they can label as fiber on the nutrition facts but act just like sugar in your bloodstream.

We have both tested the effect these candies had on our blood sugar, and the results were ridiculous. In Anthony's case, about 14 SmartSweets gummy bears literally broke his continuous blood glucose monitor. In Chris's case, his blood sugar nearly *doubled* after eating a serving of the gummies. This is all from a company marketing their products as a low-fat, low-sugar, "healthy option."

The moral of the story is that sugar-free snacks can be consumed on occasions but typically have no health benefits and may lead to unwanted side effects. Be careful which you choose and be sure to experiment.

? CAN I DRINK DIET SODA ON KETO?

While diet sodas may not contain any sugar or carbohydrates, as is the case with sugar-free snacks, these drinks contain a long list of strange ingredients and no-calorie but extremely sweet sweeteners.

Overconsumption of diet soda is linked to dozens of unwanted health problems, including headaches, dehydration, obesity, decrease in bone density, and more. However, much of the research demonstrating that the sweeteners used in these drinks are harmful is in animals and in amounts that are equivalent to ridiculous serving sizes in humans. Still, these drinks provide no added health benefit; the risk-reward for including them is up to you.

If you are looking for a soda replacement, healthier alternatives include sparkling water and stevia-sweetened soda.

While there are a lot of options on a keto diet, you may find that you are still bored and want to try some new recipes. We are especially seeing more recipes that may be used in place of your favorite carbohydrate-based meals. These include things like keto pizza, keto pasta, keto pancakes, etc. Similar to desserts, these foods should not become staples in your diet and fall more into the dirty keto lifestyle, meaning they can make good options for a more keto-friendly cheat. To find these recipes, visit perfectketo.com or check out various keto recipe books, blogs, and Pinterest accounts.

? CAN I DRINK ALCOHOL ON KETO?

While alcohol in moderation can be consumed on a keto diet, it has no health benefits and will slow down your results. Alcohol will always have the first priority in your body, before any other fuel sources can be used because your body cannot store alcohol. It has to be burned off and removed from the blood before your body will return to using fat for fuel. This means that all other fuel sources must be stored until the alcohol has been used. Simply put, over-consuming alcohol will often stall your fat loss or lead to weight gain. Additionally, alcohol tolerance goes down on keto, which can cause you to get drunk quicker and have tougher hangovers.

With that being said, it's nice to enjoy a drink every now and again, and this is something that we even do on occasions. While there are *not* physiological health benefits to drinking, the social aspect does offer some psychological health benefits. If you are going to drink, it is in your best interest to choose the lowest carb choices:

SPIRITS

Consume on the rocks or with water/soda water. Note that your tolerance to spirits will be especially lower on keto so drink with caution. Here are a few acceptable options:

- Whiskey
- Tequila
- Mezcal *(Anthony's favorite)*
- Vodka
- Gin
- Rum
- Brandy
- Wine

Wine is a little trickier because the way the grapes are farmed as well as the region they come from matters. Wines made from grapes grown in hot climates contain more sugar compared to wine made of grapes from cooler climates. Region also matters for the quality of wine. Most US grown grapes contain many pesticides and are grown in nutrient deficient soils. Finding wine that is organically grown, biodynamically farmed (Demeter certified), or dry farmed is the gold standard. Due to climate and soil, two of the best regions for wine are Austria and Loire Valley in France.

The dryness of wine refers to the sugar content of the wine. The dryer the wine, the lower the sugar. The percent of alcohol can also help you determine the sugar content of wine. A higher percent alcohol wine is generally going to contain more sugar compared to a lower percent alcohol wine. For this reason, look for wines with under 13 percent alcohol.

Another general rule is that red wines are going to be drier than whites. Of the popular red wines, Cabernet Sauvignon and Pinot Noir are of the driest red wines along with Merlot and Malbec falling in the middle range. However, there are some white wines with low sugar content such as Muscadet, Sauvignon Blanc, and Pinot Grigio. Most sparkling wines are also higher in sugar; however, sparkling wines that say brut nature on the label are classified as the lowest sugar of sparkling wines.

BEER

Beer is typically the least keto-friendly of alcohols but there are some light beers that can be okay in moderation. Aim for under 5 grams of carbs per beer. Here are a few of the most popular:

- Michelob Ultra
- Corona Premier
- Miller Light
- Miller 64
- Select 55
- Genesee Light
- Beck's Premier Light

Remember, the keto diet provides its most robust results when it is followed long term. To do this, you need to learn how to adopt this diet as a lifestyle. No one wants to feel like they are dieting all the time, and no one wants to constantly deal with the stresses of dieting in their day-to-day life. Adopt some of the principles in this chapter to help make this diet work with your life so that you can take control of your health for the long haul.

To further drive this point home, remember that if you are new to the ketogenic diet, we do not recommend taking the easier, lifestyle approaches in this chapter. It is important that you stick to the keto diet the way we mapped it out in Chapters 6 and 7 to get your health under control. Once you have done this, these strategies can be better implemented into your keto lifestyle.

CHAPTER 13

SELF-EXPERIMENTATION AND TRACKING

S elf-experimentation is the practice of testing with your own body to learn how it responds in different situations. As it relates to nutrition, self-experimentation helps you determine how different nutritional strategies can be used to achieve specific personal goals.

Tracking is recording various markers to help you determine how your body is responding to the nutrition strategies you are following and to better help you decide what improvements can be made.

By now you should have realized that nutrition should be personalized. There is no one-size-fits-all approach; even different goals require some nutritional tweaking. Since health is so individualized, treating your body a bit like a science experiment can allow you to optimize and tailor your diet. There are plenty of studies out there that you can reference to help guide you, but these studies are hard to interpret and finding which studies were conducted correctly can be even more challenging. Furthermore, no study done on large groups of people will ever directly apply to you. While this may seem discouraging, it is support for the benefits of self-experimenting and tracking.

It is important to test, not guess. However, we want to be very clear: testing is a foundational strategy to help you understand what works. It is not, and should not become, a way of life. When you first start a ketogenic diet, self-experimentation and tracking should not be the primary focus. During this time, your attention should be on cutting out the foods you shouldn't eat and consuming the foods that you should. While tracking during this time may have its benefits, it can also be an extra stressor that, in combination with such a big diet change, may make sticking to keto harder. For this reason, we recommend saving the experiments and tracking for when you are more experienced with keto. Besides, you probably need to give traditional keto a try to establish a baseline before you start experimenting with tweaking the diet.

Even after adapting to keto, many of the strategies in this chapter are not for everyone. Some people, who are seeing improvements in their health and are achieving their goals, may decide not to bother with the strategies mentioned in this chapter, and that is completely okay. However, if your goal is complete health optimization, then this chapter is for you. Below is a breakdown of what we will be discussing in this chapter:

TRACKING:

- Macronutrients
- Ketones
- Glucose
- Body composition
- Blood labs

- Self-experimentation
- Responses to foods
- Carb tolerance
- Dairy tolerance

While we do put emphasis on tracking and self-experimentation being a choice, it is worth noting that this suggestion changes under therapeutic conditions. If you are following keto for therapeutic reasons, you may need to be a little stricter and more precise, which is where tracking and self-experimentation can come in.

MACRONUTRIENTS

? SHOULD I TRACK MACRONUTRIENTS?

Earlier in the book we discussed macronutrients and whether or not you should track them. In that chapter we emphasized that if you are new to keto, put your focus on eating high-quality, keto-approved foods and avoid the foods you should not be eating. For most people, this is enough to show progress and start improving their health. We also recommend this because when most people start tracking macros, they put too much of an emphasis on a small piece of the puzzle, which takes away from the focus on food quality, which we feel should be at the core of any diet. However, once you are adapted to the ketogenic diet, tracking your macros can provide valuable insight into what is going on with your diet and help make more educated adjustments.

While each macronutrient is important, we know that keeping carbs in the appropriate range for your body and goal is of particular importance on a keto diet. For this reason, some people may benefit from simply tracking carbs. This is not the most optimal tracking approach, since fat and protein also play a big role in your success on keto, but if you do not want to track all of the macronutrients, keeping your eye on carbs is at least a good place to start.

? WHEN SHOULD I TRACK MY MACROS?

If you are more advanced or have been following keto for a longer period of time, then there are many instances where tracking your macronutrients could be beneficial, such as the following:

TO CHECK IN

It's always a good idea to check in and see what your macros are. When we talk to people who do not track macros, we frequently find that they are over-consuming carbs, under-consuming protein, or their calories aren't quite where they should be. Doing a little macronutrient check-in can be a great strategy for ensuring you are still on the right track.

YOU WANT TO BEGIN SELF-EXPERIMENTING

If you are going to start any self-experiments, such as testing different types of ketogenic diets, like those mentioned in Chapter 10, you will want to track your macros so you can see exactly what changes you are making.

YOU ARE STUCK AT A PLATEAU

If you are stuck at any plateau, such as a weight loss plateau, you could benefit from assessing your macronutrients to see if you are making any mistakes, or to see what changes you can make to start making progress again.

YOU DO NOT FEEL LIKE YOU ARE GETTING THE BENEFITS OF KETOSIS

If you do not feel like you are experiencing the benefits of ketosis, such as increased energy, satiety, mental clarity, weight loss, etc., then something could be off with your macros.

Tracking them is the first place to start. You can see where your macros actually are and make changes accordingly.

One of the biggest culprits is hidden carbs. There are so many times we have had someone tell us they are eating 30 grams of carbs, yet after tracking they find out they are actually consuming closer to 50-75! Hidden carbs can add up!

YOU ARE MAKING A GOAL SHIFT

Different goals require different dietary strategies. If you started keto for weight loss, but now you want to optimize the diet for muscle gain, that will require some tweaking. Track to establish what you have been doing with your diet so you can determine what to change going forward toward your new goal.

YOU ARE MAKING A DIETARY CHANGE

Remember that foods all vary in macronutrient makeup and each macronutrient impacts the body differently, so consuming different ratios of macronutrients will lead to different responses from the body. If you start making changes in your food choices, you will want to track your macros so you can see how they vary from what you have typically been eating and then record how your body is responding to these new foods.

? HOW DO I TRACK MY MACRONUTRIENTS?

Tracking macronutrients does not have to be difficult and it doesn't require a pen and paper. Plenty of apps allow you to easily track your macros by searching for or scanning the barcodes of the foods you are eating. Our preferred app is Cronometer. Some apps, like MyFitnessPal, are not as vetted, meaning that some of the info submitted is incorrect. That can make things pretty confusing.

If you are eating a lot of whole foods that do not have labels, tracking is a little harder. In these situations, you can search for the food you are eating and manually enter the amount into a tracking app like Cronometer. The numbers you get may not be 100 percent accurate, since foods can vary from source to source, but this method will allow you to get close enough to provide a good idea of what your daily macronutrient intake looks like.

Do not allow tracking to control your life. While recording your food when you eat may be the best strategy for ensuring you don't leave anything out, this method is annoying and prevents you from being able to enjoy your meal. We prefer entering our food at some point in the afternoon and then again in the evening, when it is convenient.

You do not have to track everyday. Unless your diet varies dramatically from day to day, you can simply track a few days a week to make a good assessment of where you are. When you do track, to get an accurate measurement, try to keep your food intake as normal as possible. Don't let the fact that you are tracking make you more disciplined for a day; that will prevent you from getting an accurate assessment of what your diet truly looks like, making it more difficult to infer anything or accurately make changes.

? HOW DO I ADJUST MY MACRONUTRIENTS?

Remember, if you are a beginner, we recommend sticking to the list of foods from Chapter 6 and eating until full. While this may lead to overeating at first, you may actually benefit from the extra energy as your body adapts. Once adapted, you can determine if you want to start tracking for any of the reasons listed earlier in this chapter.

At this point, since you have been following the diet for a bit, you have a baseline you can start making adjustments to. It is difficult to give an exact prescription since everyone is different, but this is how we suggest adjusting macros.

STEP 1: DETERMINE CURRENT CALORIE/MACRO INTAKE

Start recording your food in a macro tracking app while eating as similarly as the way you have been.

STEP 2: CALCULATE YOUR COMPUTED MACROS

Visit https://perfectketo.com/calculator and follow the instructions to calculate your macros and calories.

STEP 3: COMPARE

Compare the calories from Step 1 and Step 2. If the difference is less than 200 calories, then switch to Step 2 macro/calorie recommendations and record what happens. If the difference is greater than 200 calories, we recommend slowly transitioning to your new macronutrients by adding 200 calories per week until you reach the recommendations from Step 2.

Once you have reached the recommended macronutrients from Step 2, follow them for a couple of weeks to let your body adjust. If you are looking to adjust your macros because of any issues you are experiencing, you may notice that they disappear during this time. If they do not or you are looking to achieve a certain goal, then move to the next step.

STEP 4: DETERMINE YOUR WHY

Once you have completed the above steps and followed your new macros for a while, it is time to decide what your goal is. You need to have a clear goal to determine in which direction to start adjusting your macros.

STEP 5: ADJUST TO YOUR GOAL

Start making adjustments to your macros according to the deter-mined goal. This will be all experimentation since everyone responds to macronutrient adjustments differently. The good thing is you are now tracking, so you are getting a lot of data you can use to help make your decisions and more closely understand how your body is responding to adjustments you are testing.

Some people can adjust to their goal without tracking through what is known as intuitive eating. An example of intu-itive eating is knowing that you want to increase your protein intake and lower your fat intake and making this adjustment by choosing leaner cuts of meat that are higher in protein. This is not the most accurate approach but may be a little easier to stick to for some people. Someone who is experienced with keto and has tracked in the past can better follow an approach like this.

KETONE TESTING

SHOULD I TRACK KETONES?

> *Short Answer:* Tracking ketones can be beneficial to see how your body responds to different foods, but our understand-ing of ketone levels is limited.

Ketone testing, which can be done through urine, blood, and breath, is very popular amongst the keto community and is commonly used as an objective measure of ketosis. However, it is crucial to point out a few things here:

INTERPRETING KETONE LEVELS IS NOT EASY

When you test your ketones, you are simply testing to see how many ketones are currently present in your blood, urine, or breath. This does not tell you how effectively you are using those ketones. Furthermore, you are just getting a snapshot of what is going on currently, which is not indicative of what may have been happening previously or will happen in the future.

WE DO NOT KNOW THE OPTIMAL LEVEL OF KETONES

Despite what you may hear in research or the keto community, we do not know the optimal ketone level. Again, just because you have a certain level of ketones in your body does not mean that we know how those ketones are being used. Furthermore, everyone will have different ketone requirements, so the optimal level of ketones is dependent on the person and the goal.

HIGHER KETONES ARE NOT NECESSARILY BETTER

Many people prioritize getting their ketone levels as high as possible, yet it is not clear that higher ketones are necessarily better. It is possible that for some therapeutic reasons, higher ketone levels may be more advantageous, but for the average person this likely isn't the case. We theorize that as you become more keto-adapted, you become a more efficient ketone producer *and* utilizer, meaning the amount of ketones your body produces closer aligns with how much it actually needs. This would lead to lower ketones readingsin your blood, breath, or urine. While this is a theory, we have frequently found in our research that long-term keto dieters tend to have lower ketone levels compared to beginners.

KETONES SHOULDN'T BE THE PRIMARY GOAL

Having elevated levels of ketones doesn't necessarily mean you're getting all the benefits of a ketogenic diet. This is similar to our conversation about macros. It is just a small piece of the puzzle. You can get ketones in your blood by eating grain-fed burgers without the bun, cooked in vegetable oil, with processed dairy on top. That doesn't mean it's healthy.

Don't take any of this to mean we think testing ketones is bad. Testing is great for determining if you are consuming a diet allowing for ketone production to occur. Plus, if you have some data on what your ketone levels typically are, then you can better assess how you are responding to specific nutritional strategies.

As is the case for tracking macros, testing ketones when first starting a keto diet could be beneficial. However, if this is going to be an added stressor, which it very well could be for a new keto dieter, then sticking to the approved keto food list will do just fine for ensuring that you are getting into ketosis.

However, the key here is if you are sticking to the approved keto food list. We have talked to plenty of people who start keto, eat foods they believe to be low-carb, report not feeling the benefits of keto—and when we test their ketones the readings come back very low. When we ask about their diet, we find they are making a mistake somewhere, with hidden carbs being a common culprit. That means if you aren't going to stick to the approved food list, the importance of tracking both ketones (and macros for that matter) becomes greater.

Like macros, ketone testing is not something that needs to be done all the time. Ketone testing is a good method for making sure you are on the right track and that any changes you make allow you to maintain a state of ketosis. This can be done by simply testing ketones a few times throughout the week.

? WHAT ARE THE DIFFERENT WAYS TO TEST YOUR KETONES?

Short Answer: Ketones can be tested through urine, blood, and breath.

URINE TESTING

Acetoacetate, one of the three ketones produced in the body, can be measured through your urine. The way metabolic substrates (things your body uses for energy), like ketones, get into your urine is if they are "spilling over." If there is an excess of a certain metabolic substrate, your blood dumps it into your kidneys, to be excreted through urine. This is a good thing, but it can make interpreting urine ketone tests difficult.

Remember, when you shift from relying on carbs to relying on ketones for energy your body goes through keto-adaptation, meaning it needs to get used to using ketones for energy. This takes a while at first. Until then, your body is not efficient at using the ketones it is producing and will excrete a lot of them through your urine. You can measure these excess ketones with a simple urine strip. The strip changes color relative to the number of ketones in your urine and, *bam*, you can tell roughly what level of ketones are in excess.

When you first start keto, this method can be a great way to ensure that you are on the right track with your diet and producing ketones. However, as you become keto-adapted, your body will have fewer excess ketones and the strips will typically show a lower reading. This is misleading. You may actually be in a deeper state of ketosis, but the strip says you have fewer ketones. You are simply using the ketones now, lowering excess ketones that would be detected in the urine.

Other factors that can impact acetoacetate levels in your urine are electrolyte and hydration levels, which can produce variable readings. This is important to consider since many people are dehydrated when they first start keto, further drawing into question the accuracy of urine testing.

Another problem with testing ketones in urine is interpretation. The strip turns a shade of a color, which you have to match up with examples on the back of your urine strip bottle. There is a lot of room for user error here.

While urine testing is not the most accurate, it is cheap and can be a good starting point for a new ketogenic dieter. Pee on the stick, tap any excess urine off, then wait a few moments (usually 45 seconds) to see if there are detectable ketone levels in your urine. Refer to the package for instructions on how to interpret your results. Usually the darker purple the strip, the more ketones.

- **Advantages:** Quick and easy. Strips are affordable. You can purchase a pack of 100 strips for about $8.
- **Disadvantages:** Can get messy. Only accurate sometimes. Not a precise measurement.

BLOOD TESTING

The main ketone body used for energy is beta-hydroxybutyrate, or BHB. BHB is produced in the liver or taken as a supplement. In both cases it is released into the bloodstream where it can enter the cells and be converted to acetoacetate, which can then ultimately be converted to acetyl-CoA and used by mitochondria in your cells to produce energy. Unnecessary biochemistry aside, you can test your level of beta-hydroxybutyrate by sampling blood. This can be done easily at home the same way individuals with diabetes check their blood glucose, except testing ketones requires an actual ketone strip similar to the glucose strip.

Unlike your urine, your blood is a tightly regulated system and doesn't get diluted or change with different levels of hydration. This makes blood ketone testing a more direct way to measure ketosis.

There are still limitations to blood ketone readings. As we mentioned before, you are still simply getting a snapshot of what is available in the blood, which is not a clear indicator of what your body is utilizing. This is why it is also common to see blood ketone levels go down over time as people become further keto-adapted. Also, since this is only a snapshot, the time when you test is critical, which we will get more into in a bit. Despite this, since BHB is the primary ketone that is used for energy, testing circulating levels can be a good way to determine what is available to your brain and rest of the body, and a good way to make sure you are on the right track with your ketogenic diet.

The downside to this test is some people may have a strong aversion to pricking themselves with a tiny needle and using their own blood for a measurement. Plus, ketone testing strips can be expensive. If either of these factors are a concern for you, avoid testing regularly.

To test your blood ketones, get a meter (we recommend Keto-Mojo) and some ketone strips. Use an alcohol swab to cleanse the area you are testing (your finger) to minimize the risk of infection. Make sure this alcohol is completely rinsed and wiped off to ensure it does not skew the results. Use a fresh lancet (the needle that pokes you) every time; using the included spring-loaded tool, prick your finger. After you prick your finger, wipe the first drop of blood away to further ensure alcohol isn't in your reading, and place the next drop of blood on the strip. Wait 10 seconds for a reading. The blood level of BHB is measured in millimolar concentration (mmol).

Remember, blood ketone testing is a snapshot of what is currently going on in your body, so when you test is important. If you want to collect and compare data as scientifically as possible, you must establish a reliable baseline. To do this, limit as many factors as possible. We recommend testing under the following conditions:

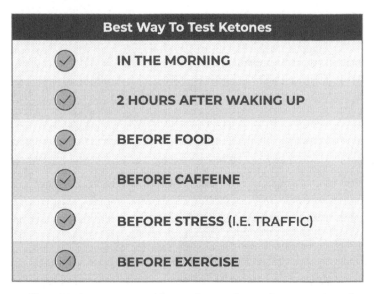

Best Way To Test Ketones
✓ IN THE MORNING
✓ 2 HOURS AFTER WAKING UP
✓ BEFORE FOOD
✓ BEFORE CAFFEINE
✓ BEFORE STRESS (I.E. TRAFFIC)
✓ BEFORE EXERCISE

Yes, this is a very specific testing regimen, but morning circadian systems, food, caffeine, exercise, and stress hormones can all impact your readings. It will be extremely difficult to establish a baseline if these factors vary each time you test.

We also understand that these conditions are not always possible, which is another reason why we do not recommend testing ketones every day. Pick one day per week where you know you can test under these conditions and use that to establish a baseline for your week, then compare week to week.

If you use ketone testing as a method for testing your responses to food, you will want to measure at different checkpoints, which we get into a little later in this chapter.

- **Advantages:** Pretty accurate measurement. In our opinion, the most reliable and effective measurement of ketone levels.
- **Disadvantages:** Expensive strips. Some may not like drawing blood.

BREATH TESTING

Acetone, or acetate, is a ketone produced by gas exchange in your lungs. You breathe out a detectable level of this particular ketone. Breath acetone has been found to be as reliable a predictor of ketosis as urine strips;[132] however, a lot more research is required to determine how reliable it is compared to blood ketone testing. Since acetone is not the primary ketone used by the body but rather a by-product of fat burning, it is an indirect method of measuring ketones. However, research has indicated that breath acetone is a reliable way to monitor rate of fat loss.[133]

Breath acetone, or BrAce, can be recorded with devices like LEVL. BrAce is measured in parts per million, or ppm, and measurements can range from 1 ppm to over 1250 ppm. Interpreting your breath acetone levels may vary depending on which software you are using.

One of the key advantages of a breath meter is that it is a reusable, one-time purchase. Once you buy the breath meter, you can test as many times as you want. This is not the case with urine or blood strips, which are one-time use.

A huge downside we've noticed is the inconsistency with breath meters. Anthony has found that he can register 2.5 mmol blood levels, yet only show trace acetone levels by breath.

Ketone breath meters are relatively new to the market and it appears may require some improvements. If you use them, testing alongside a blood meter is recommended.

---

132 K. Musa-Veloso, S.S. Likhodii, and S.C. Cunnane, S. C., "Breath Acetone is a Reliable Indicator of Ketosis in Adults Consuming Ketogenic Meals," *The American Journal of Clinical Nutrition* 76, no. 1 (2002): 65-70.

133 J.S. Anderson, J. C., "Measuring Breath Acetone for Monitoring Fat Loss," *Obesity* 23, no. 12 (2015): 2327-2334.

- **Advantages:** Reusable device. Doesn't use bodily fluids. Good option for kids managing seizures with a ketogenic diet as you don't have to prick their finger all the time.
- **Disadvantages:** Indirect and potentially inaccurate measurement. Often inconsistent readings.

? WHAT IS THE BEST WAY TO TEST KETONES?

Currently, we believe that blood ketone meters are the best way to test your ketones. While there are pros and cons to each method, we feel that the blood meters are the most accurate and allow you to gather better data to use for your personal assessments.

However, for beginners or someone who is just dabbling with keto, urine strips may be a better option, since they do not require a significant financial commitment and can be a good way to see if you are on the right track.

If you want to be a data collecting machine and help us best answer these discrepancies in ketone testing, get all three and get to testing! But your pocketbook may not thank you.

? WHAT IS THE OPTIMAL KETONE RANGE?

It is impossible to determine the optimal ketone range. There are so many factors that affect ketone levels, and interpreting the results is difficult. For example, if you have been following keto for a while, we hypothesize that your ketone levels will be lower because you are now a more efficient ketone producer and utilizer.

Research on blood ketone testing has reported that 0.5 mmol is considered being "in ketosis," while 1.5-3.0 mmol is considered "optimal ketosis"[134] Since these studies may fail to

---

134 P. Taboulet, N. Deconinck, A. Thurel, L. Haas, J. Manamani,...

account for the various factors that impact these results, we recommend aiming for being at least above 0.5 mmol in your morning-controlled blood ketone test.

Since interpreting your ketone levels is a struggle, recording your perceived feelings may be a better indicator of whether you are in an optimal ketone range. These measurements could include:

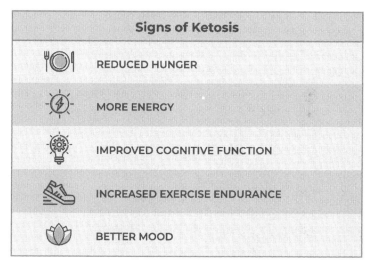

Signs of Ketosis
REDUCED HUNGER
MORE ENERGY
IMPROVED COGNITIVE FUNCTION
INCREASED EXERCISE ENDURANCE
BETTER MOOD

If you are experiencing some of these signs of ketosis, then chances are you are in your own "optimal ketone range." Even if you are recording ketone levels, record these perceived feelings with your ketone levels to see how they match up.

While the majority of ketogenic dieters put a huge emphasis on testing ketones, we think that testing your blood glucose or blood sugar is of greater importance.

...R. Porcher, R. et al., "Correlation Between Urine Ketones (acetoacetate) and Capillary Blood Ketones (3-beta-hydroxybutyrate) in Hyperglycaemic Patients," *Diabetes & Metabolism* 33, no. 2 (2007): 135-139.

BLOOD GLUCOSE TESTING

? WHY SHOULD I TEST MY BLOOD GLUCOSE?

Blood sugar is just as important, if not more important, than ketone levels because to get your body to produce ketones, your blood glucose levels must lower. Plus, fasted morning blood glucose readings are a huge indicator of overall health, especially as it relates to avoiding diabetes.

On keto, you want your blood sugar to be consistently under control. Glucose levels change constantly, depending on what environment you're in, what food you've eaten, what your workouts are, how stressed you are, and much more.

Everyone responds to stimuli differently. As Robb Wolf points out in his book *Wired to Eat*, people respond very differently even in controlled conditions. In one study, participants tracked their blood glucose in response to eating bananas versus eating cookies. One set of people had enormous blood glucose spikes from eating cookies and not much from eating the bananas. Another group had an astonishingly high blood glucose spike from the bananas and *not* the cookies.[135]

In this particular case, the best explanation is that the sugar fructose is much higher in bananas and some people react differently to fructose than they do glucose. Regardless, the point is that everyone will have different responses in blood sugar from the foods they eat, which makes testing blood glucose important.

---

135 David Zeevi, Tal Korem, Niv Zmora, David Israeli, Daphna Rothschild, Adina Weinberger, et al., "Personalized Nutrition by Prediction of Glycemic Responses," *Cell* 163, no. 5 (2015): 1079.

Keep in mind, your blood sugar will not go to zero on a ketogenic diet and even after the consumption of a keto-friendly meal, you may even see an increase in blood glucose to some degree. Thus, it is important to determine what your baseline blood glucose is and how you typically respond to various foods.

? HOW DO I TEST MY BLOOD GLUCOSE?

Testing your blood glucose is just like testing your blood ketones. In fact, they can be done on the same device, they just require a different testing strip. Luckily, glucose testing strips are much cheaper than ketone strips.

Similar to blood ketones, your blood glucose can be impacted by numerous factors and is only a snapshot of what is currently going on in your body. For this reason, establishing a controlled baseline, just as you do for ketones, is equally important. Later in this chapter we will describe how to test blood glucose responses to food.

? WHAT IS THE OPTIMAL BLOOD GLUCOSE RANGE?

The general recommendation for optimal blood glucose range is between 80-120 mg/dl fasted in the morning; however, on a keto diet, your morning blood glucose should be in the 80s or lower. Note that if you are new to keto, it may take a while to get your morning blood glucose levels this low. That's okay, Rome wasn't built in a day.

Acceptable increases in blood glucose as a response to food is very individualized. Typically, we would not like to see anything greater than a 20-point increase, and even this is pushing it.

PUT THEM TOGETHER:
GLUCOSE KETONE INDEX

The glucose ketone index, or GKI, is the ratio of glucose to ketones in the blood. The GKI was created by Dr. Thomas Seyfried, a scientist specializing in cancer metabolism and treatment who has been using the GKI in both his fasting and ketogenic diet studies.

Dr. Seyfried has demonstrated impressive therapeutic outcomes from lowering GKI. His research shows incredible results in managing tumor growth in patients with a GKI of 1.0.[136] Other specific examples of his findings are a 22 percent reduction in tumor metabolism going from 27.5 to 1.1 GKI for 56 days, an 88 percent reduction in tumor dry weight going from 15.2 to 3.7 GKI for 13 days, and a 5x (!) survival time (200+ days vs 41 days) when combining radiation treatment and lowering GKI from 32.3 to 5.7 for only 13 days.[137] We will discuss the therapeutic potential of keto for cancer in the next chapter.

The glucose ketone index isn't just for cancer treatment though. This value is important for people who have blood sugar issues, people who want to optimize their health, those looking to get the most out of their ketogenic diet, and those looking to measure how effective the results of fasting are.

If you've had a history of diabetes, obesity, or other metabolic problems, track this index and try to get it as low as possible. Here is a step by step for calculating GKI.

---

136 T.N. Seyfried and L.M. Shelton, "Cancer as a Metabolic Disease," *Nutrition & Metabolism* 7, no. 1(2010): 7.

137 T.N. Seyfried, R.E. Flores, A.M. Poff, and D.P. D'agostino, "Cancer as a Metabolic Disease: Implications for Novel Therapeutics," *Carcinogenesis* 35, no. 3 (2013): 515-527.

Calculating Your GKI

1	**MEASURE GLUCOSE** Example: 80 mg/dl glucose	
2	**MEASURE KETONES** Example: 1.5 mmol ketones	
3	**DIVIDE GLUCOSE BY 18** Example: 80/18= 4.4 mmol glucose	
4	**DIVIDE THE NUMBER YOU GET FROM STEP 3 BY KETONES** Example: 4.4/1.5=2.96 GKI	

Where Do You Stack Up?

GKI **<9**	**NOT IN KETOSIS**
GKI **6-9**	**LOW LEVEL OF KETOSIS**
GKI **3-6**	**MODERATE KETOSIS**
GKI **1-3**	**HIGH KETOSIS**
GKI **<1**	**THERAPEUTIC KETOSIS**

Anthony has been in deep ketosis for a while, and while he can sometimes sneak his GKI below 1.0, it's tough to stay in that range for long when eating. Your ketones don't get high enough and your blood sugar doesn't stay low enough for long enough. For certain therapeutic uses having an extremely low

GKI is necessary, but otherwise being in the moderate GKI range is enough to experience a lot of keto benefits!

If you are already tracking your ketone levels and not calculating your GKI, spend the extra few bucks on some glucose strips and do quick calculations to see a larger picture of your metabolism and health.

BODY COMPOSITION

On a ketogenic diet you will make positive improvements in body composition. While you should not fall victim to over obsessing about this aspect of keto, it is great to be able to track the improvements you are making to get a better picture of what is and isn't working for you.

Notice that we are saying "body composition" and not "weight." Measuring your weight is far too simple for assessing the changes happening in your body and results can often be deceiving. For example, weight loss is rapid when you first start keto due to water and glycogen loss, but you did not lose six pounds of fat your first week of keto.

Also, remember that the ketogenic diet will help burn fat and spare or build muscle, which isn't true for most other diets. Many studies comparing weight loss on keto vs. non-keto diets demonstrate similar weight loss between both diets, but when the composition of that weight loss is measured, the results demonstrate greater fat loss and less muscle loss on keto.[138] Just measuring weight on a scale won't be a good representation

---

138 C.M. Young, S.S. Scanlan, H.S. Im, and L. Lutwak, "Effect on Body Composition and Other Parameters in Obese Young Men of Carbohydrate Level of Reduction Diet," *The American Journal of Clinical Nutrition* 24, no. 3 (1971): 290-296.

of this. Even more, if you increase your muscle mass, it could actually be reflected negatively on the scale.

? SHOULD I TRACK MY BODY COMPOSITION ON KETO?

Tracking your body composition is *not* essential. However, for those who have a primary goal that is related to aesthetics (fat loss and/or muscle gain), tracking your body composition can be a good idea.

Remember, keto is a muscle sparing diet, but if the diet is not dialed in for you as an individual, muscle loss can occur. Tracking your body composition can help you determine if the keto diet is causing you to lose muscle, allowing you to make adjustments to your diet accordingly.

This isn't just important to someone worried about how their biceps look. For people with cancer, cachexia, or muscle wasting, is a common cause of disease progression and death and very important to limit. Measuring body composition can help ensure that you are on the right track in this regard as well.

If you have the means, we recommend testing body composition every once in a while to determine if you have tailored your diet to ensure that you are progressing as you would like to.

? WHAT ARE THE DIFFERENT WAYS TO TEST BODY COMPOSITION?

SCALE
This method only measures weight but does not measure the composition of that weight. It can provide some data but limited data that is hard to interpret. Don't obsess over what the scale says.

CALIPERS

Calipers measure subcutaneous fat (fat directly under your skin). While this is not a very accurate measurement technique, it is useful for tracking trends in changing body composition. Always test under the same conditions and have the test completed by the same person.

BIOIMPEDANCE

This form of measurement uses an electrical current to measure body composition. The machine estimates body composition based on how quickly the current is conducted through the body. The accuracy of bioimpedance depends greatly on hydration levels. As with the calipers, always test under the same conditions and using the same machine.

DEXA

Dual-energy X-ray absorptiometry measures body composition using two X-ray beams, with different energy levels, to determine several different components of body composition, including muscle, fat, and bone mineral density. DEXA scans are pretty accurate but can be a little skewed by changes in muscle glycogen and hydrogen status.

PROGRESS PHOTOS

Progress photos are a great way to track visual changes in body composition. Try to keep lighting and the clothes you are wearing consistent when taking progress photos. This approach won't give you measurable metrics but can capture just how far you've come in your health and fitness journey. This approach is recommended for most people.

? WHAT IS THE BEST WAY TO TEST BODY COMPOSITION?

The DEXA scan is the gold standard. DEXA scans can provide lean mass percentage, body fat percentage, bone density, muscle symmetry, and regional composition. While results from this test are not perfect and can still be misleading under certain circumstances, it is the most accurate method. DEXA machines are expensive, so few gyms have them. More advanced gyms and weight loss clinics may have a DEXA machine that you can use by appointment. You can find this by simply searching for "DEXA testing near me" on Google. DEXA scans do not have to be done frequently; once a quarter is plenty.

TROUBLESHOOTING FAILURE TO LOSE WEIGHT

Hitting a weight loss plateau can happen on keto. Usually this means that some adjustments need to be made. If this happens to you, here are a few things to consider:

#1: YOU'RE NOT ACTUALLY IN KETOSIS

Have you been following the ketogenic diet for a while but have no idea if you're in ketosis? This is where testing your ketone levels comes in. You'll only truly know whether you're in a ketogenic state when you test your ketone levels.

#2: YOU'RE OVEREATING ON CARBS/ MISSING HIDDEN CARBOHYDRATES

Certain vegetables, dairy, and nuts are on the keto-approved food list but may have a higher carbohydrate count than you think. Dairy and nuts are two of the biggest culprits of overeating carbs and carbs found in vegetables like cabbage, cauliflower, broccoli, brussels sprouts, fennel turnips, eggplant, tomatoes, peppers, onion, and squash can also add up. Count your carbs and make sure they are in check if you are stuck at a weight loss plateau.

#3: YOU'RE EATING TOO MUCH

Some new keto dieters think they can eat an endless amount of fat. Fats contain over twice the amount of calories as carbs or protein, so it is very easy to overeat it and stall weight loss. If you are stuck at a weight loss plateau, track your calories to see if you are in the right range.

#4: YOU'RE NOT EATING ENOUGH

Not getting enough calories can also stall weight loss. If you are in an extreme calorie deficit for too long, whether from undereating or excessive exercise, your metabolism slows down. If you go to the extremes and create a deficit too large, your metabolic rate will drop significantly in order to protect organs and normal bodily functions. Track your calories and if too low, start taking strategies to increase.

#5: YOU'RE GETTING TOO MUCH EXERCISE

You know the saying "too much of a good thing can be a bad thing"? That includes exercise. Exercise is great for improving overall health, but there is a limit for everyone. The main type of exercise abused by those with a goal of weight loss is cardio. Again, if you are creating too great of a caloric deficit for too long, your body may respond by slowing weight loss. Additionally, while all effective exercise creates some type of acute inflammation, chronic over exercising can create chronic, systemic inflammation as well as oxidative stress. All of which will not only slow weight loss, but also damage health. If you are over exercising, try scaling it back a bit and letting your body catch up and recover.

#6: YOU'RE EXPERIENCING STRESS

Stress is a significant factor in weight loss. Cortisol, commonly considered the stress hormone, actually has beneficial purposes in the body. The problem arises in chronic elevations in cortisol. When we're stressed out, our body produces cortisol, and when cortisol is constantly elevated you will again experience not only slow weight loss, but also damaged health. If you are experiencing a lot of stress, take steps toward reducing it such as meditation.

#7: YOU'RE NOT SLEEPING ENOUGH

Often an underestimated factor, lack of sleep can stall or prevent weight loss. Inadequate sleep can throw off your circadian rhythms and mess with your body's biological clock. All of your organs are set up for certain timing; messing with your sleep can put you at a severe disadvantage. As it relates to weight, sleep deficiency has been shown to increase the risk of obesity.

Sleep has also been shown to be a contributing factor in the balance of hormones—especially hunger hormones. Ghrelin (the hormone that makes you feel hungry) and leptin (the hormone that makes you feel full) are both affected by lack of sleep.[139] Messing with these hormones can stimulate appetite and cravings, thus making weight loss more difficult.

---

139 K. Spiegel, E. Tasali, P. Penev and E. Van Cauter, "Brief Communication: Sleep Curtailment in Healthy Young Men is Associated with Decreased Leptin Levels, Elevated Ghrelin Levels, and Increased Hunger and Appetite," *Annals of Internal Medicine* 141, no. 11 (2004): 846-850.

#8: YOU HAVE FOOD SENSITIVITIES

Even if you are following your macros and tracking your calories, something may still seem off. Many people have food sensitivities that they don't even know of, the most common of which is dairy (more tips to come on this topic). When your body is sensitive to a particular property in certain foods such as dairy or gluten, it can cause imbalances in the gut, which then leads to overall inflammation. Again, inflammation will not only slow your weight loss but also damage your health. If you think you may be sensitive to a certain food, experiment with removing it from your diet and seeing how you respond.

#9: LEPTIN RESISTANCE

Leptin is an appetite-regulating hormone produced by fat cells in the body. It's mainly responsible for regulating how many calories we eat, how many we burn, and how much fat we carry on our bodies.

Leptin resistance occurs when you have plenty of leptin, but the messages aren't being received by the brain, resulting in appetite stimulation. The major causes of leptin resistance include poor sleep patterns, a diet full of processed foods, overeating, stress, and severe calorie restriction or starvation. Properly formulating your ketogenic diet using the strategies presented in this book will be effective for improving leptin signaling.

DON'T DISCOUNT SIGNS OF PROGRESS

If you are experiencing a weight loss stall, it's important to recognize the other improvements in health you are still making. Overall health should be the goal, so give yourself credit for any and all benefits you are still experiencing, including:

- Healthier hair, skin, and nails
- More mental clarity
- Reduction in cravings
- More energy throughout the day
- Less inflammation
- Eating a diet that can protect from chronic diseases
- The knowledge that you're putting health-promoting foods in your body

Although weight is a good indicator of progress and is an important marker of health (to an extent), remember that it's about more than the number on the scale (and remember that the scale is not the best way to measure body composition changes!). If you are at a weight loss plateau, stick with it and don't be afraid to make changes.

BLOOD TESTS

? SHOULD I TAKE ANY BLOOD TESTS?

The problem with all blood tests is that in most cases we are simply testing markers of something, which is not the most direct way to measure with the highest level of confidence. In some cases, we don't even have the best understanding of the markers we are measuring, like in the case of cholesterol.

Despite our lack of understanding and interpretation of these measures, there is still a lot of value in getting blood work done. For one, you can see how different nutritional strategies are impacting your readings, which is great data to record along with things like your perceived feelings of wellness. For example, recording lower numbers of CRP, a common inflammatory marker, combined with perceived feelings of improved joint health is useful information to have together.

Testing blood is not something that you have to do frequently but getting a little blood work done every quarter is a good way to keep tabs on the changes occurring in your body over time.

② WHICH MEASURES SHOULD I BE LOOKING AT?

The blood measures you should look at depend on what is important to you; this is a conversation that you should have with your doctor. Below are a few of the tests that we think are important to measure. For each measure, we will list the reference ranges; however, it is important to note that we do not believe that we have fully figured out the best ranges of these measures, especially as it relates to a ketogenic diet, which we believe changes the recommendations. Furthermore, many of these measures are important as they relate to one another, and these relationships are still not fully understood. Again, despite the confusion, there is still a lot of value in getting these tests done and having them evaluated by a professional who understands ketogenic diets.

Reference ranges can also vary by age, sex, methods of testing, and numerous other factors. Furthermore, some tests do not have nationally established reference ranges so ranges in this chapter are approximate.

COMPLETE BLOOD COUNT (CBC)
This test tells you everything you need to know about your blood cells. A CBC measures red, white, and platelet blood cells to help you determine anything from infections to hemoglobin levels to the possible risk of blood clots and more. Below are the CBC reference ranges:

- White Blood Cells: 4,500-10,000 cells/mcl
- Red Blood Cells: 4-5 million cells/mcl (women) and 5-6 million cells/mcl (men)
- Platelets: 140,000-450,000 cells/mcl
- Hemoglobin: 12-15 gm/dl (women) and 14-17 gm/dl (men)
- Hematocrit: 36-44 percent (women) and 41-50 percent (men)

COMPREHENSIVE METABOLIC PANEL (CMP)

A CMP tests fourteen different markets: glucose, calcium, albumin, protein, sodium, potassium, chloride, bicarbonate, AST, ALT, ALP, bilirubin, urea, and creatinine.

This test tells you how healthy your liver and kidneys are, any dramatic changes in blood sugar or protein levels, and acid/base balance in your body. This test can indicate chronic health issues or track the progression of certain diseases. Below are the CMP reference ranges:

- Glucose: 70-99 mg/dL fasted (should be lower on keto)
- Calcium: 8.5-10.9 mg/dL
- Albumin: 3.9-5.0 g/dL
- Protein: 6.3-7.9 g/dL
- Sodium: 136-144 mEq/L
- Potassium: 3.7-5.2 mEq/L
- Chloride: 96-106 mmol/L
- Bicarbonate: 20-29 mmol/L
- AST: 10-34 IU/L
- ALT: 8-37IU/L
- ALP: 44-147 IU/L
- Bilirubin: 0-0.3 mg/dL (direct), 0.3-1.9mg/dl (total)
- Urea: 7-20 mg/dL
- Creatinine: 0.8-1.4 mg/dL

LIPID PANEL

This test measures your cholesterol and triglycerides. It is important to note that these reference ranges may especially vary on keto and the impact of each of these measures is dependent on numerous other factors. For instance, having a higher level of LDL may not be dangerous unless CRP, which we will cover soon, is also elevated. While we are still working to better understand the best reference ranges for keto specifically, we do know the importance of keeping triglycerides under control and having elevated HDL. Here are lipid panel reference ranges:

- Triglycerides: <160 mg/dl
- Total Cholesterol: <200 mg/dl
- HDL-C: >40 mg/dl
- LDL-C: <160 mg/dl

If you have the option, opt for an NMR lipoprofile test in place of a standard lipid panel. An NMR is a particle test that gives you much more insight into your cholesterol measurements. This test helps you determine the number, size, and density of your cholesterol particles, which is a better way to predict the impact your cholesterol is going to have on your health.

HBA1C

This test is extremely important as it relates to diabetes and prediabetes. Glucose binds to hemoglobin in red blood cells in a process known as glycation. The higher our blood sugar, the more glycation occurs. HbA1c is a measure of glycated hemoglobin, which can actually tell you your average blood sugar over the last three months. This is a great way to see how the foods you have been eating impact your blood sugar results over time. This marker is a great measure for degree of insulin sensitivity. Here are HbA1c reference ranges:

- Normal: 4.0-5.5 percent
- Prediabetes: 5.6-6.4 percent
- Diabetes: >6.5 percent
- Critical Value: >7.0 percent

CRP

CRP fights infection and increases in response to chronic stress. CRP is an inflammatory marker, and inflammation is a common contributor to many chronic health conditions. For this reason, tracking CRP and taking measures to keep it low is important. Elevated CRP can change your interpretation of other blood levels, for instance LDL as we previously mentioned. For this reason, CRP should almost always be tested. The standard reference range for CRP is <3 mg/L.

VITAMIN D

Many people are deficient in vitamin D, which can result in impaired hormonal profiles as well as altered mood. Low vitamin D can also lead to chronic fatigue and a weak immune system. Testing your vitamin D levels can be a great way to determine if you should take vitamin D supplements. Reference ranges for vitamin D is 40-100 ng/dL.

In addition to the tests mentioned above, there are plenty of other tests that can be valuable depending on the person, like thyroid, endocrine, fasting insulin or c-peptide, and vitamin B12.

OPTIMIZING FOOD INTAKE

Earlier in this chapter we discussed the importance of testing glucose. Measuring blood glucose can also be a great tool for determining which foods are the best fit for you. Not everyone reacts the same way to foods. Some keto-approved foods may agree with you, others may not. The best way to find out is through testing your responses to different foods.

STEP 1: ESTABLISH A BASELINE

Establishing a baseline is essential so you can compare and contrast how your body is responding to the things you are eating. If you're trying to be as scientific as possible, try to do these experiments with as much control as you can. For instance, if you want to test the impact of different breakfast foods, start by comparing only breakfasts, at roughly the same time in the day, under the same conditions.

Remember, lack of sleep, stress, and changed environment can all play a big role in your baseline glucose levels and the impact foods have on your body. If you do test under different conditions, be sure to record that with your data.

STEP 2: TEST FOODS

Choose the food that you want to test and eat it. If you want to be even more scientific, start with just one food group and add from there. For instance, see how you respond to just one avocado. Then the next day, see how you respond to two chicken legs. Then the next day, notice how you respond to one avocado *and* two chicken legs. Did anything change here that you weren't expecting? You'll find some interesting results with some foods causing your body to respond differently when combined with other foods.

**STEP 3: MEASURE GLUCOSE IN 30-MINUTE
INTERVALS AFTER EATING FOOD**
Try not to change too much of the setting after the meal. For instance, if you eat and then you go for a light jog or hop in your car and drive somewhere else and drastically change the setting, you will get flawed results.

STEP 4: MEASURE GLUCOSE UNTIL BACK TO BASELINE
Note your blood sugar after the first 30 minutes and compare to baseline. Chances are unless the meal was almost entirely fat, your results will be different. This is normal. Keep measuring glucose until you are roughly back at your baseline measure.

If your blood sugar spikes after 30 minutes, but your body has dealt with it and is back to baseline at 60 minutes, it was responsive, and you shouldn't fear that food very much

If you have a moderate or high spike in blood sugar, and you still have that spike 2.5 hours after eating the initial meal, that food probably isn't for you. If this result is consistent across many foods, the ketogenic diet will be a very important tool for you to help get your metabolism back under control.

OPTIONAL STEP 5: CALCULATE THE GLUCOSE KETONE INDEX
If you want to get even more information, you can test your ketones and calculate your GKI after a meal to get a picture of that meals impact on your glucose-ketone relationship. The smaller the change, the better the meal!

DETERMINING CARBOHYDRATE THRESHOLD

As you know, there is no one size fits all approach to macronutrients. This is especially true for carbohydrates. While it is commonly advised to consume at or below 30 grams of carbs per day on a keto diet, certain individuals and/or goals may require more or less carbohydrates. This is why testing for your carbohydrate threshold is important. Follow these five steps for doing so:

1. Take a fasted blood glucose and ketone test in the morning, under our recommended conditions and calculate your GKI
2. Track your carbs for a week and calculate GKI every other day
3. If your GKI is falling outside of moderate range (or whatever your goal range is), you have exceeded your carb threshold; pull back 5-10 grams and repeat step 2
4. If your GKI is not falling outside of the recommended range, increase carbs by 10 grams and repeat step 2
5. Repeat until you have determined your carb threshold

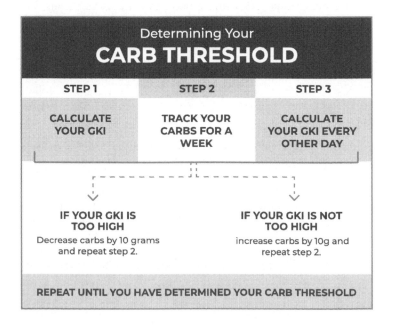

Determining Your
CARB THRESHOLD

STEP 1	STEP 2	STEP 3
CALCULATE YOUR GKI	TRACK YOUR CARBS FOR A WEEK	CALCULATE YOUR GKI EVERY OTHER DAY

IF YOUR GKI IS TOO HIGH
Decrease carbs by 10 grams and repeat step 2.

IF YOUR GKI IS NOT TOO HIGH
increase carbs by 10g and repeat step 2.

REPEAT UNTIL YOU HAVE DETERMINED YOUR CARB THRESHOLD

Note that besides certain physical performance benefits, there is no award for being able to consume more carbs.

ASSESSING DAIRY TOLERANCE

Throughout this book we have discussed dairy and how some individuals may not tolerate dairy well. While this could be a result of the quality of the dairy being consumed, assessing your dairy tolerance is a great way to determine if you have a dairy sensitivity.

To determine if you have a dairy sensitivity, you could ask your doctor to order super expensive labs for you. Companies like Cyrex will definitely help you learn if you have a sensitivity to dairy...or you could do it the old-fashioned way.

Begin by going thirty days without dairy. If you're not already keto, just start this when you go keto. If you're already in ketosis, start whenever, just start. Sometimes you may think you feel healthy...until the lights brighten a little bit and it dawns on you just how dim the room was in the first place. Some chronic symptoms that may clear up when removing dairy are:

- Fatigue
- Headaches
- Skin issues (i.e., acne, dry itchy skin, dandruff, and/or patchiness)
- Bloating or weight gain
- General inflammation
- Digestive inconsistencies

Remove dairy for thirty days. You'll live. After thirty days, hopefully you're feeling a little different and better. This will especially be the case if you've started the keto diet during this time. The trick now is to figure out if dairy was the culprit. Reintroduce dairy systematically to see if any symptoms come back. This will help you determine if you are truly sensitive to certain dairy products.

Remember, the two main reasons people react to dairy are sugars and protein. Now is the time to test to determine which you may be sensitive to. You can figure this out in a linear fashion. Add a food back in, wait one to two weeks, and see if any symptoms pop up. If nothing happens, add the next food.

Please note that this is not the extremely ridiculous "dairy reintroduction ladder" sometimes prescribed for children who appear to be allergic to dairy. This idiotic plan includes a rein-troduction phase of dairy in this order: biscuits, more biscuits, cupcakes, pancakes, pie, lasagna, pizza, chocolate, *then* yogurt, cheese, milk formula, and finally pasteurized/processed milk formula. Seriously. Seriously?!

Before you begin adding foods back into your diet, make sure you're actually getting real food dairy. Here are our recommendations:

- Go raw, whenever possible (especially milk and cheese)
- Skip skim, 1 percent, and 2 percent and go full-fat (especially milk and yogurt)
- Opt for grass-fed and organic foods whenever possible
- Look for non-homogenized milk and cream
- Buy your food local if possible
- Buy food that spoils and isn't a weird color

Add foods back to your diet in this order, paying attention to how you are feeling. Stop if you encounter problems, as these are progressively harder to tolerate:

1. BUTTER

Butter is almost entirely fat. It does have traces of lactose and milk proteins, so if you react to butter, sorry, but you should probably stop here. Dairy is not for you. Ghee and coconut oil should work just fine.

If you can tolerate butter, look for grass-fed versions to reap the benefits. Note: Stick to the most expensive butter, not the cheapest one. It should be yellow when you unwrap it (look, micronutrients!) and not white. It should also be soft(ish) when refrigerated, not rock hard.

2. CREAM

Raw cream can be purchased at a premium price. If you have the money to spend on it, spring for it. You get active enzymes, high-quality saturated fat, vitamins A, D, E, and K, among other beneficial micronutrients.

Because cream is 3 percent lactose (milk sugars) or sometimes less, depending on where get it, you may not react to this food as you would to homogenized, pasteurized milk. If you're purchasing cream in a cardboard carton, not a glass jug, you're probably not getting high-quality cream. The fats in it may be inflammatory and devoid of nutrition.

The cream should have little chunks of fat floating in it. Stay local and as raw as possible. And, no half-and-half. Cream. Real food. Feeling better after consuming cream? Then it's time to move on.

3. HARD CHEESES

Because of the fermentation process (bacteria-chomping sugars), you're looking at a very low milk sugar content, probably the lowest of any dairy. Think feta, parmesan, cheddar, gruyere, etc. Same thing here—the cheese should not be cheap or in brightly colored plastic bags or shrink-wrapped blocks. Go to a cheese counter where they are cutting it, where you can choose from raw or not, and which animals you are getting the cheese from. Your cheese should not have a nutrition facts or ingredient label.

4. FERMENTED DAIRY: KEFIR

This product shouldn't be much of an issue for those who worry about lactose because the sugar is metabolized during fermentation. In addition, the bacteria created during the fermentation process aid in digestion and supplement beneficial gut flora. However, these sources are pretty high in dairy proteins, so if you can't tolerate those, the reintroduction phase will stop here. Kefir has more probiotics and is less processed than yogurt, which is why we would try it first. Find it in the yogurt aisle but look at the ingredient list and make sure it doesn't contain a long list of strange ingredients.

5. FERMENTED DAIRY: YOGURT

Yogurt should be full-fat and unflavored. If you need it flavored go buy some berries or nuts and put those in there. This is important. Look at the ingredient list. If there are other things besides dairy on the ingredient list—skip! Not real food.

6. RAW MILK

Raw milk contains many of the enzymes and micronutrients that you need to adequately process and absorb dairy and can be thought of as an incredibly well balanced and nutritious food. We don't recommend drinking much milk if it is not raw. You are missing out on too much and it is just too far away from the real food. Some states outlaw raw milk, which is insane, but if you can get it and afford it, spring for it. As a bonus, it tastes far better than any milk you've ever had. Think milkshake.

7. SOFT CHEESES

Soft cheese like real mozzarella (comes immersed in liquid), burrata (a form of mozzarella), and the like come after raw milk in this list as they typically don't have the same nutrient and enzyme profile. Quality remains important here.

8. OTHER DAIRY PRODUCTS

This includes sour cream, cottage cheese, cream cheese, and more. This is last on the list because these foods are typically processed. It is tough to get good products from good brands, but if you want this stuff, test it separately. Look for the words "grass-fed" and "fermented" on the tub. For instance, Kalona SuperNatural has a really good grass-fed cottage cheese, and Nancy's has a really good fermented sour cream and cream cheese. Get these sources if you can.

It is important to reiterate that for the beginner, self-experimenting and tracking is not essential. For beginners, it is more important to lock down the basics of the diet and dedicate yourself to following them.

Even once adapted to the diet, the practices mentioned in this chapter still may not be for everyone. These strategies are for those who want to take things a little more serious, are very passionate about achieving a certain goal, are following the diet for therapeutic reasons, or are trying to push through a plateau. Tracking and self-experimenting will provide you more insight into what exactly is going on in your body so that you can make adjustments to optimize the diet for you.

CONCLUSION

Nutrition is at the core of health. As we have emphasized numerous times throughout this book, what you put in your body matters and determines what your life is going to look like from a physical, physiological, and psychological perspective. Knowledge is power. Knowing that you have the capability to take hold of your health and your quality of life just by changing your habits is a powerful realization. The only thing more powerful is actually implementing it into your day-to-day life.

Of course, a ketogenic diet is not the only approach that can be used to take control of your health. Furthermore, not everyone has to be on a ketogenic diet. However, the evidence is strong, a ketogenic diet hammers away at the problems rooted in our most common chronic health complications and diseases. This is why we are so passionate about keto. Keto is not the only way, but it's a pretty damn good way and we haven't found anything better yet.

It is going to be extremely important for more and more research to come out in the coming years to really help keto make the impact that it is capable of. Our current dietary recommendations are poor and based on weak evidence. While we do feel like there is plenty of research already available to make changes to these dietary recommendations, more research can only help drive the conversation forward.

Regardless of what the dietary guidelines say, you have the option to choose the best path for you to improve your health. We hope that after reading this book, the ketogenic diet is a part of your journey.

MORE TIPS FOR STARTING A KETOGENIC DIET

Starting a ketogenic diet does not have to be challenging. In conjunction with the numerous tips for getting started described throughout the book, here are a few additional short lists to help you out.

DOS AND DON'TS OF STARTING KETO

DOS

- Stick to the recommended foods from Chapter 6
- Focus on food quality when you can
- Have variety in your diet
- Stay hydrated
- Replenish electrolytes
- Move daily, even if it's just a walk
- Supplement according to your needs (see Chapter 8)
- Manage sleep and stress

DON'TS

- Weigh yourself everyday
- Count calories
- Eat vegetable oils
- Eat soy
- Eat corn
- Drink alcohol
- Eat starchy vegetables, grains, fruits
- Eat processed foods
- Drink energy drinks/diet soda

WHAT A TYPICAL DAY OF KETO LOOKS LIKE

Below is a brief breakdown of what a typical day of keto looks like for us. We have provided two examples, one for intermittent fasting days and one for non-intermittent fasting days.

INTERMITTENT FASTING DAY

- Water and electrolytes upon waking
- Black coffee, two hours after waking up
- Lunch: ¼ pound of ground beef, 2 eggs, avocado, water
- Before Workout: Perfect Keto Perform pre-workout, macadamia nuts
- After Workout: Whey protein Isolate, unsweetened coconut milk, ½ avocado
- Dinner: Salmon fillet, asparagus cooked in butter or coconut oil, side salad

NON-INTERMITTENT FASTING DAY

- Breakfast: 3 egg omelet with mushrooms, green peppers, avocado, coffee with MCT oil

- Lunch: Steak, Cobb salad
- Before Workout: Perfect Keto Perform pre-workout, almonds
- After Workout: Perfect Keto Bar, electrolytes
- Snack: Beef jerky
- Dinner: Ribeye steak, 2 eggs, brussels sprouts baked in olive oil

BRIEF SUMMARY OF WHAT OCCURS IN THE BODY WHEN STARTING A KETOGENIC DIET

You stop eating carbohydrates, so blood glucose lowers, causing a subsequent drop in insulin levels. This makes the pancreas secrete glucagon, which signals for stored fatty acids to be released from adipose tissue and into the blood where they can circulate and be taken in by various cells and used for energy. However, some fatty acids make it to the liver and are used for ketogenesis, which results in ketone molecules being produced from fat and shuttled out into the bloodstream, where they can travel to cells. Initially, these ketones have to help activate the transporters responsible for opening the doors for ketones to get in. This process can take some time and is one of the reasons why you see an increase in blood ketones, but a lag time before the benefits of ketosis are felt.

During this lag time, your body is also responding in other ways to the low insulin levels. In fact, your kidneys are responding by dumping a lot of water and electrolytes, leading to rapid weight loss, dehydration, and electrolyte depletion. Yeah, that's right, you didn't burn eight pounds of fat in four days. But that water and electrolyte loss doesn't just cause weight loss. It also causes many annoying symptoms that define the keto flu. This can be combatted through focusing on hydration and electrolyte replenishment.

You continue following a keto diet. You eat dietary fat and it gets absorbed and packaged into carriers known as chylomicrons. Chylomicrons can also travel to our cells to drop off fat for energy production and will preferentially visit just about everywhere except the liver and brain. Now more of those mobilized, previously stored fatty acids that we just talked about can go to the liver to further contribute to ketogenesis causing a greater increase in blood ketones. This is important because the brain can't use fat for fuel, it needs ketones.

After a couple of weeks, you are starting to feel better as you continue to burn more fat. Since you are becoming a more efficient fat burner and ketone producer, those transporters needed to take ketones into the cells are firing on all cylinders, making you a more efficient ketone utilizer as well. Now you are keto-adapted!

Your low insulin levels are knocking down one of the big contributors to poor health. Your brain is now running primarily on a more efficient energy source, which is leading to improved cognitive output, increased energy, and even a better mood. Greater antioxidant production and the reduction in pro-inflammatory foods are helping lower your inflammation levels, further contributing to your overall health improvements *and* allowing you to burn more fat. You keep following keto and now even your joints are starting to feel better.

As you continue to follow keto, you notice that you are not as hungry because keto, through several different mechanisms, stimulates satiety or fullness. Now you don't have the same sugar cravings you had, making it easier to follow this diet long term. However, you may notice that at some point you have lost enough weight, or you may have even lost some precious muscle. Now it is time to make some adjustments to your diet based on many of the recommendations made previously in this book.

Once you have made these adjustments, you have officially adopted the ketogenic diet as a lifestyle and are ready to either continue following the diet as long as you are seeing improvements or make adjustments to further improve your health.

EXTRA NOTES

ANCEL KEYS

We briefly mentioned Ancel Keys earlier in the book due to the impact he has had on our misunderstanding of dietary fat. Before we trash Keys for what he did to our dietary recommendations, we want to give credit where credit is due. Keys invented the K-ration during World War II, a ready to eat meal for soldiers. While he probably should have left the biscuit out of these K-rations, this was still a monumental invention.

Keys' passion for nutrition led him to start researching more on heart disease, where he found an apparent link between fat intake and risks of heart disease. Keys believed that the fat you eat affects your cholesterol levels, and that having high cholesterol levels led to heart disease.

In 1948, Keys decided to test his hypothesis by conducting the Framingham Heart Study. This study monitored over 5,000 people for six years to analyze their lifestyle habits and assess the prevalence of heart disease. Researchers involved in this study concluded that subjects at the highest risk for heart disease also had the highest cholesterol levels. So, close the book on that, right? Not so fast. What this study failed to address, just like many similar studies conducted today, are things like smoking, or lack of exercise, or, I don't know, maybe carbohydrate consumption?

Regardless, Keys trudged on, and in 1958, he conducted an experiment in which he tested saturated fat compared to unsaturated fat. He found that saturated fat led to a greater increase in cholesterol levels. This led to a hypothesis that high saturated fat intake was also a big cause of heart disease.

At this same time, the United States was seeing a dramatic increase in heart disease and a lot of pressure was being put on governing bodies to figure out what could be done about it. This is one of the reasons Keys' hypothesis was entertained in the first place; it was virtually the only starting point.

Despite the fact that cholesterol is a poor predictor of cardiovascular health, Keys' views spread like wildfire. In 1961, the American Heart Association brought Keys on their team, which led to several reports on the dangers of fat being released to the public, including a big article in *Time* magazine highlighting Keys' work. The theory of fat being the cause of heart disease began to spread globally.

All this did was further fuel the fire. Ancel Keys was conducting research left and right, intending to prove his point. The problem is that if you go back and look at these studies a little closer, you notice a few things. First of all, in a lot of the studies, such as Keys' Seven Countries Study, you find that he had a bad habit of cherry-picking his data—that is, choosing the data that supported his hypothesis. In the case of this particular study, he left out countries that did not provide data that supported his hypothesis. A big no-no in research.

Even more interesting was another Keys study where he had people consume more or less red meat, since red meat is high in saturated fat. Keys found that those consuming more red meat had higher cholesterol levels, so he concluded they must be at a higher risk for heart disease. Case closed. Except when the study was revisited years later, it was found that 26 members from the low red meat group died compared to only 6 in the high red meat group. Eight of the 26 died of heart disease, compared to 0 of the 6 in the high red meat group. There's not enough data here to conclude much, but we can say that Ancel may have missed the boat.

So why did Ancel Keys have such a strong vendetta against fat and manipulate his data? It's hard to say but many speculate that it was because he was mocked when he first presented his hypothesis on fat. Another possible explanation is that you can find whatever you want in research, and if your whole life's work is resting on finding a certain outcome, you may just find what you are looking for.

The impact Ancel had is still evident today. The fear of fat has led to low-fat dieting and an increased consumption of pro-inflammatory vegetable oils, since they were considered to be a healthy alternative to fat. Since these changes have occurred, we have seen a dramatic increase in all major chronic diseases. Simply put, Ancel Keys' hypothesis and recommendations were wrong. The truth that we have driven home throughout this book is that dietary fat should not be feared (especially when we cut out the carbs) and is essential to a healthy life.

DIFFICULTY INTERPRETING KETOGENIC RESEARCH

Throughout this book we discussed how confusing research can be sometimes. This is especially true of keto research. If this book has inspired you to start researching more, then we recommend getting a better understanding of the difficulties in interpreting ketogenic research.

Have you ever seen a headline on Facebook or Yahoo that says, "Low-carb diet leads to X, Y, Z"? If you have, then you have probably also seen headlines that really conflict, like the following:

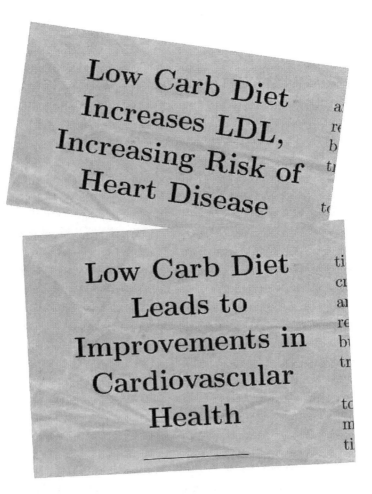

Low Carb Diet Increases LDL, Increasing Risk of Heart Disease

Low Carb Diet Leads to Improvements in Cardiovascular Health

There are several problems with these headlines, but for now we are going to tackle the "low-carb" part. One of the reasons a lot of nutrition research gets confusing is because of the way diets are classified in research. For a study to be considered low-carb, it only has to be less than 25 percent of total calories. That's really not that low-carb. If you were consuming a 2,000-calorie diet, that would be 125 grams of carbs (one gram of carbohydrate contains four calories).

While this may be low-carb compared to the standard American diet, it is clearly not as low-carb as a diet limiting you to under 30 grams of carbs like a ketogenic diet. This is important since earlier in the book we highlighted that there is a big difference in what happens in the body at different degrees of carbohydrate restriction.

In addition to failing to restrict carbs low enough, there is also a lot of confusion in studies labeled as "high-fat." You have probably also seen headlines such as, "High-Fat Diet Increases Risk of Colon Cancer." You click and it's an article that explains what this "high-fat" diet found. Now all of a sudden, keto is bad again. However, if you actually go to the study you find that just because the diet was high-fat doesn't mean it was low-carb. In many cases, these studies are actually high-fat *and* high-carb—a recipe for poor health.

There is a long list of additional difficulties with interpreting nutrition research, but the final one we want to note is the difference in study types. Many studies that are used against keto are epidemiological studies; these are also the types of studies Ancel Keys used to support his hypothesis. These studies are very weak because they are observational, meaning they follow populations for a period of time and record or have them report what they eat and try to correlate their findings with risk of disease. The problem is that these studies fail to look at health holistically. Most epidemiological studies that report high-fat diets correlating with an increased risk of a particular disease are bogus because they are not keto studies. Many of these studies simply ask a group of people questions like "how much red meat have you eaten in the last six months," or "how many eggs do you typically eat per day." The problem is that just because a person reports eating high-fat foods does not mean they are eating low-carb or keto. Furthermore, these studies do not take into account other risk factors like food quality, activity level, alcohol consumption, or sleep habits. This makes it impossible to infer from these studies.

The point is that if you are going to read research, look for randomized controlled trials or RCTs, and be sure to read past the abstract to make sure that what is reported in the abstract is actually what was found in the study.

RESOURCES

Here are our most recommended resources for learning more about and helping you better follow a ketogenic diet.

PRACTITIONERS

If you are looking to start the ketogenic diet for therapeutic purposes or you are wanting to have guidance along the way, it will be important for you to find a practitioner who understands the ketogenic diet, how to implement it, and its impact on the body. There are several resources out there that can help you search for these practitioners by location. We recommend using https://www.lowcarbusa.org/low-carb-providers/lchf-doctors/.

SCIENTISTS

If you are looking to dive more into the research on ketogenic dieting, especially for therapeutic uses, here is a list of our favorite scientists who have produced some incredible work:

- Dr. Jeffry Gerber—Weight management, general health
- Dr. Thomas Seyfried—Cancer
- Dr. Dominic D'Agostino—Cancer
- Dr. Angela Poff—Cancer
- Dr. Adrienne Scheck—Cancer
- Dr. Eric Westman—Diabetes, weight management
- Dr. Jason Fung—Diabetes, fasting
- Dr. David Ludwig—Weight management
- Dr. Ben Bikman—Weight management
- Dr. Stephen Cunnane—Neurodegenerative disease
- Dr. Mary Newport—Neurodegenerative disease
- Dr. Jong Rho—Epilepsy
- Dr. Eric Kossoff—Epilepsy
- Dr. Georgia Ede—Mental health disorders
- Dr. Jeff Volek—Human performance
- Dr. Stephen Phinney—Human performance
- Dr. Sarah Hallberg—Diabetes
- Ivor Cummins—CVD
- David Feldman—CVD
- Dr. Nadir Ali—CVD
- Dr. David Diamond—CVD
- Dr. Brett Scher—CVD
- Andrew Koutnik—Cancer, Type I diabetes
- Elena Gross—Migraines

In addition to the scientists listed above, we want to give special mention to a few educators who have produced work that has helped shape our views on nutrition:

- Gary Taubes
- Mike Mutzel
- Travis Christofferson

- Miriam Kalamian
- Robb Wolf
- Nina Teicholz

BOOKS

Below is a list of a few of the books that have helped educate us and shape our beliefs about the ketogenic diet.

- *Tripping Over the Truth* by Travis Christofferson
- *Ketogenic Diet and Metabolic Therapies* by Susan Masino
- *Keto for Cancer* by Miriam Kalamian
- *The Art and Science of Low Carbohydrate Living* by Jeff Volek and Stephen Phinney
- *The Art and Science of Low Carbohydrate Performance* by Jeff Volek and Stephen Phinney
- *The Case Against Sugar* by Gary Taubes
- *Why We Get Fat: And What to Do About It* by Gary Taubes
- *Wired to Eat* by Robb Wolf
- *The Big Fat Surprise* by Nina Teicholz
- *The Real Meal Revolution* by Professor Tim Noakes, Jonna Proudfoot, and Sally-Ann Creed

WEBSITES

Below are a few websites you can visit for more keto information resources:

- Perfectketo.com
- Dranthonygustin.com
- Theketologist.com
- Ketonutrition.org

FOUNDATIONS

If you are passionate about the ketogenic diet and want to get involved with a few of the foundations out there that are making a huge impact, check out:

- The Charlie Foundation
- The MaxLove Project
- Foundation for Metabolic Cancer Therapies
- Matthew's Friends
- Dietary Science Foundation

ACKNOWLEDGMENTS AND ABOUT THE AUTHORS

ACKNOWLEDGMENTS

The creation of this book would not have been possible without the efforts of the practitioners, researchers, scientists, and educators (mentioned in Appendix C) who have paved the way to progress the study of nutrition, especially ketogenic dieting, forward.

Anthony would like to thank his partner in crime, Martha Heymans, for continually pushing him to put out his work and her incessant support, his parents, Dennis and Lori, for never questioning his erratic path through life and believing in him the whole way, to Chris Irvin for helping push this over the many finish lines, and the Perfect Keto team for helping him push forward with making his vision of helping other people be healthier with a ketogenic diet a reality each and every day.

Chris would like to thank his wife Sara, his parents Chris and Carla, and the rest of his family for their constant, unwavering support. Chris would also like to thank Dr. Gustin for his mentorship and friendship and the Perfect Keto team for all of their support in the creation of this book. Finally, Chris would like to make special acknowledgment to the science educators he has had in his life: Jim Egelton, Ben Wittenkeller, Linda Cockerill, Dr. Elaine Chapman, Dr. Carlos Ugrinowitsch, Dr. Eduardo De Souza, Dr. Angela Poff, Dr. Shannon Kesl, and Andrew Koutnik PhDc.

ABOUT THE AUTHORS

DR. ANTHONY GUSTIN

FROM ACNE TO NASCAR TO OPTIMAL HEALTH

It is awful to feel you're living in an unhealthy body you don't want. I know. That's how my life was for a long time.

My cystic acne started early, in fourth grade. I was a complete wreck, and not just because of the zits. I was obese in grade school, depressed, irritable, and experienced constant mood swings. Doctors told me I was "overweight for my age group," and all I needed to do was run a little more to shed the pounds. My acne? A genetic problem, they said. I wouldn't be able to fix that, just had to live with it. At the time I didn't understand that my own actions were the cause of all of this.

Teenage life is hard for anyone. For me, it was flat-out miserable. I was deeply embarrassed by my acne. When my mother threw a surprise fourteenth birthday party for me, I spent half of the evening in the bathroom, grooming my erupting face. I obsessed over my skin mornings and evenings. And forget about nurturing a teen love life—sometimes I left social events because I was so embarrassed by how I looked. The lousy dermatologist I saw in central Minnesota told me this so-called genetic acne could be improved only by an expensive and painful laser treatment. It didn't work. He was wrong in more ways than one.

Luckily, I had my favorite foods. I was so attached to Cool Ranch Doritos that I kept a plastic baggy of them under my bed so I could snack whenever I wanted. (Yes, I really did. Seriously.) The food industry had me hooked on everything they wanted me to buy. Sweet snacks, savory snacks, sweet and savory snacks, Frankenfoods that caused massive damage to my body for years on end. My typical day was filled with foods so processed they could last through a nuclear winter. I had an incredible amount of gut dysfunction and issues that had me running to the bathroom in urgency—or not defecating for days while dealing with wrenching gut pain. As you can imagine, this made a normal young teen life hard to manage.

As I learned later in my functional medicine career, your skin is a reflection of your gut. I sensed it, but I didn't grasp the connection.

My doctors and the federal government's nutrition guidelines all told me that as long as a "food" was low in fat, I should eat it. Gummy Worms and Doritos are low in fat! Load 'em up! With nutritional habits like these in my formative years, it's no surprise I was embarrassingly overweight by the time I entered fifth grade.

I had numerous physical and movement problems, including severe pain in my knees and back. I couldn't even sit in a car for longer than thirty minutes without needing to extend my legs. My upper and lower back ached constantly. I didn't want to participate in any type of physical activity.

My brain didn't work, either. Not only was I slow, I thought I was stupid. I couldn't focus in class and I was extremely irritated all of the time. I would lash out at others and get none of my work done. Agitated and upset, depressed, and anxious, I was everything a young kid never should be.

THE FAT KID TRIES SCIENCE

My lightbulb moment came early in middle school as I learned how to conduct a scientific experiment. An experiment has a logical structure: a starting point, a hypothesis of the result an intervention will produce, the execution of the experiment, and then observation of the result. Did it work, or did it not work? Why or why not?

What doctors and health experts were telling me at the time wasn't fixing my health, so I decided to figure it out on my own. I used information I was learning in my biology and chemistry classes—such as how protein, fat, and carbs are metabolized and how fat is burned or stored—to run experiments on myself. I grew confident that I could systematically learn about my body by using myself as the guinea pig. This scientific method soon became second nature to me and is still baked into my brain in all decisions I make to this day.

What began with me asking, "What would happen if I started eating more vegetables?" ended up as meticulous nutrition and workout logs of every little thing I did. The more I paid attention, the more I noticed dramatic results. My first big step was to cut out all of the processed food I had been eating. Enough with the pizza, fries, and chips that were dished up as part of government-mandated school lunch! I also stopped eating vast quantities of Pizza Rolls and Toaster Treats at home. Instead I began to consume what the USDA told us at the time was healthy: low-fat, high grain diets. This meant whole wheat pasta, whole wheat bread (with low-fat mayo and lean turkey breast, of course), but ultimately a lot less refined foods and sugars and more "real" stuff. Looking back, I have to laugh, but compared to what I had been eating before the change was a vast improvement, and the results were fascinating.

Stubborn weight I had held onto for years as "the fat kid" dropped off without problem. Over the course of a single off-season I changed positions on my high school football team from offensive lineman to cornerback. If you don't play football you may not understand the significance of this: I went from one of the physically heaviest positions to one of the leanest. Offensive linemen are chosen for bulk and immovability. Cornerbacks are valued for quickness and agility. I wasn't as lean as I wanted to be, but I had made a huge change. My energy levels improved significantly, but I still experienced significant crashes day-to-day. The gut issues cleared up, but the skin problems stayed. I still suffered from irritability and mood problems. Clearly, I was on the right path, but my journey was only beginning.

Even though I had a long way to go to figure out the optimal health plan for myself, the most important light bulb had turned on: I was the one in control, the responsible one. I had learned that I couldn't rely on doctors, nutritionists, or the government to give me what I needed to be healthy. Instead, I would run test after test on myself to figure out what modifications in my life led to the result I wanted: effortless and optimal health. I would *be* the experiment.

Bingo!

Four years later, as I began a dual doctorate-plus-masters graduate program, I made another leap forward. At the time I thought I was eating super-healthy yet nagging health problems remained. Then I discovered what is now called the "paleo" diet, and it lifted me to the next level in my health journey. Here was another critical lightbulb moment, one in which I realized how much sense eating actual real food made. I started eating only high-quality foods that humans had evolved eating: meat, fish, vegetables, fruits, nuts, and seeds. If I couldn't have hunted it or harvested it, I didn't eat it. The result? My acne completely disappeared, my mood improved drastically, and I felt like a whole new person.

And yet—I knew I could do more. Nagging issues remained. My energy was still unreliable, and inflammation was causing joint pain and gut dysfunction. I realized that the years of poor nutritional habits had produced a body that does not process carbohydrates very well. This is when I turned to a ketogenic diet.

I removed carbohydrates almost entirely from my diet, so my body started burning the breakdown of fat (ketones) for energy instead of burning carbs, a state known as ketosis. By following a ketogenic approach while keeping food quality high, I brought myself to a point where I feel the best I've felt in my life. My energy finally was boundless, I could manage stress more easily and I felt, at last, that I had my health completely figured out.

RACING CARS AND NBA STARS

Nutrition wasn't the only thing I modified to earn my health back. My lifelong science experiment led to learning not only about nutrition but also movement practices, stress management, and sleep quality. These are what I call the four pillars of health; getting them right so I could solve my own problems led me to dedicate my life to helping others do the same thing: using an individualized approach to fixing health.

Now that my health was in tip-top shape, I wanted to help others. As soon as I was out of school and into practice as a sports rehab clinician, I began to learn as quickly as possible. I obsessed over the strategy behind what I was doing, breaking down how my career in healthcare could be as impactful as possible. My analysis led me to take a page from the most unexpected of places: car racing.

NASCAR is a prime example of innovation happening at the cutting edge. Racing comes down to performing at the absolute highest levels, with careers made or lost by margins of seconds. Each racing company does a massive amount of research and development in search of the slightest edge. Tweaked aerodynamics can give a car just a few more miles per gallon, brakes can be fine-tuned to perform in specific turns, a design alteration can save a pound or two. Yet drivers also have to be able to walk away from 160 mph crashes. These advances in safety and car technology trickle down to the rest of us on the showroom floor. Most of the safety and performance boosts found in everyday cars came from the front-line innovations developed at the most competitive level.

This trickle-down effect isn't limited to NASCAR. The space program gave us ballpoint pens and Teflon. The GPS in your phone was, just a few years ago, a top-secret military technology. And on and on.

I thought, "If I want to develop the best skills and innovate in health care, why not start with those at the cutting edge of competition?" This is one reason I worked with professional and elite athletes. If I could see how they move, what they eat, and how their bodies function, I could extrapolate that down to the general population. I could optimize the strategies for widespread use (and steal some of those strategies for myself).

The plan worked. I learned in a high-paced environment, running a sports medicine clinic in San Francisco that grew to accommodate the demands not only of skilled athletes but also the general population. I saw what I could do to improve the recovery time of NBA superstars, so they could play nearly 100 games per season, and I learned what it takes to bring NFL

All-Pros to a level even higher than they had achieved. As I sharpened my skills at making the best even better, I used these tools for the general population.

What fascinated me the most is that these strategies weren't just based on movement. Even the smallest tweaks in nutrition had big impacts on recovery and performance. Wanting to pull this thread further, I took what I was learning from athletes and began to apply it to individuals who were sick. This is where my functional medicine career started. This led me to working with people one-on-one to fix chronic issues that Western medicine is generally terrible at: diabetes, obesity, heart disease, gut issues, adrenal problems, etc. What surprised me was the effectiveness of the ketogenic diet to help so many of my patients. After I saw how hard it was to stick to the diet at the time, due to lack of products that were compliant and lack of clear information, I decided to leave my clinical practice and start Perfect Keto to solve those problems.

CHRIS IRVIN

FROM SHRIMP TO SPORTS TO NERD

Nutrition, health, and fitness have always been passions of mine. As a kid, I was big into sports, especially basketball. As I was finishing up middle school, I was a skinny and pretty nerdy looking kid that wasn't too bad at shooting the ball. However, I knew that as I entered high school, I needed to get bigger if I was going to be able to compete. This was the first thing that turned me to fitness.

As I entered high school, I started lifting weights and eating as much food as I could to help put on some weight. Based on what my diet was, it's safe to say I wasn't passionate about nutrition yet, but I was growing so it worked at the time. After my freshman year of high school, I shot up 6 inches and went from 5' 6" to 6'. Then after my sophomore year, I shot up another 2-3 inches. While this growth was great in theory for basketball, it made my goal of getting bigger even harder. So, I just continued to eat.

I remember the rest of my high school career consisted of lifting weights and eating every second I could. Two breakfasts, a full meal or snack between every class, lunch, a pre-practice meal, dinner, and snacks until bedtime. Of course, the foods I was eating were not the most optimal for health or performance but when you are a skinny high school kid with a ravenous appetite, you can get away with it.

Despite this, when I graduated high school, I was 6 foot 3 inches and weighed a measly 175 pounds. I was going on to play small college basketball and I had some work to do. My first semester of college, I took a nutrition class that served as my first introduction to the world of nutrition. Looking back, the information I learned in this class was very outdated and incorrect, but what it did was teach me that what you put in your body impacts the way your body functions. This led me to start following a more paleo style diet while in college. This approach, combined with me finally making it through puberty, led to some muscle gain over the course of my college career, which made a big impact on my physical performance. During my time in undergrad, my emphasis was much more on exercise science, but I had begun to see the impact nutrition has on so many factors of human performance.

When I graduated college, my goal was to become a professional strength and conditioning coach in the NBA. I set out to achieve this by taking a job as a youth, high school, and collegiate strength and conditioning coach at a small gym in central Illinois. During this time, I was still training myself and never lost the goal of trying to put on more size. The problem was that I had gotten away from nutrition and was back on eating whatever I could to put weight on, even if it wasn't good weight.

While I was working my first job after college, I was introduced to the world of bodybuilding by a coworker of mine who had recently competed in a physique competition. I thought it was a pretty interesting sport and after my roommate told me that I couldn't be that disciplined with my diet (probably because we were "bulking" by eating pizza every night), my competitiveness got the best of me and I decided to sign up for a competition myself.

At this time, I was still very naive in my understanding of nutrition, so I had that coworker who had experience in preparing for a show give me a hand. Over the course of twelve weeks, I stayed disciplined to my programmed macros, I worked out, I did cardio, and it worked. I got shredded. I also developed a mild eating disorder, hormonal complications, I was weak, and was way skinnier than I ever want to be again. Safe to say that competition was my one and only.

The diet I was following at this time was not an optimal approach for health or a healthy relationship with food, but it did work and while I regret actually putting my body through this, it did light a passion for nutrition in me that forced me to change my career path. Later that year, I turned down an opportunity to get my master's in kinesiology and instead moved down to Tampa, Florida to get a master's in exercise and nutrition science. During this time, I was first introduced to the ketogenic diet and was immediately intrigued by the physiological changes that occurred on the diet and how this could relate to human performance. During my first half of graduate school, I spent time researching the diet for human performance, which was an incredible experience that allowed me to test different keto approaches in relatively well-trained college athletes and students. This first-hand experience taught me so much.

Halfway through my graduate schooling I picked up a book called *Tripping Over the Truth* by Travis Christofferson. This book is an incredible account of the history of cancer research, treatment, our misunderstandings, and how metabolic based treatments, such as a ketogenic diet, could be used in the treatment of cancer. This was my first real introduction into the therapeutic potential of a ketogenic diet, and I was hooked. I was so passionate about this topic that I went on a six-month sprint of reading every single cancer paper I could find. During this time, I was fortunate enough to get connected to Dr. Angela Poff, who had recently published an incredible dissertation on the use of keto and other metabolic based treatments for cancer. Lucky for me, there were extra hands needed in the lab she worked in at the University of Southern Florida and I was able to come in and learn directly from brilliant educators like her, Dr. Shannon Kesl, and soon to be doctor Andrew Koutnik.

This lab was a little different from what I was used to because the subjects were animals and not humans; an incredible experience that allowed me to gain a better understanding of what the academic world of research looks like. The doctors in this lab taught me so much and I got to be a part of some really cutting-edge research, an opportunity I will forever feel grateful for.

After spending a few months in this lab, I started to realize that while my passion was definitely keto for therapeutics, I enjoyed reading and writing a lot more than I did conducting research. During this time, I became very disappointed that there were so many rock star researchers out there, like the ones I was learning from, who had research that was either not accessible to the general population or not as easily understood. This is when I decided to set out on a mission to do my part to help educate the masses on the various potentials of the ketogenic diet and highlight the research from these incredible scientists—a mission that eventually and fortunately led to me joining the Perfect Keto team.

Over the last four years, since being introduced to keto, I have had my own dietary journey. When I first started keto, I had no idea what I was doing, but over the last few years I have continued to learn from experimenting on myself and working to help others optimize their ketogenic diet. In research, if you are humble, you will have your opinion on certain topics changed frequently, and I have. Being a part of the creation of this book has also forced me to rethink some of my own conventional wisdom thanks to the brilliance of Dr. Gustin. I hope you guys enjoy what we worked so hard to put together and I hope it makes a big difference in the lives of many.

KETO ANSWERS

CHAPTER 13: SELF-EXPERIMENTATION AND TRACKING

Made in the USA
Monee, IL
29 December 2019